DIXIE CORTNER BROOKE

BORDERLINE PERSONALITY DISORDER

ETIOLOGY AND TREATMENT

BORDERLINE PERSONALITY DISORDER

ETIOLOGY AND TREATMENT

Edited by **Joel Paris, M.D.**
Sir Mortimer B. Davis—Jewish General Hospital
and Department of Psychiatry, McGill University,
Montreal, Quebec, Canada

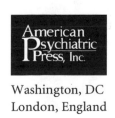

American Psychiatric Press, Inc.

Washington, DC
London, England

Note: The authors have worked to ensure that all information in this book concerning drug dosages, schedules, and routes of administration is accurate as of the time of publication and consistent with standards set by the U.S. Food and Drug Administration and the general medical community. As medical research and practice advance, however, therapeutic standards may change. For this reason and because human and mechanical errors sometimes occur, we recommend that readers follow the advice of a physician who is directly involved in their care or the care of a member of their family.

Copyright © 1993 American Psychiatric Press, Inc.
ALL RIGHTS RESERVED
Manufactured in the United States of America on acid-free paper
96 95 94 93   4 3 2 1
First Edition

American Psychiatric Press, Inc.
1400 K Street, N.W., Washington, DC 20005

Library of Congress Cataloging-in-Publication Data
Borderline personality disorder : etiology and treatment / edited by
    Joel Paris. — 1st ed.
        p.   cm.
    Includes bibliographical references and index.
    ISBN 0-88048-408-X
    1. Borderline personality disorder—Etiology. 2. Borderline personality
    disorder—Treatment. I. Paris, Joel, 1940– .
        [DNLM: 1. Borderline Personality Disorder—etiology.
    2. Borderline Personality Disorder—therapy. WM 190 B728]
    RC569.5.B67B689 1993
    616.85′852—dc20
    DNLM/DLC   92-7020
    for Library of Congress   CIP

British Library Cataloguing in Publication Data
A CIP record is available from the British Library.

CONTENTS

SECTION I: ETIOLOGY

SECTION II: TREATMENT

CONTRIBUTORS

Ingrid Boiago, Ph.D., Department of Psychiatry, McMaster University, Hamilton, Ontario, Canada

John F. Clarkin, Ph.D., New York Hospital—Westchester Division, White Plains, New York; Department of Psychiatry, Cornell University, New York, New York

Laura J. Gold, Ph.D., Department of Psychiatry, University of Michigan, Ann Arbor, Michigan

John Gunderson, M.D., McLean Hospital, Belmont, Massachusetts; Department of Psychiatry, Harvard University, Cambridge, Massachusetts

Judith L. Herman, M.D., Cambridge Hospital, Department of Psychiatry, Harvard University, Cambridge, Massachusetts

Otto F. Kernberg, M.D., New York Hospital—Westchester Division, White Plains, New York; Department of Psychiatry, Cornell University

Kelly Koerner, B.A., Department of Psychology, University of Washington, Seattle, Washington

Jerome Kroll, M.D., Department of Psychiatry, University of Minnesota, Minneapolis, Minnesota

Marsha M. Linehan, Ph.D., Department of Psychology, University of Washington, Seattle, Washington

Paul S. Links, M.D., Department of Psychiatry, McMaster University, Hamilton, Ontario, Canada

Thomas H. McGlashan, M.D., Yale Psychiatric Institute, New Haven; Department of Psychiatry, Yale University, New Haven, Connecticut

Theodore Millon, Ph.D., Department of Psychology, University of Miami, Miami, Florida; Department of Psychiatry, Harvard University, Cambridge, Massachusetts

Joel Paris, M.D., Sir Mortimer B. Davis—Jewish General Hospital; Department of Psychiatry, McGill University, Montreal, Quebec, Canada

J. Christopher Perry, M.D., M.P.H., Cambridge Hospital, Department of Psychiatry, Harvard University, Cambridge, Massachusetts

Michael Porder, M.D., Private Practice in Psychoanalysis, New York, New York

Michael Rosenbluth, M.D., Toronto East General Hospital, Department of Psychiatry, University of Toronto, Toronto, Ontario, Canada

Alex N. Sabo, M.D., McLean Hospital, Belmont, Massachusetts; Department of Psychiatry, Harvard University, Cambridge, Massachusetts

Edward N. Shearin, Ph.D., Department of Psychiatry, New York Hospital—Westchester Division, White Plains, New York

Kenneth R. Silk, M.D., Department of Psychiatry, University of Michigan, Ann Arbor, Michigan

Daniel Silver, M.D., Mount Sinai Hospital, Toronto, Ontario; Department of Psychiatry, University of Toronto, Toronto, Ontario, Canada

Paul H. Soloff, M.D., Department of Psychiatry, University of Pittsburgh, Pittsburgh, Pennsylvania

Michael H. Stone, M.D., Department of Psychiatry, Columbia University, New York, New York

Rob van Reekum, M.D., Department of Psychiatry, McMaster University, Hamilton, Ontario, Canada

Mary C. Zanarini, Ph.D., McLean Hospital, Belmont, Massachusetts; Department of Psychiatry, Harvard University,

Hallie Zweig-Frank, Ph.D., Sir Mortimer B. Davis—Jewish General Hospital; Department of Psychology, Concordia University, Montreal, Quebec, Canada

PREFACE

BOOKS ABOUT BORDERLINE PERSONALITY DISORDER (BPD) ARE AL-ways in demand among clinicians. The reason is simple: borderline patients are difficult to treat and their treatment is stressful for therapists. But the real problem is that we do not know what causes BPD. This book, therefore, differs from other texts in its commitment to empirical data as the basis for progress in understanding and treating the borderline patient. There is also room for clinical wisdom in these pages, and the psychoanalytic tradition, which introduced the idea of borderline personality, is well represented. However, there has been an explosion of research on BPD in the last 10 years. Borderline personality is the most researched Axis II disorder and is beginning to rival the functional psychoses for space in prominent journals. Although we have a long way to go to have an adequate model for the etiology of BPD, or for a comprehensive and effective treatment approach, research findings in both areas are beginning to lead us to some tentative answers.

There are a number of important questions about BPD that are dealt with only indirectly in this book. Although etiology and treatment are the most important questions about any disorder, problems of defining the boundaries of BPD, identifying subgroups, and considering the effects of comorbidity emerge in virtually every chapter. The problem of definition has bedeviled investigation of borderline personality from the very beginning. However, whatever the limitations of the DSM-III-R criteria for BPD, these criteria provide a basis for research that will allow subdefinition or reclassification of borderline cases at some future point. Those wishing to explore further the history of the borderline concept will find the subject well reviewed elsewhere.[1]

The assumption behind the present volume is that the reader is already familiar with the clinical features of BPD. However, given the heterogeneity of this disorder, theories of etiology drawn from one group of borderline patients may not apply to another, while treatments that work for some patients may be ineffective with others. Any of the research findings discussed in this book could be influenced by comorbidity and to what extent the clinical samples studied are representative of borderline patients as a whole.

---

[1] Stone MH: *Essential Papers on Borderline Disorders.* New York, New York University Press, 1986.

Another issue not addressed in detail by this book is epidemiology. This area is only beginning to be explored, although we have some preliminary data suggesting that BPD is fairly common in the community.[2] We do not know whether BPD varies in its prevalence with class or culture, or to what extent it is influenced by social and historical forces.

One area where there has been important new information on BPD in recent years is outcome research. This set of data is referred to in the book where it has implications for etiology or treatment. The natural history of BPD shows short-term chronicity and long-term recovery. Any theory of etiology has to try to account for this phenomenon. Any study of treatment needs to measure itself against naturalistic improvement.

The book is divided into separate sections on etiology and treatment, and each section concludes with a critical overview. All of the authors are authorities on BPD and among the leading researchers in their areas. Each chapter is a comprehensive literature review, but in most cases recent research by the authors is also presented.

It is striking how much new data has emerged since the empirical research on BPD was last summarized in the annual review published by the American Psychiatric Association.[3] The present volume is therefore up to date, but can expect predictable obsolescence, which is a measure of how rapidly clinical research on BPD is progressing. This is particularly true of research on etiology, and therefore Section I is the longer part of this book. When we know more about the etiology of BPD, we will be on our way toward developing rational treatments.

---

[2]Swartz M, Blazer D, George L, et al: "Estimating the prevalence of borderline personality disorder in the community." *Journal of Personality Disorders* 4:257–272, 1990.

[3]Gunderson JG (ed): "Borderline personality disorder (Section I), in *American Psychiatric Press Review of Psychiatry,* Vol 8. Edited by Tasman A, Hales RE, Frances AJ. Washington, DC, American Psychiatric Press, 1989, pp 5–125.

ACKNOWLEDGMENTS

The idea for this book originated from its publisher, American Psychiatric Press, Inc. The Editor-in-Chief, Carol Nadelson, M.D., has provided crucial support and help. The staff at American Psychiatric Press have made the book possible: Timothy Clancy with the original idea, and Claire Reinburg with nuts and bolts along the way. My work as editor has been supported by the Sir Mortimer B. Davis—Jewish General Hospital, Montreal, and its Psychiatrist-in-Chief, Dr. Philip Beck, as well as the Department of Psychiatry of McGill University, and its Chairman, Dr. Gilbert Pinard. Secretarial support for the editing was provided by the staff of the Institute of Community and Family Psychiatry of the Sir Mortimer B. Davis—Jewish General Hospital. My family has given me consistent and needed encouragement to carry this project through.

SECTION I:
ETIOLOGY

INTRODUCTION

UNDERSTANDING THE ETIOLOGY OF BORDERLINE PERSON-ality disorder (BPD) demands a biopsychosocial model. This could be even more true for BPD than for many other forms of psychopathology, because we are studying a syndrome with a complex pathogenesis that resists reduction to biological vulnerability, childhood experiences, or social forces. Although the biopsychosocial model is often accepted in principle, in practice it is often given only lip service. Multi-dimensional models can be mind-boggling, and most clinicians prefer simplicity to complexity. Attempts have been made to understand BPD reductionistically as an atypical affective disorder or a posttraumatic syndrome. However, no single etiologic factor is likely to account for BPD, and researchers and therapists need to understand that the variables we study are not single causes but risk factors in the complex pathway that leads to psychopathology.

Understanding the etiology of BPD, as with other mental disorders, should begin with constitution. As psychiatry has matured, our approach no longer considers constitution or environment in isolation. For most disorders, this means applying a *predisposition-stress model,* with the pre-disposing factors reflecting biological vulnerability. One way of looking at this model is that biological variability determines the specific disorder to which any individual is prone, while stressors determine when and to what extent that disorder will become clinically apparent. Trait variability, although genetically determined, can be adaptive or maladaptive in differ-ent environmental contexts. In the case of BPD, a reasonable hypothesis is that patients will not develop borderline syndrome without a constitu-tional predisposition, but they need not develop borderline pathology even in the presence of such a predisposition.

Although we have some strong and heuristic hypotheses, we have not clearly established which factors determine biological vulnerability to BPD. One problem may well be the heterogeneity of the syndrome: BPD is not a phenotype. We are caught in a Catch-22 in which the best way to define BPD for research would be with biological markers, but we cannot

3

identify the markers until we have a more precise boundary for BPD. Paradoxically, though we look to biology for specificity, many of the findings about the biology of BPD are not that specific. On the whole, there is more specificity for personality traits such as impulsivity (Coccaro et al. 1989), or for behaviors such as serious suicide attempts (Gardner et al. 1990). Because biological markers pick up the propensity for psychiatric disorder rather than the disorder itself, this lack of specificity is not surprising. But biological findings could help us to subgroup borderline patients.

The present state of knowledge from the point of view of genetics, brain dysfunction, and biological markers is reviewed in Chapter 1 by van Reekum, Links, and Boiago. Where do we locate the hypothesized constitutional predisposition to BPD? In the neurotransmitters, or at a higher level of neurophysiological organization? The authors present an intriguing case for the role of brain dysfunction in BPD, in parallel with developments in the understanding of the functional psychoses. However, the evidence is still soberingly tentative.

Because of the prominent dysthymia seen in BPD, it has often been suggested that BPD is best understood as an affective spectrum disorder (Akiskal 1981). The arguments for and against this position were reviewed a few years ago by Gunderson and Elliott (1985) and were recently updated by Gunderson and Phillips (1991). The key question is whether the affective instability of the borderline patient is a variant of mood disorder or an entirely different phenomenon. Gold and Silk, in Chapter 2, do not describe what constitutional factors exist in BPD but rather whether these factors can be accounted for by the affective element of the syndrome. These authors agree with van Reekum et al. that data on biological markers are too preliminary to answer this question, and they go on to review a number of recent studies on drug response in BPD that suggest, at best, a mixed verdict. The problem of BPD definition and subgrouping appears again, and Gold and Silk suggest that there could be an affective spectrum subgroup of borderline patients, even if most borderline patients do not respond to drugs in the same way as do patients with affective disorders. Findings from personality tests and from outcome studies also suggest overlap, but not equivalence, of BPD and affective syndromes. It therefore seems wrong to reclassify BPD as "subaffective dysthymia." The lack of specificity for the constitutional factors in BPD can be explained in another way: borderline patients share their biological vulnerability with a number of other conditions in which impulsivity is a characteristic symptom.

This issue is discussed in detail in Chapter 3 by Zanarini. This time the question is whether the constitutional and/or developmental factors in the etiology of BPD are common to the disorders in the impulsive spectrum. Siever (1990) has remarked that the neurotransmitters do not seem to have read the DSM-III-R criteria for mental disorders. Rather, each biological variable influences a broad range of behaviors that may turn up in any number of diagnoses. As Zanarini demonstrates, a number of lines of evidence link BPD with its near-neighbor Axis II disorders, particularly antisocial personality disorder, and with substance abuse. Both of these conditions are frequently comorbid with BPD. It was suggested many years ago by Vaillant (1975) that antisocial patients look "borderline" on a psychiatric ward, and it is also possible that the gender predominances in the two disorders (male for antisocial personality disorder and female for BPD) reflect definitional differences masking a core commonality. The concept of "impulse spectrum disorder" presented by Zanarini in her chapter is a grouping that is in concordance with a large amount of empirical work that shows that the most striking comorbidity of BPD is not in the affective spectrum, but with other disorders that have impulsivity as a predominant feature. Whether this comorbidity reflects a common biology, common family experiences, or both, remains to be seen. It is also possible that there are subgroups of BPD that have stronger impulsive or affective components (Silverman et al. 1991; also see Gold and Silk, Chapter 2).

In Chapter 4, Stone presents a different perspective on constitutional factors in BPD, suggesting that hyperirritability is "the red thread" that could account for much of the clinical picture in borderline patients. Stone's concept is more complex and more subtle than Klein's (1977) "affective instability" or the concept of impulsivity. Like van Reekum et al. in Chapter 1, Stone suggests that borderline patients have faulty limbic modulation. He also attempts an integration of biology with psychological factors during development (especially abuse) and with social factors (cultural modulation of aggression). His arguments underline that whatever the constitutional factors in the etiology of BPD, these factors can hardly explain by themselves the development of the syndrome. With a reasonably supportive environment during development, genotypic variability in such areas as impulsivity or affective instability may lead to phenotypic variability in personality traits, but by no means necessarily to severe personality disorder. Stone (1990) has suggested elsewhere that there are some borderline patients with high biological risk who develop the syndrome even in an average expectable environment, others who have normal biology but develop the syndrome due to extreme environmental insult, and still others, probably the majority, who require both factors to become borderline. Therefore, biological risk factors are only meaningful when considered in interaction with other variables. Stone links constitution, developmental trauma, and social risk factors in an interactive theoretical framework.

A similar point of view underlies Chapter 5 by Linehan and Koerner. They describe their theory as "dialectical," but psychiatrists will find it biopsychosocial. Linehan integrates a great deal of data about the etiology of BPD. In spite of being drawn from a different intellectual tradition (i.e., behavioral psychology), her conclusions about the relations between constitution and family experience are surprisingly similar to those of Stone. Linehan's views of emotional dysregulation as the primary difficulty in BPD seem fairly comparable to the affective dysphoria and impulsivity described by other constitutional theorists. Social learning theory is used to conceptualize environmental effects as various as sexual abuse and emotional neglect. Linehan's concept of the "invalidating environment" also parallels psychodynamic theory and is in concordance with the empirical findings presented in the next few chapters.

Psychoanalytic theories about BPD have only recently been operationalized sufficiently to be open to empirical testing. Nevertheless, clinical observation by psychoanalytically oriented therapists has provided most of our hypotheses on the role of family environment in BPD and has led to systematic investigation of the reports that borderline patients present about their childhood experiences. Such research also has the advantage of drawing on larger and more representative populations of borderline patients, not just those in intensive psychotherapy.

Psychotherapists have theorized that abnormal childhood experiences contribute a major share to the development of borderline personality. This does not necessarily imply failing to take into account constitutional vulnerability. However, psychodynamic theory differs from purely neo-

Kraepelian models (Cloninger et al. 1990) that attribute the specificity of psychopathology to constitution and view environment as providing only precipitating factors. A key concept in psychodynamic thinking is that there are specific factors in development associated with specific psycho-pathological constellations. In order to test this hypothesis empirically, investigators have compared the frequency of developmental risk factors in borderline patients with comparison groups of nonborderline patients.

In recent years there has been much interest in the effects of childhood trauma on adult development. In Chapter 6, Perry and Herman review this exciting and controversial area of research on the etiology of BPD. The evidence that borderline patients have a high rate of physical abuse, childhood sexual abuse, and other traumatic experiences during child-hood has been reported from so many sources and samples by now that it is overwhelming. As pointed out by Gunderson (1990), the findings for this environmental risk factor are as dramatic as any described in biological research. Of particular importance to clinicians is the association of trauma with dissociative defenses. The presence of dissociative phenom-ena is therefore a clue for the clinician to search for an abuse history.

One possible interpretation of these data is to see BPD as a posttrau-matic syndrome. Some (but not all) of the clinical features of BPD can in fact be explained by this model (Gunderson 1991). However, before adopting a theory that could be overly simplistic, we need to be cautious and take into account the interactions between trauma and constitution, and between trauma and other environmental risk factors.

Paris and Zweig-Frank, in Chapter 7, review research on a more non-specific environmental factor, parental bonding. If we take the reports of borderline patients about their childhood experience seriously, then we will believe them when they say they were abused, and we will also believe them when they say they were neglected or overprotected. But there are pitfalls in accepting retrospective data, and prospective or high-risk stud-ies are needed to establish the validity of these reports (Gunderson and Zanarini 1989). However, the retrospective data make a good deal of clinical sense and provide confirmation for psychoanalytic hypotheses about the effects of a failed holding environment during childhood.

The borderline concept derives from the psychoanalytic tradition. However, not all psychoanalysts are comfortable with the direction of research on BPD. One objection is that in the process of operationalizing both diagnostic criteria and developmental risk factors, we can lose some of the essence of concepts that were derived from clinical data. In particular, there is a respectable minority who feel that the DSM-III-R (American Psychiatric Association 1987) definition of BPD creates an artificial boundary between behavioral and intrapsychic disturbances. This is the position taken in Chapter 8 by Clarkin and Kernberg. They review empirical findings on the early experiences of borderline patients, comparing the DSM-III-R diagnosis of BPD with the larger group of impulsive personality disorders characterized by Kernberg as "borderline personality organization" (BPO). Clarkin and Kernberg consider the considerable overlap of BPD with other Axis II disorders and argue that this supports the construct of BPO.

The BPO construct also parallels theories coming out of the tradition of academic psychology. Frances and Widiger (1986) and Livesley et al. (1989) have suggested that the categorical approach to personality should be replaced by the study of traits or dimensions, and that dimensions could have more specific relations with etiologic factors. The concept of BPO seems to be on the same level of abstraction as a personality trait, and the four factors in the syndrome described by Clarkin and Kernberg parallel the subscales in the Diagnostic Interview for Borderlines—Revised (DIB-R; Zanarini et al. 1989). Because impulsivity is one of the core features of BPO, Clarkin and Kernberg can also be seen as supporting Zanarini's concept of impulse spectrum disorders.

However, there are several problems with the BPO construct. It is overly broad and includes too large a percentage of patients with personality disorders. Clarkin and Kernberg acknowledge that although reliable assessment of BPO is possible, it has not yet been fully developed with a well-validated clinical instrument. However, their point is that neither constitutional nor developmental risk factors follow the present categories. Clarkin and Kernberg also review theories based on clinical data that suggest that the developmental risk factors in borderline patients can be located in early childhood. Thus far this position has not been supported by empirical research. Even among psychoanalysts there is disagreement as to whether primitive mental structures play a crucial role in BPD.

In Chapter 9, Porder presents an alternative view. He reviews the theoretical contributions of the analysts who have studied borderline patients and goes on to suggest a more complex developmental path involving many stages of development. In his view, it is too simplistic to relate more severe levels of character pathology to earlier stages of development, because there are as many similarities as there are differences between borderline and classically neurotic character structures. Porder's ideas derive from the clinical study of borderline patients in psychoanalysis, not from empirical research, but are consistent with trends in child development to reject phase-specific theories in favor of the cumulative interaction of many factors (Rutter 1989).

One area that has been almost totally neglected in discussions of the etiology of BPD are sociocultural factors. A lack of data is certainly part of the reason. Social theories at present are speculative, although they are open to empirical testing. In Chapter 10, Millon takes some pains to make clear that the social factors in BPD are more likely to play a precipitating rather than truly causal role. However, BPD cannot be fully understood without a historical or cultural perspective.

There is a potential fallacy in theories of social change and psychiatric disorders: the assumption that humanity once lived in a state of harmony and community that has only recently been disrupted by modernization. Human society has probably always had to deal with a certain level of transgenerational discontinuity. Nonetheless, we cannot ignore cross-cultural evidence that psychiatric syndromes as important as eating disorders (DiNicola 1990) are unique to modern societies, and the same could be the case for some personality disorders. Because tradition and social control have a containing influence on impulsive behavior, rapid social change may put the "borderline-prone" individual at particular risk.

If we are in fact seeing an increase of BPD in our society, this points to the interface between child-rearing practices and the effects of social structures that come into play during adolescence and young adulthood. There are cross-cultural questions here that parallel Millon's psychohistorical perspective. For example, we need to know whether BPD occurs in traditional societies, because if it does not, this would support an emphasis on modernization as a factor in the development of BPD (Paris 1991). Millon's ideas could also be empirically tested by examining the prevalence of BPD among ethnic groups in our own society that vary in their own level of social cohesion. However, if Millon is right, then the incidence of BPD will continue to increase, and the information provided in books like this will be even more necessary in the coming century.

In Chapter 11, Kroll provides an overview of etiologic theories. Integrating all the evidence available thus far, Kroll concludes that BPD requires a multifactorial model. At present, he considers that the strongest findings are those for psychic trauma, but trauma lacks sensitivity and specificity in relation to the borderline diagnosis. Although our knowledge of BPD is still limited, there is quite a bit to guide the open-minded clinician. There is enough evidence for constitutional abnormalities to stop blaming families but not enough to consider BPD reductionistically as a biological disorder. There is enough converging evidence from psychoanalytic clinical studies, from research on trauma, and from systematic reports of the family environment of borderline patients during childhood to support the crucial role of psychological development in the etiology of BPD. Finally, there are reasonable theoretical grounds for considering that social factors may encourage the development of borderline pathology.

How does our present knowledge of the etiology of BPD help us with the treatment of this difficult syndrome? A parallel can be drawn between the need for a multivariate model for the etiology of BPD and a multifactorial treatment approach. Just as no single risk factor explains BPD, no single treatment is likely to be effective in the majority of cases. How to balance the therapeutic possibilities open to the clinician is the subject of the second half of this book.

REFERENCES

Akiskal HS: Subaffective disorders: dysthymic, cyclothymic and bipolar II disorders in the "borderline" realm. Psychiatr Clin North Am 4:25–46, 1981

American Psychiatric Association: Diagnostic and Statistical Manual of Mental Disorders, 3rd Edition, Revised. Washington, DC, American Psychiatric Association, 1987

Cloninger CR, Martin RL, Guze SB, et al: The empirical structure of psychiatric comorbidity and its theoretical significance, in Comorbidity of Mood and Anxiety Disorders. Edited by Maser JD, Cloninger CR. Washington, DC, American Psychiatric Press, 1990, pp 439–462

Coccaro EF, Siever LJ, Klar HM, et al: Serotonergic studies in patients with affective and personality disorders: correlates with suicidal and impulsive aggressive behavior. Arch Gen Psychiatry 46:587–599, 1989

DiNicola VF: Anorexia multiforme: self starvation in historical and cultural context. Transcultural Psychiatric Research Review 27:165–196, 1990

Frances AJ, Widiger T: The classification of personality disorders: an overview of problems and solutions, in Psychiatry Update: American Psychiatric Association Annual Review, Vol 5. Edited by Frances AJ, Hales RE. Washington, DC, American Psychiatric Press, 1986, p 52

Gardner DL, Lucas PB, Cowdry RW: CSF metabolites in borderline personality disorder compared with normal controls. Biol Psychiatry 28:247–254, 1990

Gunderson JG: New perspectives on becoming borderline, in Family Environment and Borderline Personality Disorder. Edited by Links PS. Washington, DC, American Psychiatric Press, 1990, pp 149–159

Gunderson JG: BPD and PTSD: phenomenology and treatment distinctions. Paper presented at the 144th annual meeting of the American Psychiatric Association, New Orleans, May 1991

Gunderson JG, Elliott GR: The interface between borderline personality disorder and affective disorder. Am J Psychiatry 142:277–288, 1985

Gunderson JG, Phillips KA: A current view of the interface between borderline personality disorder and depression. Am J Psychiatry 148:967–975, 1991

Gunderson JG, Zanarini MC: Pathogenesis of borderline personality, in American Psychiatric Press Review of Psychiatry, Vol 8. Edited by Tasman A, Hales RE, Frances AJ. Washington, DC, American Psychiatric Press, 1989, pp 25–48

Klein DF: Psychopharmacological treatment and delineation of borderline disorders, in Borderline Personality Disorders: The Concept, the Syndrome, the Patient. Edited by Hartocollis P. New York, International Universities Press, 1977, pp 365–384

Livesley WJ, Jackson DN, Schroeder NL: A study of the factorial structure of personality pathology. Journal of Personality Disorders 3:292–306, 1989

Paris J: Personality disorders, parasuicide, and culture. Transcultural Psychiatric Research Review 28:25–39, 1991

Rutter M: Pathways from childhood to adult life. J Child Psychol Psychiatry 30:23–51, 1989

Siever L: Biology of impulsivity in borderline personality. Paper presented at the 143rd annual meeting of the American Psychiatric Association, New York, May 1990

Silverman JM, Pinkham L, Horvath TB, et al: Affective and impulsive personality disorder traits in the relatives of patients with borderline personality disorder. Am J Psychiatry 148:1378–1385, 1991

Stone NH: The Fate of Borderline Patients: Successful Outcome and Psychiatric Practice. New York, Guilford, 1990

Vaillant GE: Sociopathy as a human process: a viewpoint. Arch Gen Psychiatry 32:178–183, 1975

Zanarini NC, Gunderson JG, Frankenburg FR, et al: The revised Diagnostic Interview for Borderlines: discriminating BPD from other Axis II disorders. Journal of Personality Disorders 3:10–18, 1989

Constitutional Factors in Borderline Personality Disorder: Genetics, Brain Dysfunction, and Biological Markers

Rob van Reekum, M.D.
Paul S. Links, M.D.
Ingrid Boiago, Ph.D.

A CONSTITUTIONAL ETIOLOGIC MODEL TO EXPLAIN BOR-
derline personality disorder (BPD) requires in-
trinsic factors in the individual that precede the manifest disorder. These
intrinsic factors may be the result of genetic or acquired problems leading
to brain, and therefore behavioral, dysfunction. Needless to say, focusing
on the individual separate from the environment is simplistic and reductionistic. However, to establish the building blocks of an etiologic model
of BPD, we must first examine each block, and then find its dimension and
position in the overall structure.

In this chapter we will review empirical data on genetic factors in the
etiology of BPD. Evidence suggesting acquired or developmental brain
dysfunction in the etiology of BPD will also be reviewed. Biochemical
markers in BPD will be examined because they may demonstrate possible
associations between BPD and other disorders and suggest possible biological mechanisms that explain the pathophysiology of BPD. Studies
using such approaches are an important link in understanding how genetic or acquired factors may lead to BPD. Finally, the relative strengths of
the genetic factors will be highlighted and four possible etiologic models
elucidated.

GENETIC FACTORS

Family History Studies

Family history studies are used for two scientific purposes: 1) to establish the validity of a psychiatric diagnosis and 2) to examine etiologic relationships between disorders. The validity of a psychiatric diagnosis is supported if an increased prevalence of the disorder A is found in the biological relatives of probands with the disorder A (Robins and Guze 1970). Therefore, like begets like. Etiologic relationships can be inferred if another disorder, B, is prevalent among the biological relatives of probands with disorder A. Family history studies cannot distinguish environmental from genetic factors; this requires other research designs such as twin or adoptive studies.

Diagnostic validity. A number of investigators have carried out family studies to examine whether BPD is found more frequently in the families of BPD patients. These studies (Baron et al. 1985; Links et al. 1988; Loranger et al. 1982; Pope et al. 1983; Schulz et al. 1986; Zanarini et al. 1990) are discussed in detail in Chapter 3 because they lend support to the idea that BPD lies in a spectrum of impulse disorders. In all of these studies (except for Pope et al. 1983) there was an increased prevalence of BPD in the families of BPD patients. The findings from these studies therefore provide robust support for the validity of the BPD diagnosis.

However, it is also possible that some of the dimensions or traits in BPD could be studied using the family history method. For example, Silverman et al. (1991) focused on dimensions of BPD and examined relatives of BPD patients for increased levels of chronic affective instability and chronic impulsivity. The first-degree relatives of probands with definite BPD were compared with the first-degree relatives of probands with other personality disorders and the first-degree relatives of male schizophrenic patients. The morbid risks of relatives of BPD patients were not significantly different from those in the comparison groups for major affective disorders, schizophrenia-related disorders, alcoholism, substance use disorder, or antisocial personality disorder. However, chronic affective instability and chronic impulsivity were significantly more common in the relatives of BPD patients compared with the relatives of a restricted group of patients with other personality disorders and the relatives of schizophrenic patients. The authors suggested that future investigations should focus on traits rather than on the diagnosis of BPD.

Etiologic relationships between disorders.   Family history studies can shed light on the controversy about which other psychiatric disorders are most closely related to BPD. Is the borderline syndrome most related to schizophrenia (Hoch and Polatin 1949), to affective disorders (Stone 1977), or to substance abuse and antisocial personality disorder (Gunderson and Zanarini 1989)?

A modern review will have to exclude studies that were done prior to the establishment of DSM-III-R (American Psychiatric Association 1987) criteria for the disorder (e.g., Stone et al. 1981). There are a number of studies using established diagnostic criteria that report prevalence rates of disorder in first-degree relatives. These reports, some of which were mentioned above, are discussed in detail in Chapter 3 and summarized in Table 3–2.[1] There are a number of consistent findings that shed light on the etiologic relationship of BPD to other disorders:

1. BPD is found more frequently in the families of BPD patients than in the families of schizophrenic, bipolar, schizotypal, antisocial, or dysthymic patients.
2. There is no increase in the prevalence of schizophrenia in the families of BPD patients.
3. Alcoholism and substance abuse are found frequently in the first-degree relatives of BPD patients.

The relationship of BPD to major depression is the most difficult to resolve. (This question is discussed in detail in Chapter 2.) The majority of evidence seems to support the hypothesis that there is no specific relationship between BPD and affective disorder except when BPD probands have either concurrent or lifetime histories of major depression.

---

[1] In addition to those mentioned previously, the studies include Loranger and Tulis 1985; Schulz et al. 1989; and Soloff and Millward 1983b.

Twin Study, Adoptive Studies, and Segregation Analyses

Torgersen (1984) has published the only report of a twin study done with the aim of examining the contribution of genetic factors in the development of schizotypal personality disorder (SPD) and BPD. This report was part of a larger Norwegian study of same-sexed twins with nonpsychotic functional psychiatric disorders. Twins were diagnosed using DSM-III (American Psychiatric Association 1980) criteria, and the rater was blind as to the zygosity of the twins. Of the 69 probands receiving personality disorder diagnoses, only 10 were considered to have BPD, and another 15 were diagnosed as having both BPD and SPD. The results were not felt to support a genetic etiology for BPD because none of 3 monozygotic co-twins of probands with BPD and only 2 of 7 dyzygotic co-twins had BPD. Unfortunately, the prevalence of BPD was low in this sample, leaving the possibility of a type II error.

Adoptive studies are the other designs that have been used to examine the contributions of heredity and environment to abnormal behavior (Bohman 1981). Several specific designs exist:

1. *Adoptees family study.* In this study, the biological relatives of affected adoptees and unaffected control adoptees are compared. The prevalence among relatives of biological and control families allows for an estimation of genetic and environmental factors.
2. *Adoptees study method.* In this method the prevalences of disorder among adoptees born to affected and unaffected parents are compared.
3. *Cross-fostering methods.* In this approach adoptees born of affected parents are contrasted with adoptees born of unaffected parents but reared by an adoptive parent who was affected by the disorder under study.

Adoptive studies, as summarized by Bohman (1981), have supported genetic factors as being important in the etiology of alcoholism, but there is less evidence that antisocial behavior is genetically determined. As of yet, there are no published reports of adoptive studies that have examined parents or adoptees diagnosed with BPD. Although adoptive status is not uncommon in borderline cohorts (see Links et al. 1988, in whose study approximately 10% of the cohort was adopted), and borderline mothers often have children removed from their care, focusing on the specific diagnosis may not be as valuable as focusing on specific traits that may be inherited. Torgersen (1984) examined heritability of different personality traits in his sample of same-sexed twins. As a result, he was able to identify hereditary and environmental factors. For example, the factor named "aggressive impulsiveness" was selected as an environmental factor resulting from upbringing, family pattern, and cultural style rather than genetic factors.

A crucial question remains to be determined: What is the phenotype that may be an expression of the inherited defect in BPD?

Four genetic models (autosomal dominant, recessive, polygenic, and X-linked) of inheritance were tested using segregation analyses (Links and Boiago, in press). The proposed models were fitted to data on the occurrence of psychiatric illness in the first-degree relatives of BPD patients. None of the models was supported when the observed and expected proportions of affected siblings and offspring were compared based on the genetic hypotheses outlined. The frequent occurrence of the possible phenotypic behaviors of impulsivity (39% of offspring of affected parents) and suicide attempts (38% of offspring) and the unequal sex distribution of affected offspring were most compatible with an environmental etiologic model rather than with the proposed genetic hypotheses.

Summary

This review suggests the need for further twin and adoptive studies to clarify the contribution of genetic factors in BPD. The consistent finding of the increased occurrence of BPD in the families of BPD patients needs to be explained. We remain uncertain about whether there is a specific phenotype that is expressed as the inherited defect in BPD.

The possible implications of environmental traumata in the causation of BPD seem more supported by current research (see Links and Munroe Blum 1990), but the actual mechanisms involved will require further elaboration. Previous work in this area indicates that family psychopathology may create an environment where abuse and childhood traumata occur (Links and Boiago, in press). In summary, most of the evidence to date suggests that BPD is the result of "living under the same roof" with a psychiatrically ill parent(s), in which context the parental psychiatric illness, instability, and resulting traumata lead to impaired development and an adult personality disorder.

ACQUIRED AND DEVELOPMENTAL BRAIN DYSFUNCTION

In this section we examine the evidence supporting a causal role for brain dysfunction in producing BPD. Brain dysfunction, in this context, is based on the relationship of both acquired and developmental neurologic (or "organic") brain injuries, as well as on the evidence provided by neurologic and neuropsychological testing, neurobehavioral models of brain functioning, and response to treatments. The evidence is summarized in Table 1–1.

The strength of the association between BPD and brain dysfunction has been examined in case-control design studies that 1) compare the prevalence of acquired and developmental brain injuries in BPD patients with the prevalence of such injuries in patients with other diagnoses; or 2) employ investigative tools to attempt to detect brain dysfunction in BPD patients.

Prevalence of Brain Injuries in Patients With Borderline Personality Disorder

Andrulonis et al. (1981) presented preliminary data suggesting that a significant proportion of BPD patients (29% of the females and 56% of the males) had a history of "organicity." This "organic" group was composed of two subgroups. A minimal brain dysfunction subgroup was composed of patients with histories of attention-deficit disorder or a learning disability. A second subgroup was composed of patients who had suffered acquired brain injuries, including trauma, encephalitis, and epilepsy. Those patients with histories of "organicity" had earlier onset of illness, acted out more frequently, and had stronger family histories of substance abuse. This study, however, which involved a treatment-resistant group at the Institute of Living, did not include a control group and study personnel were not blinded (Cornelius et al. 1989).

Andrulonis et al. (1982) did a follow-up study in which BPD patients

Table 1–1. Summary of evidence supporting an association between borderline personality disorder and brain dysfunction

Authors	Evidence	Findings BPD	Controls	Findings Controls	P
Andrulonis et al. (1981)	Prevalence of brain injuries	38%	None	—	—
Andrulonis et al. (1982)	Prevalence of brain injuries	40% 14%	Schizophrenia	25.5%	—
Andrulonis et al. (1984)	Prevalence of brain injuries	40% 14%	Affective disorders	7%	—
Soloff and Millward (1983a)	Complications of pregnancy	17.8%	Schizophrenia	0.0%	< .03
		17.8%	Major depression	4.8%	< .03
van Reekum et al. (submitted)	Prevalence of brain injuries	81%	Mixed psychiatric	22%	< .001
Cowdry et al. 1985	EEG (sharp abnormalities)	59%	Major depression	25%	< .02
Snyder and Pitts (1984)	EEG	19%	Dysthymia	0.0%	< .05
van Reekum et al. (submitted)	EEG	23.5%	Mixed psychiatric	6.3%	NS
Cornelius et al. (1986)	EEG	18.8%	Mixed psychiatric (Axis II)	9.1%	NS
Snyder et al. (1983)	CT scan (ventricular enlargement)	0.0%	—	—	—
Schulz et al. (1983)	CT scan (ventricle: brain ratio)	2.9%	Schizophrenia	8.4	< .004
		2.9%	Normal subjects	2.7	NS
Lucas et al. (1989)	CT scan: Ventricle:brain ratio	3.4	Normal subjects	4.1	NS
	Gross anatomical change	13%	Normal subjects	14%	NS
Chapin et al. (1987)	Reaction time test: Point of crossover	19.0	Schizophrenia	7.3	< .001
			Schizotypal	10.9	< .001
			Major depression	18.5	NS
			Normal subjects	24.0	NS
	Latency	420	Schizotypal	424	< .02
			Normal subjects	298	< .02
			Schizophrenia	370	NS
			Major depression	267	< .02

Table 1–1.   Summary of evidence supporting an association between borderline
             personality disorder and brain dysfunction *(continued)*

Authors	Evidence	Findings BPD	Controls	Findings Controls	P
Kutcher et al. (1987)	Auditory P300:				
	Latency	340	Schizophrenia Normal, depressed, and	341	< .05
		340	non-BPD Axis II	316	< .01
	Amplitude	5.7	Schizophrenia	5.46	Similar at *P* < .01
			Normal, depressed, and		
		5.7	non-BPD Axis II	6.9	< .01
Gardner et al. (1987)	Soft signs (2 or more)	65%	Normal	32%	< .05
van Reekum et al. (submitted)	Soft signs (2 or more)	60%	None	—	—
Cornelius et al. (1989)	Neuropsychological test battery (nonfrontal)	Normal	Historical	—	—
van Reekum et al. (submitted)	Neuropsychological test battery (nonfrontal)	78% abnormal	None	—	—

Note. NS = not significant.

were matched for age and sex with patients meeting DSM-III criteria for
schizophrenia. The proportion of BPD patients, both male and female,
who had suffered a brain injury did not change significantly from the
authors' previous study. Schizophrenic males and females both suffered
fewer brain injuries than did patients in the BPD groups.

Andrulonis and Vogel (1984) also presented the above data but with
the addition of a control group of patients with affective disorders. Approximately the same relative proportions of BPD patients (40% and 14%
of males and females, respectively) fell into one of the two "organic"
subgroups, whereas 25% of the schizophrenic patients and only 7% of the
patients with affective disorders had histories of developmental or acquired brain injuries. The increased prevalence of brain injuries observed
in BPD males compared with BPD females was not found in the control
populations, in which no sex differences were observed.

Soloff and Millward (1983a) studied patients who scored positive on the Diagnostic Interview for Borderlines (DIB) (Gunderson et al. 1981), predominantly young, female, Caucasian, and from a lower- to middle-class catchment area, who were admitted to a university-operated in-patient facility. They were compared with patients meeting Research Diagnostic Criteria for major depression and meeting criteria for schizophrenia. Patients with BPD were significantly younger than depressed control subjects. Because patients were excluded if they had chronic disorders that had required more than 2 years of hospitalization within the previous 5 years, a less severely ill group was selected. Furthermore, patients with a history of "organic brain syndrome," seizure disorder or "any known CNS abnormality," borderline mental retardation, substance abuse, or "any medical disorder with known psychiatric sequelae" were excluded. Not surprisingly, given that patients with CNS lesions were excluded, a significant prevalence of brain injuries in the BPD population was not found. Only complications of pregnancy (17.8% of patients with BPD vs. 0.0% of schizophrenic patients and 4.8% of depressed control subjects) were significantly more common in BPD probands. Soloff and Millward's study also suffered many of the same pitfalls as the work by Andrulonis et al.—namely, lack of observer blindness, a heavy reliance on retrospectively obtained data, and poorly defined diagnostic criteria for neurodevelopmental disorders.

Van Reekum et al. (unpublished observations) had the opportunity within the Veterans Affairs (VA) hospital system to study a group of patients who, for the most part, derive from a relatively low socioeconomic level. Veterans tend to remain with the VA system, so complete medical and psychiatric histories were easily obtained, often dating to entry into the armed services. Developmental histories were present, in most cases, on the basis of routinely obtained second-person informants. A case-control study involving retrospective chart review included 48 (primarily male) DIB-positive veterans with BPD who had been hospitalized on the acute psychiatry wards of the Bedford VA Hospital in Massachusetts. The probands were compared to 50 age-matched veterans, with a mixed set of psychiatric diagnoses, derived from the same wards. Formal criteria for neurodevelopmental diagnoses were established. BPD patients and control patients were not statistically different on age, gender, demographic variables, onset and duration of illness, and prevalence of substance abuse.

The study showed that 81% of BPD patients compared with 22% of control patients ($P < .0001$) had a definite history of developmental delay (44% of BPD patients) or acquired CNS injury (58% of BPD patients). Developmental delay diagnoses included attention-deficit disorder, learning disorder, or other developmental delay. Acquired CNS injuries included traumatic brain injury, seizures, and other CNS lesions (e.g., tumors, hydrocephalus, encephalitis). This study, while agreeing with the work of Andrulonis et al. (see above), also suffered from lack of blindness and selection bias.

Van Reekum et al. also compared the chart-review diagnoses of brain insults with diagnoses based on prospective interview in a subgroup of 10 patients with BPD and found that the prevalence of brain insults did not change significantly. Prospective neurologic soft sign assessment and neuropsychological screening were also completed in this subgroup. (These results are discussed below in the section –Neuropsychological Evidence.") Findings from this prospective component of the study lent further support to diagnoses made on the basis of chart review.

The specific association between BPD and epilepsy has received attention. Two case reports (Messner 1986; Schmid et al. 1989) documented cases of patients diagnosed as "borderline" who later were discovered to have seizure disorders felt to be causative of the behavioral disturbance. In a more thorough study of this relationship, Mendez et al. (1989) examined subjects who had attempted suicide by overdose identified from patients admitted to University Hospitals of Cleveland from 1981 through 1987. Of the epileptic patients, 45.5% received the BPD diagnosis compared with 13.6% of control subjects ($P < .01$). There was a trend toward a greater prevalence of psychosis ($P = .06$), as well as fewer adjustment reactions ($P < .05$) in the epileptic group compared with the control group. The prevalence of major depression did not significantly differentiate the two groups.

Borderline Personality Disorder and Prospective Neurologic Methods

The second approach to establishing an association between BPD and brain dysfunction is to prospectively investigate current brain functioning in BPD patients. One study found a higher prevalence of abnormalities on the electroencephalogram (EEG) in patients with BPD compared with control subjects with major depression (Cowdry et al. 1985); another study also found an increased prevalence of EEG abnormalities in patients with BPD compared with control subjects with dysthymia (Snyder and Pitts 1984). Trends toward a higher prevalence of EEG abnormalities were found in two other studies that compared groups of BPD patients with mixed groups of patients having other psychiatric diagnoses, including Axis II diagnoses (Cornelius et al. 1986; R. van Reekum, C. Conway, D. Gansler, et al, submitted for publication). The prevalence of all EEG abnormalities in BPD subjects ranged from 18.8% to 59% (Cornelius et al. 1986). When only the more specific, or severe, EEG abnormalities are considered, the prevalence decreases, ranging from 13% (Cornelius et al. 1986) to 41% (Cowdry et al. 1985). No pattern of localization is obvious, nor is the nature of the EEG abnormalities. The significance of these abnormalities in terms of behavioral change is not known. Larger studies employing standardized, and perhaps quantitative, EEG assessments are, however, indicated by the uniformly high prevalence of EEG abnormalities found in the four studies described above.

Cowdry et al. (1985) further examined the prevalence of complex partial seizure symptoms in their BPD population. Most, but not all, symptoms were frequently found in the BPD group. Although the authors did not feel that their patients suffered from "classical complex partial seizures," the reporting of increased clinical evidence of seizure phenomena does lend increased credibility to the electroencephalographic findings.

Evidence of structural brain abnormalities in patients with BPD has been sought in studies using computed tomography (CT) (Lucas et al. 1987; Schulz et al. 1983; Snyder et al. 1983). Snyder et al. (1983) reviewed CT scans of BPD patients in an uncontrolled study and found no evidence of abnormalities. Schulz et al. (1983) compared the CT scans of BPD patients with those of a schizophrenic group and a normal population. The schizophrenic group had significantly larger ventricular-brain ratios than did either of the other two groups. BPD patients and normal control subjects did not differ. Lucas et al. (1989), in a blinded study of BPD patients compared with normal control subjects, found no differences in ventricular-brain ratios, nor did they find evidence of increased gross anatomical changes in the BPD group. A trend toward increased CT scan abnormalities had been found in the small subgroup of van Reekum et al.'s (submitted for publication) BPD patients who had received CT scans. Given the lack of significant findings in these studies, further CT scan studies in BPD are not recommended.

The absence of findings does not, however, rule out the possibility of a more subtle brain pathophysiology underlying BPD. Indeed, CT scan findings are often absent in those brain disorders most frequently associated with BPD, such as traumatic brain injury, idiopathic epilepsy, attention-deficit disorder, and learning disabilities.

Other neurologic investigative studies have been reported. Chapin et al. (1987) used a reaction time test to compare BPD patients to patients in four other diagnostic categories. BPD patients differed on the point-of-crossover component of the study (i.e., "a measure of ability to benefit from preparatory intervals of different lengths" [p. 949]) from a group of schizophrenic patients and a group of patients with schizotypal personality disorder. On the latency measure, the BPD subjects differed from the schizotypal and the normal control subjects. BPD subjects did not differ from the patients with major affective disorder on point of crossover or latency measure. The authors concluded only that the BPD subjects were different from the schizotypal subjects. The difference on the latency measure between the BPD subjects and the normal control subjects was felt to reflect the inpatient status of the BPD patients.

Kutcher et al. (1987), using P300 and other long-latency auditory event–related electroencephalographic potentials, demonstrated that BPD subjects and schizophrenic patients share a "dysfunction of auditory neurointegration." The P3 latency was longer, and the amplitude smaller, in the BPD group. These measures were similar in the BPD and schizophrenia groups, distinguishing these two categories from normal, depressed, and non-BPD Axis II disorders. The results do not help to localize the brain dysfunction, and the significance of the biological similarity with schizophrenia "awaits further study and clarification."

Gardner et al. (1987) examined BPD females using a battery of neurologic soft signs and compared them to normal control subjects. The assessment was not blinded to BPD status. BPD subjects as a group had significantly more soft signs than did the control subjects ($P < .02$, one-tailed). Using a cut-off score of two or more soft signs revealed a significant difference between BPD subjects (65%) compared with control subjects (32%, $P < .05$). In another study (van Reekum et al., submitted for publication), 6 out of 10 BPD patients who received a soft-sign assessment were found to have two or more soft signs.

Taken as a whole, the neurologic investigation studies reviewed above suggest subtle, nonlocalizable (using today's technology) brain dysfunction in the absence of gross structural change. Clearly, there remains a paucity of data and an inability to interpret the results of abnormal investigations. Both replication studies and studies involving more sensitive brain imaging and brain functioning technologies are needed.

Neuropsychological Evidence of Association

The effects of brain dysfunction on BPD patients may be better discerned by examining the neuropsychological functioning of these patients. Surprisingly few studies have been reported to date. Cornelius et al. (1989) have the only published study. Again, however, as with their EEG data, Cornelius et al. have selected out those patients in whom brain dysfunction is most likely to occur—that is, chronically ill patients and patients with "overt organicity," physical disorders of known psychiatric consequence, or borderline mental retardation. The remaining BPD subjects were compared with historical controls only. The subjects performed normally on measures of memory, language, motor, and visuospatial functioning. Cornelius et al. make two conclusions that appear unwarranted. They suggest that neuropsychiatric abnormalities are "at most an uncommon etiology" of BPD. Again, one cannot exclude such patients and then hope to find them. Second, the authors conclude that "no consistent pattern of abnormalities" was found. This lack of a consistent pattern is, however, to be expected when one considers the choice of neuropsychological functions that were assessed. Nothing about the behavior of BPD patients would suggest an abnormality in language, motor, memory, and spatial functioning. What is most obvious about BPD patients is their impulsive, often self-mutilative behavior, their affective disinhibition, and their frequent failure to put into effect gains made in psychotherapy. This behavioral pattern suggests dysfunction in limbic and frontal sites.

Van Reekum et al. (submitted for publication) studied the previously mentioned subgroup of 10 BPD subjects with a neuropsychological screening battery. The results were interpreted by a neuropsychologist blinded to BPD status. None of the patients was suffering from an affective, psychotic, or confusional state that would have influenced the results of testing (based on the assessment of the attending psychiatrist and on screening measures for attentional functions and affective state). Seven of nine patients who completed interpretable testing showed evidence of frontal system dysfunction. Deficits most often included impulsivity, cognitive inflexibility, poor self-monitoring, and perseveration. These were noted most often in the Wisconsin Card Sort (Berg 1948), the Trails B (Army Individual Test Battery 1944), and the Rey-Osterreith Complex Figure (copy and recall) (Osterreith 1944). Other neuropsychological tests were performed normally. These data suggest that larger controlled assessments utilizing further measures of frontal functioning should be made. The pattern of cognitive deficits is consistent with the behavioral disturbance that defines BPD and with the poor response to psychotherapy seen in some BPD patients.

Summary of the Evidence

How strong is the association between brain dysfunction and BPD? To determine this, we will use the rules of causation set forth by Sir Bradford Hill (1965). These criteria include the strength of the association, consistency of the evidence, specificity of causation, temporal relationship, biological gradient, biological plausibility, and experimental and analogous evidence.

1. As discussed above, prevalence studies, neurologic investigations, and neuropsychological tests suggest some association between brain injury and BPD.
2. Except for the data generated at the Western Psychiatric Institute (Cornelius et al. 1986, 1989; Soloff and Millward 1983b), and the CT scan findings (Lucas et al. 1989; Snyder et al. 1983), most studies to date have been consistent in finding evidence for brain dysfunction in a significant number of BPD patients.
3. Evidence for a specific causal relationship is lacking at this time. The models of etiology in BPD, presented herein, reflect a complexity of variables and of their interactions. Brain deficits have been postulated for other disorders such as antisocial personality disorder and schizo-

phrenia. The elaboration and identification of models specific to these disorders comprise a potentially fruitful area of study.

4. Evidence for a temporal relationship between brain dysfunction and subsequent onset of BPD awaits prospective cohort studies. It is possible that impulsive behavior (e.g., substance abuse) of BPD patients leads to the high prevalence of traumatic brain injury. Independent of the direction of causality, acquired brain insults may exacerbate underlying BPD traits and will likely have treatment ramifications.

5. Evidence for a biological gradient in which increasing brain dysfunction is associated with increasing severity of BPD is limited to the findings of van Reekum et al. (submitted for publication). They found that a score generated by totaling the number of both developmental and acquired brain insults correlated highly with the score on the DIB for the total group of subjects studied.

6. Biological plausibility for a role of brain dysfunction in BPD is provided by the known behavioral effects of traumatic brain injury (Benson and Blumer 1975; Cummings 1985; Rosenbaum and Hoge 1989), epilepsy (especially with temporal lobe foci) (Bear and Fedio 1977; Fedio 1986; Wender et al. 1985), and developmental disturbance (Baron et al. 1985; Bellak 1979; Cowdry et al. 1985; Lou et al. 1989; Menkes et al. 1967; Rapin 1982). Of note, scales developed to assess the behavioral sequelae of these types of brain insult exhibit remarkable overlap with the behaviors found in the DIB (Alves et al. 1986; Ruff et al. 1986). Neuropsychological test results suggested that the primary deficits in a BPD population reflected frontal and possibly primarily orbital-frontal system dysfunction (van Reekum et al., submitted for publication). This is consistent with the cognitive and physiological effects of traumatic brain injury (Benson and Blumer 1975) and attention-deficit disorder (Boucugnani and Jones 1989; Mattes 1980; Rosenthal and Allen 1978). Cummings' (1985) description of the behavioral sequelae of orbital-frontal lesions is striking in its similarity to the behaviors of patients with BPD: "Lesions in this region appear to divorce frontal monitoring systems from limbic input, resulting in a disinhibited behavioral syndrome where impulses are acted on without consideration of consequences, antisocial actions occur, and emotional lability is marked" (p. 63). It is biologically plausible that orbital-frontal system dysfunction underlies BPD in at least a subgroup of patients.

7. Experimental verification of the role of brain dysfunction in BPD is limited to pharmacological studies. Hooberman and Stern (1984) noted the efficacy of methylphenidate in a patient with BPD and attention-deficit disorder. In a controlled study, Wender et al. (1985) found behavioral and subjective improvement in a group of patients with adult attention-deficit disorder. However, BPD patients had been excluded. It should be noted that dysphoria (Lucas et al. 1987) and psychosis (Schulz et al. 1985) have been demonstrated in BPD subjects given methylphenidate and D-amphetamine, respectively. Cowdry demonstrated clinical improvement, as evidenced by observer ratings, with carbamazepine in a double-blind, randomized clinical trial of 16 female BPD subjects (Cowdry et al. 1985). The case for causality of underlying brain dysfunction would be strengthened by studies that document improvement in brain function coincident with improvement in behavioral functioning. Analogous evidence for causation is provided by the evidence supporting a role for brain dysfunction in antisocial personality disorder (Cowdry and Gardner 1988), a disorder that frequently overlaps with BPD (Pope et al. 1983).

Implications of the Evidence Supporting a Causal Role for Brain Dysfunction in Borderline Personality Disorder

The evidence suggests that brain dysfunction may quantitatively affect behavior (i.e., by increasing the severity of a behavioral disturbance). Whether brain dysfunction also qualitatively shapes behavior cannot be addressed with the findings to date but might, on the basis of orbital-frontal lesion studies (Cummings 1985), be expected to do so. Of greater certainty is the fact that brain dysfunction must interact with environmental and psychodynamic factors in producing behavioral change. Determining how this interaction occurs will await prospective studies that incorporate measures of brain dysfunction and measures of environmental and psychodynamic factors.

However, evidence for underlying brain disorders and cognitive limitations in patients with BPD should be looked for. Abnormalities will be found frequently, especially in those patients whose behavioral disturbance is severe.

There are a number of implications for treatment of brain dysfunction in BPD. Linehan's model (1989) may provide a basis for behavioral rehabilitative efforts, with modification based on each patient's pattern of cognitive and behavioral deficits. Pharmacological treatment of underlying neurobehavioral syndromes, such as with methylphenidate in patients with attention-deficit disorder (Schulz et al. 1985) or with carbamazepine in patients with an underlying seizure disorder (Cowdry and Gardner 1988), may be considered. Preventing behavioral outcomes in identified high-risk, brain-disordered persons might be possible through treatment of the brain disorder or through treatment of the family. Finally, recognition of cognitive limitations and adaptation of existing traditional forms of therapy to reflect these limitations may follow.

BIOLOGICAL MARKERS IN BORDERLINE PERSONALITY DISORDER

Various biochemical measures have been assessed in BPD as possible markers. The purpose behind these investigations is twofold:

1. Associations between BPD and other disorders may be studied. If an association can be established based on the presence of similar biological markers, then an argument for an analogous pathophysiology can be presented. Unfortunately, such arguments tend to be rather weak but are a starting point for investigating BPD.
2. The development of an understanding of the biological mechanisms explaining the pathophysiology and resulting phenomenology can lead to the development of psychopharmacological approaches for the treatment of the disorder.

Three basic methods have been employed in studying biological markers in BPD. The most common method is to study the prevalence of biological markers in various diagnostic groups compared with their prevalence in BPD. This work has been summarized by Steiner et al. (1988) and again by Lahmeyer et al. (1989). The second method is to use psychopharmacological probes as a way to understand the pathophysiology of BPD. Gardner and Cowdry (1989) have argued that this is the most appropriate method to understand BPD and hypothesize that progress will come from the study of dysregulation in biological functions. Finally, psychopharmacological trials and response to medication have been used to try to understand the pathophysiology of the disorder. This approach has recently been summarized by several authors (see, e.g., Links and Steiner 1988). The present discussion will focus mainly on examining the success of using biological markers in establishing possible etiologic associations between BPD and other disorders.

Affective Disorders

As reviewed by Gold and Silk in Chapter 2, the relationship between BPD and affective disorders has been the most studied. The principal markers have included the dexamethasone suppression test (DST), sleep studies, and pharmacological trials.

Steiner et al. (1988) have summarized that the DST has a fairly low sensitivity in samples of BPD patients, with the sensitivity ranging anywhere from 10% to 85% and the specificity ranging from 37.5% to 92.3%. In addition to the low sensitivity, the DST is not a very useful marker in the BPD patient because of the frequency with which technical problems and exclusion criteria for the DST occur. For example, borderline patients often have coexisting eating disorders or drug and alcohol abuse that renders the DST invalid and impractical as a clinical test.

Sleep studies have been carried out in samples of patients with BPD. BPD and major depression together seem to be associated with more significant abnormalities of rapid eye movement (REM) latency and density. A history of affective disorder is related to decreased REM latency, and this area of study seems to comprise the most robust biological marker relating affective disorders to BPD (Lahmeyer et al. 1989). Other biological markers, such as DST and drug response, have been used to argue against a close association between BPD and affective disorders (Lahmeyer et al. 1989).

The psychopharmacological trials of the response of depression in BPD to antidepressants have been unsupportive of a relationship between BPD and affective disorders. Previous studies of BPD patients have not shown a specific response of depressive symptoms to tricyclic antidepressants. One study, by Cowdry and Gardner (1988), did show some response of affective symptoms to monoamine oxidase (MAO) inhibitors. However, there seems to be a lack of relationship between target symptom response and drug type (see Soloff, Chapter 15).

Schizophrenia

Various markers have been studied to connect biological markers for schizophrenia to BPD. These include monitoring smooth pursuit eye tracking, auditory evoked potentials, electroencephalographic recording, and platelet MAO. Kutcher et al.'s (1989) studies are perhaps most interesting because auditory P300 long-latency auditory event–related potentials in BPD patients have been found that are similar to those found in schizophrenic individuals. However, the BPD group was significantly differentiated from the depressive control group. This relationship was not explained by the presence of schizotypal traits. However, Kutcher et al. did find that the BPD patients had similar evoked-potential responses to the schizotypal control sample.

There is some evidence from challenge studies of a possible dopaminergic action in patients with BPD. For example, Schulz et al. (1985) found a dysphoric response to amphetamines, and, similarly, Lucas et al. (1987) found dysphoria from the administration of methylphenidate. Adding to this evidence is the consistent finding of the effectiveness of low-dose neuroleptics in BPD patients. This seems to be a nonspecific but consistent improvement.

In summary, the evidence suggests that there may be an association between the biological markers found in schizophrenia and BPD. It is possible that a third factor related to the presence of schizotypal features or that some other factors may be producing this relationship. Future studies may need to examine whether the third factor is a specific aspect of the phenomenology that creates the bridge between schizophrenia and BPD.

Impulse Disorders

Gunderson and Zanarini (1989) have postulated that BPD may be characterized by an underlying impulse disorder (see Chapter 3). A recent report by Coccaro et al. (1989) showed a reduced prolactin response to fenfluramine in patients rated with impulsive aggressiveness. These results seemed to indicate a reduced central serotonergic function in this subgroup of patients. The evidence for an abnormality of serotonergic functioning is consistent with the recent finding in our own study (Links et al. 1990) of the effectiveness of lithium versus placebo and desipramine. The lithium tended to decrease anger and suicidal symptoms, whereas desipramine increased these symptoms (Links et al. 1990). We interpreted these results as indicating that lithium may be acting on the impulsive aspects of BPD. Similarly Cowdry and Gardner (1988) showed that carbamazepine was an effective agent, specific for the behavioral dyscontrol aspects of this syndrome.

Conclusions

1. No clear associations have been established between major Axis I disorders and BPD based on biological markers. This method of study may have reached its pinnacle, at least until new technologies develop new biological tests.
2. Future studies of biological markers must address such aspects as outcome, drug response, and rating changes that capture the fluctuating clinical state of these patients.
3. Biological markers should be related to environmental events. For example, the attempts to relate early traumata and the resulting dissociative states to biological abnormalities may prove a useful way to proceed in the study of these issues.

CONSTITUTIONAL FACTORS AND MODELS OF ETIOLOGY

Our review might suggest four possible etiologic models for BPD:

1. Brain injury, especially to orbital-frontal cortex and other limbic sites, could cause a disorder of impulse control, affective dysregulation, cognitive disability, and predisposition to psychotic decompensation. Neuronal misconnections may be the intermediary pathological step (Goodman 1989). Alternatively, a specific set of cognitive dysfunctions may lead to the alteration in behavior. Other possible mediators include

limbic hyperactivity, possibly through seizure activity (Cowdry et al. 1985), and altered monoamine metabolism (Cloninger 1987). Social and interpersonal dysfunction follows secondarily. Behaviors are moderated by preexisting social, educational, and psychodynamic factors.

2. In patients with developmental disturbances, other family members, notably parents, may also suffer developmental disturbance. Thus, patients are more frequently exposed to aberrant behaviors such as substance abuse, erratic parenting, marital discord, and physical/sexual abuse. Exposure to these behaviors contributes to injury to the self, alters normal psychosexual development, and, through learning/modeling, may directly affect behavioral development. The effects of developmental disturbance in the patient and of the exposure to aberrant behaviors produced by developmentally disturbed family members may be additive.

3. BPD is a primary disorder of impulse control, perhaps with genetic predisposition to developmental disturbance. Poor impulse control leads to a higher risk of traumatic brain injury and substance abuse, both of which exacerbate the preexisting impulse control disorder (Woodcock 1986), and contribute to the development of cognitive limitations. In a subgroup of patients, traumatic brain injury or other CNS illness occurs in the absence of preexisting impulse control disorder and is the primary cause of impulsivity in the patient. Impulsive behavior and impulsively formed cognitions, in the absence of self-monitoring and modulation, lead to repeated personal failures and aberrant self-other images, and secondarily to depressed/angry affects and predisposition to psychosis.

4. Normal personality development may require a critical mass of cognitive functioning, which is dependent on an intact brain. Any combination of insults to cognitive functioning that surpasses the critical mass required leads to a final common pathway of "borderline" personality development. For example, it has been observed that brain injuries in previously highly functioning individuals have lesser impact on behavior than do otherwise equivalent brain insults in individuals with fewer cognitive and ego strengths. In many patients, then, there will be an absence of brain and cognitive dysfunction. BPD behavior can result from a genetic predisposition shared with affective disorder or psychotic illness, as well as from experiential effects on ego functioning.

REFERENCES

Alves WM, Colohan ART, O'Leary TJ, et al: Understanding posttraumatic symptoms after minor head injury. Journal of Head Trauma Rehabilitation 1:1–12, 1986

American Psychiatric Association: Diagnostic and Statistical Manual of Mental Disorders, 3rd Edition. Washington, DC, American Psychiatric Association, 1980

American Psychiatric Association: Diagnostic and Statistical Manual of Mental Disorders, 3rd Edition, Revised. Washington, DC, American Psychiatric Association, 1987

Andrulonis PA, Vogel NG: Comparison of borderline personality subcategories to schizophrenic and affective disorders. Br J Psychiatry 144:358–363, 1984

Andrulonis PA, Glueck BC, Stroebel CF, et al: Organic brain dysfunction and the borderline syndrome. Psychiatr Clin North Am 4:47–66, 1981

Andrulonis PA, Glueck BC, Stroebel CF, et al: Borderline personality subcategories. J Nerv Ment Dis 170:670–679, 1982

Army Individual Test Battery: Manual of Directions and Scoring. Washington, DC, Ward Department, Adjutant General's Office, 1944

Baron M, Gruen R, Asnis L, et al: Familial transmission of schizotypal and borderline personality disorders. Am J Psychiatry 142:927–934, 1985

Bear DM, Fedio P: Quantitative analysis of interictal behavior in temporal lobe epilepsy. Arch Neurol 34:454–467, 1977

Bellak LP (ed): Psychiatric Aspects of Minimal Brain Dysfunction in Adults. New York, Grune & Stratton, 1979

Benson DF, Blumer D: Psychiatric Aspects of Neurologic Disease. New York, Grune & Stratton, 1975

Berg RA: A simple objective technique for measuring flexibility in thinking. J Genet Psychol 39:15–22, 1948

Bohman M: The interaction of heredity and childhood environment: some adoption studies. J Child Psychol Psychiatry 22:195–200, 1981

Boucugnani LL, Jones RW: Behaviors analogous to frontal lobe dysfunction in children with attention deficit hyperactivity disorder. Arch Clin Neuropsychol 4:161–173, 1989

Chapin K, Wightman L, Lycaki H, et al: Difference in reaction time between subjects with schizotypal and borderline personality disorders. Am J Psychiatry 144:948–950, 1987

Cloninger CR: A systematic method for clinical description and classification of personality variants: a proposal. Arch Gen Psychiatry 44:573–588, 1987

Coccaro EF, Siever LS, Klar HM, et al: Serotonergic studies in patients with affective and personality disorders: correlates with suicidal and impulsive aggressive behavior. Arch Gen Psychiatry 46:587–599, 1989

Cornelius JR, Brenner RP, Soloff PH, et al: EEG abnormalities in borderline personality disorder: specific or nonspecific. Biol Psychiatry 21:977–980, 1986

Cornelius JR, Soloff PH, George AWA, et al: An evaluation of the significance of selected neuropsychiatric abnormalities in the etiology of borderline personality disorder. Journal of Personality Disorders 3:19–25, 1989

Cowdry RW, Gardner DL: Pharmacotherapy of borderline personality disorder: alprazolam, carbamazepine, trifluoperazine and tranylcypromine. Arch Gen Psychiatry 45:111–119, 1988

Cowdry RW, Pickar D, Davies R: Symptoms and EEG findings in the borderline syndrome. Int J Psychiatry Med 15:201–211, 1985

Cummings JL: Clinical Neuropsychiatry. Orlando, FL, Grune & Stratton, 1985

Fedio P: Behavioral characteristics of patients with temporal lobe epilepsy. Psychiatr Clin North Am 9:267–281, 1986

Gardner DL, Cowdry RW: Borderline personality disorder: a research challenge (editorial). Biol Psychiatry 26:655–658, 1989

Gardner D, Lucas PB, Cowdry RW: Soft sign neurological abnormalities in borderline personality disorder and normal control subjects. J Nerv Ment Dis 175:177–180, 1987

Goodman R: Neuronal misconnections and psychiatric disorder: is there a link? Br J Psychiatry 154:292–299, 1989

Gunderson JG, Zanarini MC: Pathogenesis of borderline personality, in American Psychiatric Press Review of Psychiatry, Vol 8. Edited by Tasman A, Hales RE, Frances AJ. Washington DC, 1989, pp 25–48

Gunderson JG, Kolb JE, Austin V: The diagnostic interview for borderline patients. Am J Psychiatry 138:896–903, 1981

Hill AB: The environment and disease: association or causation? Proc R Soc Med 58:295–300, 1965

Hoch P, Polatin P: Pseudoneurotic forms of schizophrenia. Psychiatr Q 23:248–276, 1949

Hooberman D, Stern TA: Treatment of attention deficit and borderline personality disorders with psychostimulants: case report. J Clin Psychiatry 45:441–442, 1984

Kutcher SP, Blackwood DHR, St Clair D, et al: Auditory P300 in borderline personality disorder and schizophrenia. Arch Gen Psychiatry 44:645–650, 1987

Kutcher P, Blackwood DHR, Gaskell DF, et al: Auditory P300 does not differentiate borderline personality disorder from schizotypal personality disorder. Biol Psychiatry 26:766–774, 1989

Lahmeyer HW, Reynolds CF, Kupfer DJ, et al: Biologic markers in borderline personality disorder: a review. J Clin Psychiatry 50:217–225, 1989

Linehan MM: Cognitive and behavior therapy for borderline personality disorder, in American Psychiatric Press Review of Psychiatry, Vol 8. Edited by Tasman A, Hales RE, Frances AJ. Washington, DC, American Psychiatric Press, 1989, pp 84–102

Links PS, Boiago I: Borderline personality disorder as an impulse disorder: evidence from family and genetic studies. Journal of Personality Disorders (in press)

Links PS, Munroe Blum H: Family environment and borderline personality disorder: development of etiologic models, in Family Environment and Borderline Personality Disorders. Edited by Links PS. Washington, DC, American Psychiatric Press, 1990, pp 1–24

Links PS, Steiner M: Psychopharmacologic management of patients with borderline personality disorder. Can J Psychiatry 33:355–359, 1988

Links PS, Steiner M, Huxley G: The occurrence of borderline personality disorder in the families of borderline patients. Journal of Personality Disorders 2:14–20, 1988

Links PS, Steiner M, Boiago I, et al: Lithium therapy for borderline patients: preliminary findings. Journal of Personality Disorders 4:173–181, 1990

Loranger AW, Tulis EH: Family history of alcoholism in borderline personality disorder. Arch Gen Psychiatry 42:153–157, 1985

Loranger AW, Oldham JM, Tulis EH: Familial transmission of DSM-III borderline personality disorder. Arch Gen Psychiatry 39:795–799, 1982

Lou HC, Henriksen L, Bruhn P, et al: Striatal dysfunction in attention deficit and hyperkinetic disorder. Arch Neurol 46:48–52, 1989

Lucas PB, Gardner DL, Wolkowitz OM, et al: Dysphoria associated with methylphenidate infusion in borderline personality disorder. Am J Psychiatry 144:1577–1579, 1987

Lucas PB, Gardner DL, Cowdry RW, et al: Cerebral structure in borderline personality disorder. Psychiatry Res 27:111–115, 1989

Mattes JA: The role of frontal lobe dysfunction in childhood hyperkinesis. Compr Psychiatry 21:358–369, 1980

Mendez MF, Lanska DJ, Manon-Espaillat R, et al: Causative factors for suicide attempts by overdose in epileptics. Arch Neurol 46:1065–1068, 1989

Menkes MD, Rowe JS, Menkes SJH: A twenty-five year follow-up study on hyperkinetic child with minimal brain dysfunction. Pediatrics 39:393–399, 1967

Messner E: Covert complex partial seizures in psychotherapy. Am J Orthopsychiatry 56:323–326, 1986

Osterreith PA: Le test de cope d'une figure complexe. Archives Psychologie 30:206–356, 1944

Pope HG Jr, Jonas JM, Hudson JI, et al: The validity of DSM III borderline personality disorder: a phenomenologic family history, treatment response, and long-term follow-up study. Arch Gen Psychiatry 40:23–30, 1983

Rapin I: Children With Brain Dysfunction: Neurology, Cognition, Language and Behavior. New York, Raven, 1982

Robins E, Guze SB: Establishment of diagnostic validity in psychiatric illness: its application to schizophrenia. Am J Psychiatry 126:983–987, 1970

Rosenbaum A, Hoge SK: Head injury and marital aggression. Am J Psychiatry 146:1048–1051, 1989

Rosenthal RH, Allen JW: An examination of attention, arousal, and learning dysfunctions of hyperkinetic children. Psychol Bull 85:689–715, 1978

Ruff RM, Levin KS, Marshall LF: Neurobehavioral methods of assessment and the study of outcome in minor head injury. Journal of Head Trauma Rehabilitation 1:43–52, 1986

Schmid EM, Handleman MJ, Bidder TG: Seizure disorder misdiagnosed as borderline syndrome (letter). Am J Psychiatry 146:400–401, 1989

Schulz SC, Koller MM, Kishore PR, et al: Ventricular enlargement in teenage patients with schizophrenia spectrum disorder. Am J Psychiatry 140:1592–1595, 1983

Schulz SC, Schulz PM, Dommisse C, et al: Amphetamine response in borderline patients. Psychiatry Res 15:97–108, 1985

Schulz PM, Schulz SC, Goldberg SC, et al: Diagnoses of the relatives of schizotypal outpatients. J Nerv Mental Dis 174:457–463, 1986

Schulz PM, Soloff PH, Kelly T, et al: A family history of borderline subtypes. Journal of Personality Disorders 3:217–229, 1989

Silverman JM, Pinkham L, Horvath TB, et al: Affective and impulsive personality disorder traits in the relatives of patients with borderline personality disorder. Am J Psychiatry 148:1378–1385, 1991

Snyder S, Pitts WM Jr: Electroencephalograph of DSM-III borderline personality disorder. Acta Psychiatr Scand 69:129–134, 1984

Snyder S, Pitts WM Jr, Gustin Q: CT scans of patients with borderline personality disorder. Am J Psychiatry 140:272, 1983

Soloff PH, Millward JW: Developmental histories of borderline patients. Compr Psychiatry 24:574–588, 1983a

Soloff PH, Millward JW: Psychiatric disorders in the families of borderline patients. Arch Gen Psychiatry 40:37–44, 1983b

Steiner M, Links PS, Korzekwa M: Biological markers in borderline personality disorders: an overview. Can J Psychiatry 33:350–354, 1988

Stone MH: The borderline syndrome: evolution of the term, genetic aspects, and prognosis. Am J Psychother 31:345–365, 1977

Stone MH, Kahn E, Flye B: Psychiatrically ill relatives of borderline patients: a family study. Psychiatr Q 53:71–84, 1981

Torgersen S: Genetic and nosological aspects of schizotypal and borderline personality disorders: a twin study. Arch Gen Psychiatry 41:546–554, 1984

Wender PH, Reimherr FW, Wood D, et al: A controlled study of methylphenidate in the treatment of attention deficit disorder, residual type, in adults. Am J Psychiatry 142:547–552, 1985

Woodcock JH: A neuropsychiatric approach to impulse disorders. Psychiatr Clin North Am 9:341–352, 1986

Zanarini MC, Gunderson JG, Marino MF, et al: Psychiatric disorders in the families of borderline outpatients, in Family Environment and Borderline Personality Disorder. Edited by Links PS. Washington, DC, American Psychiatric Press, 1990, pp 67–84

Exploring the Borderline Personality Disorder–Major Affective Disorder Interface

Laura J. Gold, Ph.D.
Kenneth R. Silk, M.D.

PERHAPS THE MOST STRIKING FEATURE OF THE TERM *BOR-derline personality disorder* (BPD) is the transformation that has taken place from its initial association with schizophrenia to its current association with affective disorders (Kroll 1988; Stone 1979). Recently, there has been significant debate concerning the high concurrence of BPD and affective illness. The available evidence suggests a 40% to 60% overlap between major affective disorder (MAD) and BPD among hospitalized and clinic patients (Gunderson and Elliott 1985). Some researchers conclude that BPD is simply a variant of MAD and not a discrete diagnostic entity. In their comprehensive review of the literature, Gunderson and Elliott (1985) critically evaluated three prevailing conceptualizations of the relationship between BPD and MAD. Akiskal (1981) and others such as Liebowitz and Klein (1981) posit that borderline character pathology arises secondarily from an affective disorder. This theory attributes borderline symptoms such as suicide attempts, poor object relations, and sexual promiscuity to, respectively, despair, poor self-esteem, and efforts to alleviate depression. Kernberg (1975) and others such as Masterson (1976), on the other hand, suggest that affective illness develops as a consequence of the BPD patient's failed relationships, impulsive behavior, and hypersensitivity to separation and loss. Thus depression, according to this conceptualization, is secondary to the personality disorder. A third hypothesis postulates that the two syndromes are unrelated and only coincidentally occur simultaneously, with no causal or meaningful relationship.

After closely examining the merits of each hypothesis in terms of issues such as general prevalence, phenomenology, course, family prevalence, psychodynamic factors, biological factors, and drug response, Gunderson and Elliott (1985) concluded that none of the three hypotheses satisfactorily accounts for the data. They offer a fourth hypothesis: that both borderline personality and affective disorder arise from many sources and that "the observed concurrence of affective and borderline symptoms results from that heterogeneity" (p. 286). They explain:

> For either disorder, individuals may start with a bio-physiological vulnerability that increases their risk of being psychologically impaired in early development. Such early traumas may create vulnerability to either or both disorders, but the actual presentation varies as a function of later physiological and psychological reactions to environment and temperament. The key to the overlap and dissimilarities between these two disorders, then, may be a constellation of innate and external factors that are inconsequential individually but combine to shape depression, chronic dysphoria, or borderline behavior—alone or in any possible combination. (p. 286)

Although similar to the third hypothesis, Gunderson and Elliott's hypothesis suggests that the *same* etiologic base of biophysiological and environmental factors that shape depression can shape borderline pathology *or* a combination of the disorders. Thus, either disorder can be, but does not have to be, primary. Further, these authors, as well as Widiger (1989), suggest that BPD and MAD are not in actuality sharply discontinuous categorical diagnostic concepts as implied by the Axis I–Axis II division in DSM-III-R (American Psychiatric Association 1987).

Recently, Gunderson and Phillips (1991) reviewed the literature since 1985 and concluded more strongly that BPD is *not* simply an affective disorder. They are unimpressed with the comorbidity between BPD and major depression or dysthymia, because it also exists for all other personality disorders. Moreover, there is a qualitative difference between the empty, environmentally responsive mood of borderline patients and classic depression. Family history studies (see Zanarini, Chapter 3) do not support the link, and borderline patients do not have the same response to antidepressants as those patients with affective disorder. Biological markers are shared with depression only when dysthymia is present. Finally, there is stronger evidence for environmental causation in BPD. Gunderson and Phillips therefore conclude that although BPD and depression coexist, these disorders are not otherwise related.

In this chapter we attempt to explore further the BPD and MAD interface. Studies that have often been used to support a strong connection between BPD and MAD are reevaluated to focus on the fact that the data can also be interpreted to refute a connection between BPD and MAD. We have focused our discussion initially on biological "tests," because it is from this research that much of the argument that BPD is a variant of MAD arises. We then look at the Minnesota Multiphasic Personality Inventory (MMPI) data as representative of psychological approaches, the other dominant perspective applied to the study of borderline personality. Other methodological approaches are then briefly discussed. The chapter concludes with an attempt to suggest why an empirically based, comprehensive view of the interface of BPD with affective illness still eludes us.

BIOLOGICAL APPROACHES

Since the introduction of psychotropic medications to treat schizophrenia in the 1950s, psychiatry has searched for biological etiologies for and somatic treatments of a range of mental disorders. Hypotheses concerning problems with synthesis, functioning, and breakdown of neurotransmitters and receptors have been proposed to explain many psychiatric disorders, including affective disorder. Although clinical and laboratory tests have been suggested to explore possible biological markers of depression, no such biological hypotheses for or markers of BPD have been proposed.

A strategy of examining studies of clinical markers of depression in patients with BPD and depressed patients as well as studies of how BPD patients respond to antidepressants and other medications has been developed with the hope of gaining a greater understanding of the relationship between BPD and MAD. This chapter will not be a comprehensive review of the biological studies of BPD (which are covered by van Reekum et al. in Chapter 1). Rather, it will look at specific studies in an attempt to review their methodology and conclusions in light of the question of the relationship between BPD and MAD.

Biological Markers

Studies in which biological tests for depression were administered to BPD patients have yielded inconsistent results. A positive (i.e., nonsuppressing) result on the dexamethasone suppression test (DST), believed to indicate the presence of endogenous depression (Carroll et al. 1981a), has been reported in 20% to 75% of patients with BPD (Baxter et al. 1984; Carroll et al. 1981b; Silk et al. 1985; Soloff et al. 1982; Sternbach et al. 1983; Val et al. 1983). When both prospective and retrospective studies are considered, 44% of BPD patients on average have a positive DST; the average drops to 24% when only prospective studies are considered (Silk et al. 1985).

This substantial percentage of BPD subjects with positive DSTs does not lead, however, to a clearer understanding of the BPD-MAD interface. In some studies, a positive DST closely follows the affective comorbidity of the BPD subject. Of the 19 patients with BPD in Baxter et al.'s (1984) sample who had a positive DST, 18 met some concurrent affective diagnosis, and only 1 BPD patient without a concurrent MAD diagnosis had a positive DST. Krishnan et al. (1984) found that 7 out of 8 of their patients with BPD who had a positive DST also had a DSM-III (American Psychiatric Association 1980) Axis I mood disorder (though none met the criteria for melancholic depression), while only 1 out of 12 of the BPD patients without a mood disorder failed to suppress cortisol.

On the other hand, other studies show a much lower percentage of positive DSTs even among BPD patients who are comorbid for affective disorder. Soloff et al. (1982) found that only 16% of BPD inpatients in their study had a positive DST even though 73% of the BPD subjects had concurrent Research Diagnostic Criteria (RDC) (Spitzer et al. 1975) major depressive disorder (MDD), with 37% meeting the criteria for endogenous depression. Only 3 out of 8 of the endogenous patients had positive DSTs, and none of the other 8 depressed BPD patients had a positive DST. Similarly, Nathan et al. (1985) found only 2% of borderline patients with a positive DST.

In other studies, a positive DST does not follow comorbidity for depression among BPD patients. Our own data reveal that 38% of 50 patients with BPD had a positive DST. Yet a positive DST did not correspond to a concurrent diagnosis of major depression. Of the 6 BPD patients who met RDC criteria for endogenous depression, only 1 had a positive DST; of the 20 who met the criteria for nonendogenous MDD, 9 had a positive DST; and of the 24 BPD patients who did not have concurrent MDD, 9 had a positive DST (Silk et al. 1990a).

Thus, a careful look at the DST studies that in the past have been used to support the idea that BPD is closely related to MAD reveals inconsistent and, at times, contradictory results. While 25% to 50% of all BPD patients have been found to have positive DSTs, it is not possible on these data alone to conclude the type of relationship between BPD and MAD patients. Among the former, the DST does not correspond well to endogenous/nonendogenous or melancholic/nonmelancholic divisions in patients who are concurrently depressed. In fact, in some studies of BPD patients, the DST does not correspond well at all, even to the depressed/nondepressed distinction (Beeber et al. 1984; Silk et al. 1990a).

Thyrotropin (thyroid-stimulating hormone; TSH) response to thyrotropin-releasing hormone (TRH) has also been suggested as a useful diagnostic aid for endogenous depression (Loosen and Prange 1982). Although Garbutt et al. (1983) found 7 out of 15 BPD patients with a blunted TSH response to TRH, 5 out of 7 of the "blunters" were concurrently depressed. Sternbach et al. (1983) found *no* significant difference between BPD patients with and without concurrent MDD with regard to the presence of an abnormal DST or TRH test. Nevertheless, they concluded that many BPD patients have a genuine affective component to their illness, and they viewed their findings as supporting the concept of BPD being more closely related to affective illness.

The latency of onset of rapid eye movement (REM) sleep, observed in sleep electroencephalographic studies, is another biological marker frequently associated with primary depressive illness that has also been studied in patients with BPD (Kupfer and Thase 1983). But again, the issue of whether the sampled BPD patients were concurrently depressed complicates the interpretation of the results. Only one study (Benson et al. 1990) found that BPD patients had significantly longer REM sleep onset (66.5 minutes) when compared with MDD control subjects (54.6 minutes). Yet the REM latency among depressed BPD patients was not significantly different from that of the nondepressed BPD patients. However, this study stands in contrast to at least six other studies (Akiskal et al. 1985; Bell et al. 1983; Lahmeyer et al. 1988; McNamara et al. 1984; Reynolds et al. 1985; Silk et al. 1988) that found essentially no difference in REM latency between BPD patients and depressed patients. These studies, like the DST studies above, are confounded by comorbid Axis I diagnoses of the BPD subjects. The BPD patients had more internight variability in their REM latency than did the depressed patients. McNamara et al. (1984) contend that similar electroencephalographic sleep measures between two cohorts with different diagnoses do not dictate that the samples represent the same illness and that "dissimilar underlying etiologic mechanisms could result in similar biologic signs" (p. 185).

Akiskal et al. (1985) then attempted to solve this problem by studying BPD patients specifically when the patients were not depressed. The patients with DSM-III BPD in this study were free from definite or probable depressive episodes for at least a year before the sleep study. This group was compared with patients with major depression, patients having personality disorders other than BPD, and nonpatient control subjects. The borderline and major depressive cohorts, while not significantly different from each other with respect to REM latency, did have significantly shorter REM latencies when compared with the two control groups. The authors concluded that "borderline patients seem to share a fundamental neurophysiologic characteristic of primary affective patients not observed in a group of patients who had mixed personality disorders with predominantly histrionic and somatization attributes" (p. 195).

However, although the BPD patients in Akiskal et al.'s sample had not experienced major affective illness in the year preceding the sleep study, they differed substantially from the non-BPD personality-disordered control subjects with regard to lifetime diagnoses. As Akiskal et al. (1985) themselves point out, 71% of the BPD subjects had some form of chronic affective illness (dysthymia, atypical bipolar disorder, or cyclothymia), which contrasts with only 31% of control subjects with personality disorders other than BPD (all dysthymic). Furthermore, 46% of the BPD patients had histories of major depression before the year preceding the study compared with only 19% of the control subjects who had personality disorders other than BPD. Of particular importance is that 76% of the

BPD subjects with lifetime affective diagnoses had REM latencies below the median for the entire BPD group, and their REM latencies were significantly different from the REM latencies of borderline subjects without affective lifetime diagnoses. Perhaps the REM latency findings for the entire BPD group may have been unduly influenced by the significant presence of chronic or lifetime affective illness within the group, despite the precautions taken to exclude BPD patients with recent major depressive episodes. As Akiskal et al. remind us, and as Perry (1985) confirms, it is very difficult to completely exclude this confounding variable from a sample of BPD patients, given that both DSM-III and DIB (Gunderson et al. 1981) criteria for BPD give positive weight to depressive symptomatology. Thus, we think that Akiskal et al.'s conclusion that BPD is a "subtle subsyndromal expression of affective illness" (p. 196) is premature. Akiskal et al.'s results could support the hypothesis proposed by Gunderson and Elliott (1985): that overlapping heterogeneous etiologies of both BPD and MAD could potentially include or result in certain overlapping biological signs as well as clinical symptoms.

Reynolds et al. (1985) analyzed the electroencephalographic sleep data of four groups of subjects: prospective BPD subjects, retrospective BPD subjects, subjects with major primary depression, and normal control subjects. Again, however, there were no significant differences in Hamilton Rating Scale for Depression (HRSD; Hamilton 1960) scores between the depressed and BPD groups. Similar REM latency sleep abnormalities were found in the BPD and depressed patients, a finding that is consistent with results reported in the other studies described above. Yet the sleep abnormalities were independent of the level of depressive symptom severity in the BPD samples, a finding we confirm (Silk et al. 1988) and that is consistent with Akiskal et al.'s reports of EEG sleep abnormalities in clinically nondepressed BPD patients (Akiskal et al. 1985). This lack of relationship between severity of depression and REM latency is not found in outpatient and inpatient non-BPD patients with major depression, whose REM latencies are significantly inversely correlated with HRSD scores (Reynolds et al. 1985). Reynolds et al. are careful in drawing conclusions from the data. While the data "suggest a convergence of diagnostic and EEG sleep measures (notably REM latency), supporting the concept of an intrinsic relationship between the borderline disorder and affective illness," the authors acknowledge that the data "do not, however

. . . . answer the question of whether there is a unique characterologic vulnerability to affective disorder in the borderline, or whether the borderline may itself be an affective disorder" (p. 13).

Lahmeyer et al. (1988) also found that it was difficult to tease apart the effects of concurrent depression in BPD patients based on sleep EEG results. Of the 7 BPD patients who had REM latencies of less than 60 minutes, 4 met the RDC criteria for MDD. Of the 10 BPD patients who had REM latencies of greater than 60 minutes, 3 met the RDC criteria for MDD. In our study of BPD patients, we found no significant difference in REM latency when the BPD patients were compared with our MDD control subjects. More important, the REM latency of those BPD patients who did not have MDD (40.1 minutes) was not significantly different from that of the BPD patients who also had MDD (42.1 minutes) (Silk et al. 1988).

Thus, sleep EEG data yield no clearer results than do DST data. In some studies the shortened REM latency among BPD patients seems to closely follow concurrent comorbidity of affective disorder. In other studies, the shortened REM latency does not correspond to comorbid affective disorder. These inconsistencies do not allow us to draw any conclusions about the BPD-MAD interface.

Using a technique related to sleep EEG analysis, Kutcher et al. (1987) measured long-latency auditory event–related electroencephalographic potentials (ERPs) in subjects with BPD, in subjects with other personality disorders, in schizophrenic individuals, in subjects with major depression, and in volunteer control subjects. The borderline subjects were carefully diagnosed based on the Diagnostic Interview for Borderlines (DIB; Gunderson et al. 1981), DSM-III, and the Borderline Ego Function Inventory (Perry and Klerman 1980). Auditory P300 (P3), the long-latency ERP that occurs 300 milliseconds after the onset of an auditory stimulus when the subject is attending to a two-tone discrimination task, has been found to be abnormal in a high proportion (up to 70%) of schizophrenic patients. Kutcher et al. found alterations in P3 latency and amplitude in the BPD patients that significantly differentiated their ERPs from the ERPs of patients with MDD, as well as from those of other personality-disordered subjects with or without MDD. In fact, the ERP abnormalities in the BPD patients were indistinguishable from those found in the schizophrenic subjects. Thus, Kutcher et al.'s results do not promote the hypothesis that

BPD is a variant of depressive illness but instead provide support for the notion that, at least at this particular physiological level, BPD is closer to schizophrenia than to affective illness. (This important study is also discussed by van Reckum et al. and Stone in Chapters 1 and 4, respectively.)

As Steele (1983) aptly points out, major depression is currently defined by clinical symptoms (such as those in the RDC and DSM-III) and *not* by laboratory tests like the dexamethasone suppression test, the TRH test, or electroencephalographic sleep studies. Thus, the merit of using such tests to investigate the relationship of one clinical syndrome to another is questionable.

Drug Responses

Since Gunderson and Elliott published their review in 1985, a number of pharmacotherapeutic studies have been devised to test the efficacy of medications on the borderline condition (see Chapter 15). In general, these studies do not support a strong link between BPD and MAD. Although current thinking holds that the BPD patient's "border" is with affective rather than schizophrenic illness, most pharmacological studies, if they support a relationship to an Axis I disorder at all, tend to support the "old" notion of a relationship between BPD and schizophrenia. (A number of these studies are reviewed in detail by Soloff in Chapter 15.)

Schulz et al. (1985) found in a small sample of BPD patients an exacerbation of symptoms with amphetamine that was more typical of schizophrenia than depression. Goldberg et al. (1986) reported on the effectiveness of thiothixene for the psychotic-like symptoms of BPD, although his sample consisted of volunteers and not patients. In a series of studies, Soloff et al. (1986a, 1986b) found that not only is amitriptyline ineffective with BPD patients, but it also makes some of these patients worse, prompting the comment that "the interpretation of the diagnosis of depression in patients with borderline disorder warrants closer review" (Soloff et al. 1986b, p. 696). Furthermore, the same studies showed that low-dose haloperidol was clearly superior to antidepressants in controlling the symptoms of BPD. The superiority of low-dose neuroleptic medication speaks against the hypothesis put forward by Akiskal and others that BPD is a subaffective disorder. This finding is more consistent with a view that the relationship between the two disorders is incidental or that the disorders are too heterogeneous to predict drug response (Gunderson 1986), or that there may be some relationship to schizophrenia.

When Soloff et al. (1986a) examined more closely the paradoxical effects of amitriptyline among patients with BPD, they found that subjects who responded to either amitriptyline or placebo improved in global functioning, depression, and psychoticism but not in self-rated hostility. Those patients who responded to amitriptyline alone improved in all areas of impulsive behavior on the ward, specifically in temper tantrums and assaultive and manipulative behavior. Those patients who did not respond to amitriptyline actually *worsened* in global functioning, paranoid ideation, and all areas of impulsive ward behavior. Amitriptyline nonresponders were more demanding, made more suicide threats, and were more physically assaultive toward others than were the placebo nonresponders. However, the amitriptyline nonresponders *improved* more than the placebo nonresponders on the affectively loaded scales, thus suggesting that "treatment failure" on amitriptyline was largely attributable to its paradoxical *behavioral* effects and not to any failure to improve depressive affect.

Soloff et al.'s studies suggest, then, that BPD may be a distinct entity and not representative of an atypical affective disorder. The differing pharmacological responses in Soloff et al.'s subjects suggest that BPD differs from affective disorder in that it has at least three components, each with a different pharmacological response: 1) an affective (perhaps atypical) component that may respond to a tricyclic and/or an antipsychotic medication, 2) a behavioral (impulsive) component that may respond to or get worse with a tricyclic, and 3) a psychotic-like/paranoid component that may respond to antipsychotics. (This fails to account for the defect in interpersonal relationships, but we have no data that would suggest any primary pharmacological effect in this area.)

Cowdry and Gardner's study (1988) may provide further evidence for selective responsiveness of different components of BPD to different pharmacological agents. Although they found that some patients responded well to the monoamine oxidase (MAO) inhibitor tranylcypromine, this response was primarily in the area of mood rather than behavior. On the other hand, some patients had a positive response to carbamazepine, but this response was primarily in the area of behavior and impulse. If improvement in mood did occur with carbamazepine, it was difficult to quantify, and it seemed qualitatively different from the mood improvement found with the MAO inhibitor. Low-dose neuroleptics appeared helpful, particularly in areas of mood and anxiety (as rated by the patient) and suicidality.

Lastly, Links et al. (1990) compared responses of BPD patients to lithium, desipramine, and placebo. Although only 10 subjects completed the full double-blind crossover trial, Links et al.'s results again question the relationship of BPD to affective disorders. Active medication had little benefit over placebo in improving depressive symptomatology. Yet lithium was felt, at least based on observer ratings, to cause a decrease in irritability, anger, and suicidality. Links et al.'s subjects did not show increasing behavioral problems on the tricyclic desipramine as some of Soloff et al.'s subjects had shown on the tricyclic amitriptyline. Still, lithium seemed primarily to improve behavior and not mood.

The pharmacological studies, then, do not clarify the relationship between BPD and MAD. Some BPD patients may respond to antidepressants (e.g., tricyclics, MAO inhibitors, lithium), but the response is not always in the area of improved affect (e.g., lithium). Some BPD patients reveal worsening of symptoms on tricyclic antidepressants. Antipsychotics also appear to improve mood. Medications that improve behavior do not necessarily improve mood.

A review of the current biological literature suggests that the hypothesis stating that BPD is a form of affective disorder is supported by some and contradicted by much of the evidence collected to date. From DST, REM latency, and ERP studies to pharmacological studies, an overview of the empirical data implies that despite the great overlap of symptomatology and the high rate of concurrent diagnoses, many patients meeting criteria for BPD are different from those with affective disorder in some fundamental, biophysiological way. Other BPD patients do appear to share enough biological characteristics with depressive patients to suggest that there exists a subtype of BPD that is a variant of affective disorder.

Personality Assessment Approaches

One avenue for exploring the relationship between BPD and MAD has focused on comparing the personality profiles of patients diagnosed with each of the disorders using standardized personality tests. Several investigations have used the MMPI (Hathaway and McKinley 1943) to compare the personality profiles of patients diagnosed with BPD, MAD, and other affective, personality, and residual disorders (Evans et al. 1984; Lloyd et al. 1983; Snyder et al. 1982; Widiger et al. 1986). However, before reviewing this literature, it will be helpful to discuss a few studies that have tried to evaluate 1) the effects of the depressive state on personality assessment and 2) how personality disorder and traits might affect the assessment and clinical picture of depression.

Hirschfeld et al. (1983) evaluated the influence of the clinically depressed state on personality assessment by comparing self-report personality inventories of clinically depressed patients and at follow-up 1 year later. Patients completed a personality battery during intake evaluation and again at 1-year follow-up. The personality battery consisted of 17 scales drawn from 5 different self-report personality inventories, including 2 from the MMPI. Subjects were instructed to answer questions according to the person's "usual self." The "recovered" group had been free of all affective residual symptoms for at least 2 weeks at the time of the 1-year follow-up personality assessment. The "unrecovered" group experienced some symptoms of major depressive disorder during the 2 weeks before the follow-up assessment.

The effect of the clinical state of depression on personality trait assessment was analyzed by comparing entry personality scores with those at 1-year follow-up. In the recovered group, statistically significant shifts toward health were observed in increased emotional strength and decreased interpersonal dependency. When compared with assessment during a depressive episode, patients when well had lower scores on neuroticism, orality, emotional reliance on another person, and lack of social self-confidence, and higher scores on emotional stability and objectivity. The unrecovered group did not demonstrate any significant changes in personality between assessment at entry into the study and at 1-year follow-up. Hirschfeld et al. (1983) concluded that the clinical state of depression does influence selected areas of patients' self-perceptions, particularly "assessments of emotional strength and interpersonal dependency [that] reflect the clinical state of depression rather than enduring personality traits" (p. 698). However, those scales assessing impulsivity, submissiveness, demandingness, and obsessionality appeared to remain stable over time despite the remission of depressive symptoms, and these scales may be reliable indicators of underlying personality characteristics rather than measures of clinical state.

Hirschfeld et al.'s conclusions raise interesting questions as to the overlap between MAD and BPD. The intense, unstable interpersonal relationships that are a hallmark of BPD are frequently characterized by emotional reliance on another person, a trait found by Hirschfeld et al. to be state dependent. Thus, psychiatric patients who are depressed may present themselves as more dependent and unhealthy than when they are asymptomatic, and some patients may be misdiagnosed as having BPD because of the distorting effect of the depressive state. On the other hand, some characteristically borderline traits such as impulsivity, submissiveness, and demandingness appeared to remain constant regardless of a state of clinical depression.

Charney et al. (1981), considering personality traits and personality disorder as distinctly separate concepts, investigated the relationship of each to major subtypes of depression in inpatients who met DSM-III criteria for a major depressive episode. Personality disorder was assessed by using the DSM-III definition of a chronic pattern of maladaptive behavior resulting in impaired functioning or repeated subjective distress, as well as by assessing the degree of functional impairment present throughout adulthood. Although 11 personality traits were rated, only the 4 that achieved sufficient interrater reliability (i.e., borderline, compulsive, histrionic, and hostile) were examined further. The authors found that personality disorder was significantly more common in the unipolar nonmelancholic depressed patients (61%) than in the unipolar melancholic (14%) and bipolar depressed (23%) patients. Because of low frequency in the other groups, the relationship of personality disorder to patient characteristics and treatment outcome was determined only in the unipolar nonmelancholic group. In this group, personality disorder was associated with an earlier onset of depressive illness and a poorer response to treatment. The character of the depressive episode was different in only 3 of 28 symptoms, with personality-disordered subjects having more suicidal ideation, more depersonalization, and less ruminative thinking. Nonmelancholic patients, when compared to melancholic patients, were more histrionic and hostile and had more borderline features.

The finding of an early age of onset and poor treatment outcome of the depressive syndrome in patients with personality disorder suggests two possibilities.

1. An earlier onset of depression may result in early functional impairment that is later viewed as personality disorder. While this hypothesis may be similar, though not identical, to Akiskal's hypothesis that BPD is a form of affective disorder, Charney et al.'s finding could imply that depression is one component related to the etiology of BPD.
2. Conversely, character disorder that causes repeated subjective distress and significant problems with work and relationships may predispose the individual to depressive illness.

The significantly lower frequency of personality disorder in the unipolar melancholic patients compared with nonmelancholic depressed patients was replicated by Davidson et al. (1985), who found that personality disorder occurred in approximately two-thirds of nonmelancholic patients as compared with one-third of melancholic patients. Thus, melancholic depressed patients may have a clearer biological vulnerability to depression than do nonmelancholic depressed patients, who may have more of a "characterologic" propensity toward depression.

In most of the studies exploring the relationship between BPD and affective illness, "major affective disorder" has been treated as a single entity rather than broken up into the subtypes of DSM-III or RDC. The Charney et al. (1981) study points to the importance of analyzing the relationship of BPD to individual subtypes of affective disorder, as there appears to be a fundamental difference in the occurrence of personality disorder in nonmelancholic (nonendogenous) compared with melancholic (endogenous) depression.

Several studies have explored the MMPI profiles of patients with BPD and compared them with profiles in other diagnostic groups, including patients with affective disorder. Snyder et al. (1982) compared the MMPI profile of BPD patients with that of patients with dysthymic disorder (or "depressive neurosis"), a chronic, nonmajor depression. The inclusion criteria for BPD were stricter than those of DSM-III, requiring that six out of eight rather than five out of eight criteria be fulfilled. Patients with other Axis II disorders were excluded, and patients in the dysthymic comparison group had no additional Axis I disorders. The MMPI was administered to the patients upon admission.

While borderline patients' two highest mean scores were on the Psychasthenia and Schizophrenia Scales, the scales that best discriminated BPD patients from dysthymic patients were two of the validity scales, the Lie (L) Scale (on which BPD patients scored low) and the Frequency (F) Scale (on which BPD patients scored high). Using these two scales as a discriminant model, the authors correctly classified 21 of the 26 BPD subjects. When the validity scales were eliminated from the discriminant analysis, the authors found the Hypochondriasis and Schizophrenia Scales to be almost as powerful as the Lie and Frequency Scales in classifying subjects as having BPD (20 out of 26). Clinically, the borderline MMPI profile was interpreted as indicating psychological turmoil with anger and projection employed to defend against feelings of being mistreated. Subjects with BPD appeared to have superficial interpersonal relationships without warm attachments. Compared with the dysthymic subjects, the BPD subjects were more conflicted about sexual identity, had a greater propensity toward homosexual behavior, were more impulsive, and felt boredom and emptiness more intensely.

Snyder et al. thus provide some evidence that BPD can be differentiated from at least one type of affective disorder, dysthymia, on the basis of a personality profile. However, one must question Snyder et al.'s findings based on their patient sample, which consisted of male Veterans Administration inpatients, certainly not the most generalizable of patient samples for a disorder found predominantly in females. Thus, it would be helpful to repeat the study with other diagnostic/comparison groups, particularly patients with other mood disorders, such as bipolar, unipolar melancholic, and unipolar nonmelancholic depression, and with other personality disorders as well.

Lloyd et al. (1983) used an abbreviated form of the MMPI, the MMPI-168, to assess the validity of the borderline construct by exploring whether patients with BPD would demonstrate a pattern distinguishable from other psychiatric patients. The authors also wished to examine the specific nature of these differences. They compared personality profiles in DSM-III borderline outpatients with those of other psychiatric outpatients. Nonborderline patients were divided into three groups: those patients having affective disorders, those having personality disorders other than

BPD, and those patients with adjustment disorders, marital problems, or anxiety disorders who formed a residual group. Both the BPD and the non-BPD patient groups were elevated on the Psychopathic Deviate and Psychasthenia Scales. These two groups, however, showed significant differences on two of the three validity scales, with BPD patients rating higher on the Frequency and Correction (K) Scales. Significant differences also occurred in 3 out of 10 clinical scales, with BPD patients scoring higher on the Psychopathic Deviate Scale, the Paranoia Scale, and the Schizophrenia Scale. Importantly, the BPD patient profile was most similar to the affective patient profile, least similar to the residual category profile, and intermediate in similarity to the non-BPD personality-disordered group. Unlike Snyder et al., Lloyd et al. found it more difficult to differentiate between BPD and affective disorder than to differentiate between BPD and either non-BPD personality disorders or adjustment and anxiety disorders. However, Lloyd et al. failed to identify subtypes of affective disorder or other comorbid diagnoses among their BPD patients. Perhaps if groups could be defined by strict criteria to make them mutually exclusive, a difference in MMPI profiles could be found. When there is naturally occurring comorbidity in group membership, "clean" profiles do not emerge.

Evans et al. (1984) conducted an investigation similar to those described above in which the MMPI profiles of inpatients meeting DSM-III criteria for BPD were compared with those of chronic schizophrenic inpatients and inpatients with acute psychotic illness. Because Evans et al. did not use an affective comparison group, we will not discuss the specific intergroup results but will turn our attention to analysis of their findings in comparison with those of Snyder et al. (1982) and Lloyd et al. (1983). Evans et al. found that the MMPI profiles in their BPD patients did not match the profiles of BPD patients in either Snyder et al.'s or Lloyd et al.'s study, even after taking subgroups of their sample that would correspond to the demographics of the sample of BPD patients in each of the other two studies.

In summary, one MMPI study reveals a different profile for BPD patients and dysthymic patients (Snyder et al. 1982). Another MMPI study fails to find a different profile for BPD patients and affective disorder patients (Lloyd et al. 1983). And a third study reveals MMPI profiles for BPD patients different from the MMPI profiles of borderline patients in each of the other two studies (Evans et al. 1984). Thus, a clear MMPI profile of BPD still eludes us.

The disparity among the findings of those MMPI studies may reflect the heterogeneity of the borderline construct, but the differences could also be related to severity of symptoms or illness. Thus, homogeneous subgroups (based on, for example, severity of affective symptomatology) may still be able to be identified within the broader, heterogeneous category of BPD.

The heterogeneity in symptomatology in BPD is thought by Widiger and his colleagues (1986) to result from a prototypic or polythetic rather than a "classical" model of categorization found in DSM-III (Cantor et al. 1980). In a prototypic or polythetic model, members of the category are heterogeneous with respect to symptomatology; symptoms are only correlated with category membership, and there are overlapping boundaries. In the classical model, however, members share all of the defining features, boundaries are distinct, and symptoms are considered to be singly necessary and jointly sufficient (Widiger et al. 1986). In BPD as defined by DSM-III (and DSM-III-R), possession of any five of the eight specified symptoms qualify a patient for inclusion in the BPD diagnostic group. Thus, substantial heterogeneity exists within the diagnosis.

Another feature of DSM-III-R that hampers efforts to identify a specific MMPI profile for BPD is the abundance of multiple diagnoses at the same level of classification that a prototypic or polythetic model permits. That is, in addition to the frequent concurrence of an Axis I diagnosis of affective disorder, DSM-III-R allows for overlapping diagnoses within the Axis II personality disorders category as well. BPD has been shown to overlap especially with schizotypal, histrionic, and antisocial personality disorders, as well as with dependent, narcissistic, and passive-aggressive personality disorders (Gunderson 1984; Hyler et al. 1989; Loranger et al. 1987; Stangl et al. 1985; Zanarini et al. 1987). As was pointed out earlier, when studies use BPD samples in which patients are not necessarily "purely" borderline and when overlaps with other Axis I and Axis II diagnoses are not identified, one cannot determine if the profile seen in a group of BPD patients is the result of the BPD diagnosis, an overlapping diagnosis, or a combination of disorders. It is precisely this problem that has made it difficult to take advantage of the potential the MMPI has for shedding light on the relationship of BPD to MAD. Perhaps, however, a group of "purely" borderline patients would be less representative of the typical borderline group that is "naturally" heterogeneous, and the MMPI profile of a group of purely borderline patients would not be very helpful in the diagnosis of BPD in most populations, wherein multiple diagnoses are the norm (Widiger et al. 1986).

Research into the relationship between affective disorder and BPD thus continues to be hindered by concurrent and multiple diagnoses that make it difficult to distinguish the symptoms, etiologies, treatment effects, etc., of each. The issue seems to be particularly problematic in the personality research conducted in recent years, and future research employing tools like the MMPI will need to use more fully diagnosed (if clinically accurate, multiply-diagnosed) subjects, in whom the specific personality disorders and types of affective disorders are identified. Recent studies by Perry and Cooper (1986) and Westen et al. (1990) that empirically explore psychodynamic aspects of borderline object relations and their association to quality of depression and to object relations in depressed patients offer unique approaches aimed at clarifying the BPD-MAD connection.

CRITIQUE OF METHODOLOGY

As has been evident in our discussion, a variety of methodological tools have been brought to bear on the investigation of the relationship between BPD and MAD. Biological markers, drug response, and personality tests have been used to try to discriminate the disorders and discern their relationships to one another. Other research strategies have examined patterns of psychopathology in the relatives of patients, as well as the course of each disorder. These diverse instruments and strategies have strengths and limitations that must be considered both when interpreting the results of past studies and when designing future studies.

Inquiries that have relied on biological markers for illuminating the relationship between BPD and MAD presume that a marker for depression that is positive in a patient diagnosed with BPD indicates that the patient suffers from an underlying affective disorder. Yet a careful review of the sensitivity and specificity of the DST, for example, suggests that the DST is better able to identify non-MDD patients than to screen for patients with MDD, a factor that must be considered when evaluating the DST as an indicator of depression (Arana et al. 1985). When one tries to understand the confusing and inconsistent results found with the DST in BPD patients, the following explanations need to be considered. Perhaps BPD patients present themselves in peculiar ways clinically so that their borderline features obscure depressive symptoms, and clinicians are unable to uncover or fail to appreciate endogenous symptoms underlying borderline pathology and identified by the DST. Alternatively, the negative response to the DST among a sample of BPD patients may reflect the limited sensitivity of the DST. A third possibility is that major depression diagnosed in BPD patients is fundamentally different from "standard" affective illness marked by a positive DST, and represents instead secondary results of the borderline character state.

A more important question than how well biological markers "mark" is whether utilizing such markers is a sound method for investigating the interrelationship of BPD and MAD. The presence of affective illness in roughly half of all BPD patients has been fairly well established by numerous studies, as reported by Silk et al. (1985), and it seems that biological markers of depression can do little more than address the issue of overlap of markers but not overlap between the disorders. Certainly markers cannot be used to clarify the relationship between the disorders. If we reduce diagnosis to the response to a laboratory test, then we remove the complexity and richness of human presentation and experience. Although it is this very heterogeneity that poses problems to diagnosticians, the solution should not be to make homogeneous that which is heterogeneous and variable.

Another biological approach to understanding the relationship between BPD and MAD is analyzing drug treatment response. Like laboratory tests, this method poses significant problems. Some patients with BPD have evidenced improved functioning following treatment with antidepressants, suggesting an affective component to their illness (Soloff et al. 1986a). Again, this finding is consistent with the broad overlap between BPD and MAD found in other studies, but it does not address the nature of the concurrence. The failure of a BPD patient to respond to antidepressant medication does not necessarily imply that the patient does not have an affective component to his or her illness; similarly, one would err to assume that a positive response to antidepressant medication indicates that the BPD patient "really" has an affective disorder. To retrospectively diagnose a patient according to drug response seems as ill advised and as invalid as diagnosing as "borderline" those patients who are "incurable" by psychoanalysis. As McNamara et al. (1984) stated in reference to EEG sleep measures, similar drug responses in two differently diagnosed samples do not necessarily mean that the samples represent the same illness. Different underlying etiologic factors could result in a similar drug response. This understanding of the variability of drug response would be in accordance with Gunderson and Elliott's (1985) hypothesis.

Personality studies have revealed that certain borderline features are stable despite the abatement of depressive symptoms (Hirschfeld et al. 1983), and that borderline conditions are more likely to prevail in nonmelancholic depressed patients than in melancholic depressed patients (Charney et al. 1981). These studies lend support to the idea that there exists a BPD that is distinguishable from MDD. Studies assessing personality with the MMPI have failed to identify one specific profile unique to BPD patients, although patients with BPD have been differentiated from depressed patients based on the MMPI (Evans et al. 1984; Lloyd et al. 1983; Snyder et al. 1982; Widiger et al. 1986). The problem most likely lies not in the MMPI itself but in the heterogeneity of the borderline picture and the multiplicity of codiagnoses that are possible with DSM-III-R. It is unusual for a patient to present only with discrete borderline symptoms; rather, there is typically overlap with at least one other personality disorder (Widiger et al. 1986) and/or Axis I clinical syndrome such as affective illness (Koenigsberg et al. 1985).

The identification of a sensitive and specific MMPI profile for BPD would serve as a kind of "marker" for BPD, much as markers may exist for MAD, that could aid in diagnosis and consequently in treatment. It seems unlikely, however, that the MMPI will be capable of identifying such a profile given the present system of classification according to the prototypic model of DSM-III-R. Nevertheless, unlike biological markers, which may indicate the presence or absence of a specific clinical syndrome, the MMPI may be better able to identify personality features with specific clinical and etiologic implications.

As researchers struggle to understand how depression and borderline behavior are shaped and how they are related, it seems imperative that longitudinal investigations be conducted. Tracing the development of children in at-risk families as they grow into adolescence and adulthood would enable diagnostically "blind" raters to observe factors that contribute to the eventual formation of a particular diagnostic syndrome. Developmental theories offer cogent explanations for the formation of personality disorders as well as for certain kinds of clinical depression (nonmelancholic or nonendogenous). Retrospective approaches taken by the few empirical studies that have explored pathological personality development have serious pitfalls that render their findings inconclusive. Prospective, methodologically sound studies need to be devised.

One research method that may help identify "at-risk" families is the study of family prevalence of the disorder in question (see Zanarini, Chapter 3). Although Loranger et al. (1982) used retrospective data, this study nevertheless provided tentative support for the validity of the BPD syndrome as distinct from affective illness. Both Links et al. (1988) and Baron et al. (1985) found high prevalence rates for BPD as well as MAD in first-degree relatives of BPD patients.

Soloff and Millward (1983) also investigated psychiatric disorders in the families of BPD patients (see Chapter 3). This study supports a relationship of criteria-defined borderline disorders to affective disorders, but it does not resolve the varying diagnostic perspectives represented by the four hypotheses described at the beginning of this chapter. Further, in Soloff and Millward's study, approximately half of the borderline probands had concurrent affective disorder. This is not different from the findings of Pope et al. (1983), who noted that significantly more first-degree relatives of BPD patients with concurrent MAD had affective disorders than did first-degree relatives of BPD patients without MAD.

A final methodological approach is that of long-term follow-up of BPD and depressed patients. Pope et al. (1983) followed up after 4–7 years 27 patients meeting DSM-III criteria for BPD. The BPD patients who also had MAD had significantly better outcome on social functioning and freedom from residual symptoms. In all areas, the patients with BPD and MAD demonstrated a better outcome than did the patients with "pure" BPD. In several cases of BPD with MAD, the borderline symptoms seemed to remit with the remission of affective symptoms. This suggests that for some of the BPD patients with concurrent MAD, the symptoms of BPD may have been secondary to the affective disorder.

Thus, Akiskal's (1981) hypothesis may apply to certain ostensibly "borderline" patients. If all cases of BPD actually represented affective disorder, however, one would expect patients with primary BPD who did not have MAD to display a frequent tendency for episodes of MAD to develop during the follow-up interval, which was not observed in any of Pope et al.'s cases, but which has been observed by Perry (1985). Pope et al.'s (1983) conclusion is consistent with Gunderson and Elliott's (1985) hypothesis: ". . . the most parsimonious explanation of the observations seems to be that BPD and MAD are separate diagnostic entities, although they coexist in many patients, and symptoms suggestive of either disorder may occasionally be secondary to the coexisting disorder" (p. 29).

McGlashan's (1986) retrospective long-term outcome study of borderline personalities involved patients who were "purely" borderline and not overlapping with any other diagnostic category. Based on outcome data collected an average of 15 years after discharge, McGlashan found that BPD patients were comparable with unipolar depressed patients and scored significantly better than schizophrenic patients on most indexes of outcome. His finding stands in contrast to that of Pope et al. (1983), whose "pure" BPD cohort registered the poorest outcomes along with their schizophrenic group. McGlashan revealed a trend in the direction opposite that of Pope et al. when he found that adding a diagnosis of MAD to BPD resulted in a poorer long-term outcome.[1]

In a recent study (Silk et al. 1990b), we followed up 2 to 5 years posthospitalization nine BPD patients who were comorbid for RDC MDD at the time of index hospitalization. To be chosen for follow-up, the subject could no longer meet RDC MDD and had to have a HRSD score of less than 10. While eight of the nine patients improved, seven of the nine remained borderline based on the DSM-III, and five of the nine remained borderline based on the DIB. Thus, while some subjects seemed to lose their borderline symptoms coincident with the remission of the depression, most did not. Decreased use of substances as well as more

---

[1] It has been proposed that the difference in these two studies may have to do with length of time between index hospitalization and follow-up. McGlashan (1986) has shown that patients with BPD do poorly in the first decade posthospitalization, the period within which Pope et al. were assessing their patients. McGlashan's patients did not improve until the second decade posthospitalization.

limited interpersonal activity also seemed to be related to improvement and to loss of the borderline diagnosis.

CONCLUSIONS

We conclude that while there is some evidence to favor the hypothesis that at least one subtype of BPD belongs in the realm of affective illness, this subtype certainly does not include all borderline patients.

A major limitation when attempting to integrate the findings of the many studies in this area concerns the disparate samples being compared. There are frequently differences in the populations from which samples are drawn (inpatient vs. outpatient, male vs. female vs. mixed gender groups), and diagnoses are often based on different criteria systems. "Borderline personality disorder" may be diagnosed by DIB or DSM-III criteria. "Affective illness" can refer to any of several DSM-III diagnoses (major depressive disorder or episode with or without melancholia, bipolar disorder, cyclothymic disorder, dysthymic disorder, or atypical bipolar disorder), which may or may not be congruent with RDC diagnoses (delusional or nondelusional primary unipolar depression, endogenous or nonendogenous depression, bipolar depression, bipolar type II depression). Such diagnostic differences must be taken into account when comparisons are made between investigations that purportedly study the "same" diagnostic groups.

Moreover, studies do not always clarify whether their samples are "pure" or include subjects who meet criteria for more than one diagnosis. The distinction is important not only for the sake of comparisons among studies but also for the generalizations that can be made from any single study. It is ironic that while a homogeneous borderline cohort may demonstrate important features of the borderline condition, it may not represent the borderline personalities typically found in the population, which present heterogeneously and usually amid other diagnostic syndromes. Despite recent increased agreement over the diagnosis of BPD, in large part due to the established reliability of the DIB (Cornell et al. 1983; Gunderson et al. 1981), the diagnosis of BPD continues to include a broad, heterogeneous range of symptoms and patients that may represent different subtypes of BPD that may eventually be delineated into more specific, homogeneous groups. If current and future research endeavors can further delineate a "pure" BPD from a subtypical BPD that is more a part of the affective spectrum, treatments could be developed and administered appropriate to the kind of borderline disorder a patient has.

With the advent of psychopharmacology used adjunctively with psychotherapy, great strides have been made in the psychiatric treatment of a wide range of affective disorders. However, treatment of characterologic problems has remained difficult and often ineffective. Identification of "borderline" patients whose affective symptoms represent an underlying affective disorder can allow clinicians to provide more effective treatment, because those patients will presumably be amenable to standard treatments for affective disorder. Identification of patients who are "purely" borderline will pave the way for researchers to compare the efficacy of various treatment interventions with a homogeneous cohort. As future studies are conducted, the goals of improved understanding of and more effective treatment for seemingly entrenched pathologic personality disorders may increasingly come within the reach of mental health professionals.

REFERENCES

Akiskal HS: Subaffective disorders: dysthymic, cyclothymic and bipolar II disorders in the "borderline" realm. Psychiatr Clin North Am 4:25–46, 1981

Akiskal HS, Yerevanian BI, Davis GC, et al: The nosologic status of borderline personality: clinical and polysomnographic study. Am J Psychiatry 142:192–198, 1985

American Psychiatric Association: Diagnostic and Statistical Manual of Mental Disorders, 3rd Edition. Washington, DC, American Psychiatric Association, 1980

American Psychiatric Association: Diagnostic and Statistical Manual of Mental Disorders, 3rd Edition, Revised. Washington, DC, American Psychiatric Association, 1987

Arana GW, Baldessarini RJ, Ornsteen M: The dexamethasone suppression test for diagnosis and prognosis in psychiatry: comments and review. Arch Gen Psychiatry 42:1193–1204, 1985

Baron M, Gruen R, Asnis L: Familial transmission of schizotypal and borderline personality disorders. Am J Psychiatry 142:927–934, 1985

Baxter L, Edell W, Gerner R, et al: Dexamethasone suppression test and Axis I diagnoses of inpatients with DSM-III borderline personality disorder. J Clin Psychiatry 45;150–153, 1984

Beeber AR, Kline MD, Pies RW, et al: Dexamethasone suppression test in hospitalized depressed patients with borderline personality disorder. J Nerv Ment Dis 172:301–303, 1984

Bell J, Lycaki H, Jones D, et al: Effect of preexisting borderline personality disorder on clinical and EEG sleep correlates of depression. Psychiatry Res 9:115–123, 1983

Benson KL, King R, Gordon D, et al: Sleep patterns in borderline personality disorder. J Affective Disord 18:267–273, 1990

Cantor N, Smith EE, French RD, et al: Psychiatric diagnosis as prototype categorization. J Abnorm Psychol 89:181–193, 1980

Carroll BJ, Feinberg M, Greden JF, et al: A specific laboratory test for the diagnosis of melancholia: standardization, validation, and clinical utility. Arch Gen Psychiatry 38:15–22, 1981a

Carroll BJ, Greden JF, Feinberg M, et al: Neuroendocrine evaluation of depression in borderline patients. Psychiatr Clin North Am 4:89–99, 1981b

Charney DS, Nelson JC, Quinlan DM: Personality traits and disorder in depression. Am J Psychiatry 138:1601–1604, 1981

Cornell DG, Silk KR, Ludolph PS, et al: Test-retest reliability of the Diagnostic Interview for Borderlines. Arch Gen Psychiatry 40:1307–1310, 1983

Cowdry RW, Gardner DL: Pharmacotherapy of borderline personality disorder: alprazolam, carbamazepine, trifluoperazine and tranylcypromine. Arch Gen Psychiatry 45:111–119, 1988

Davidson J, Miller R, Strickland R: Neuroticism and personality disorder in depression. J Affective Disord 8:177–182, 1985

Evans RW, Ruff RM, Braff DL, et al: MMPI characteristics of borderline personality inpatients. J Nerv Ment Dis 172:742–748, 1984

Garbutt JC, Loosen PT, Tipermas A, et al: The TRH test in patients with borderline personality disorder. Psychiatry Res 9:107–113, 1983

Goldberg SC, Schulz SC, Schulz PM, et al: Borderline and schizotypal personality disorders treated with low-dose thiothixene vs placebo. Arch Gen Psychiatry 43:680–686, 1986

Gunderson JG: Borderline Personality Disorder. Washington, DC, American Psychiatric Press, 1984

Gunderson JG: Pharmacotherapy for patients with borderline personality disorder. Arch Gen Psychiatry 43:698–700, 1986

Gunderson JG, Elliott GR: The interface between borderline personality disorder and affective disorder. Am J Psychiatry 142:277–288, 1985

Gunderson, JG, Phillips, KA: A current view of the interface between borderline personality disorder and depression, Am J Psychiatry 148:967–975, 1991

Gunderson JG, Kolb JE, Austin V: The diagnostic interview for borderline patients. Am J Psychiatry 138:896–903, 1981

Hamilton M: A psychiatric rating scale for depression. J Neurol Neurosurg Psychiatry 23:56–62, 1960

Hathaway SP, McKinley JC: The Minnesota Multiphasic Personality Inventory Schedule. Minneapolis, MN, University of Minnesota Press, 1943

Hirschfeld RMA, Klerman GL, Clayton PJ, et al: Assessing personality: effects of the depressive state on trait measurement. Am J Psychiatry 140:695–699, 1983

Hyler SE, Rieder RO, Williams JBW, et al: A comparison of clinical and self-report diagnoses of DSM-III personality disorders in 552 patients. Compr Psychiatry 30:170–178, 1989

Kernberg O: Borderline Conditions and Pathological Narcissism. New York, Jason Aronson, 1975

Koenigsberg HW, Kaplan RD, Gilmore MM, et al: The relationship between syndrome and personality disorder in DSM-III: experience with 2,462 patients. Am J Psychiatry 142:207–212, 1985

Krishnan KRR, Davidson JRT, Rayasam K, et al: The dexamethasone suppression test in borderline personality disorder. Biol Psychiatry 19:1149–1153, 1984

Kroll J: The Challenge of the Borderline Patient. New York, WW Norton, 1988

Kupfer DJ, Thase ME: The use of the sleep laboratory in the diagnosis of affective disorders. Psychiatr Clin North Am 6:3–25, 1983

Kutcher SP, Blackwood DHR, St Clair D, et al: Auditory P300 in borderline personality disorder and schizophrenia. Arch Gen Psychiatry 44:645–650, 1987

Lahmeyer HW, Val E, Gaviria FM, et al: EEG sleep, lithium transport, dexamethasone suppression, and monoamine oxidase activity in borderline personality disorder. Psychiatry Res 25:19–30, 1988

Liebowitz MR, Klein DF: Interrelationship of hysteroid dysphoria and borderline personality disorder. Psychiatr Clin North Am 4:67–87, 1981

Links PS, Steiner M, Huxley G: The occurrence of borderline personality disorder in the families of borderline patients. Journal of Personality Disorders 2:14–20, 1988

Links PS, Steiner M, Boiago I, et al: Lithium therapy for borderline patients: preliminary findings. Journal of Personality Disorders 4:173–181, 1990

Lloyd C, Overall JE, Kimsey LR, et al: A comparison of the MMPI-168 profiles of borderline and nonborderline outpatients. J Nerv Ment Dis 171:207–215, 1983

Loosen PT, Prange AJ Jr: Serum thyrotropin response to thyrotropin-releasing hormone in psychiatric patients: a review. Am J Psychiatry 139:405–416, 1982

Loranger AW, Oldham JM, Tulis EH: Familial transmission of DSM-III borderline personality disorder. Arch Gen Psychiatry 39:795–799, 1982

Loranger AW, Susman VL, Oldham JM, et al. The Personality Disorder Examination: a preliminary report. Journal of Personality Disorders 1:1–13, 1987

Masterson J: Psychotherapy of the Borderline Adult. New York, Brunner/Mazel, 1976

McGlashan TH: The Chestnut Lodge follow-up study, III: long-term outcome of borderline personalities. Arch Gen Psychiatry 43:20–30, 1986

McNamara E, Reynolds CF III, Soloff PH, et al: EEG sleep evaluation of depression in borderline patients. Am J Psychiatry 141:182–186, 1984

Nathan RS, Soloff PH, George A, et al: DST and TRH tests in borderline personality disorder, in Proceedings of the IV World Congress of Biological Psychiatry. New York, Elsevier, 1985, p 564

Perry JC: Depression in borderline personality disorder: lifetime prevalence at interview and longitudinal course of symptoms. Am J Psychiatry 142:15–21, 1985

Perry JC, Cooper SH: A preliminary report on defenses and conflicts associated with borderline personality disorder. J Am Psychoanal Assoc 34:863–893, 1986

Perry JC, Klerman GL: Clinical features of the borderline personality disorder. Am J Psychiatry 137:165–173, 1980

Pope HG Jr, Jonas JM, Hudson JI, et al: The validity of DSM-III borderline personality disorder: a phenomenologic, family history, treatment response, and long-term follow-up study. Arch Gen Psychiatry 40:23–30, 1983

Reynolds CF III, Soloff PH, Kupfer DJ, et al: Depression in borderline patients: a prospective EEG sleep study. Psychiatry Res 14:1–15, 1985

Schulz SC, Schulz PM, Dommisse C, et al: Amphetamine response in borderline patients. Psychiatry Res 15:97–108, 1985

Silk KR, Lohr NE, Cornell DG, et al: The dexamethasone suppression test in borderline and nonborderline affective patients, in The Borderline: Current Empirical Research. Edited by McGlashan T. Washington, DC, American Psychiatric Press, 1985, pp 99–116

Silk KR, Lohr NE, Shipley JE, et al: Sleep EEG and DST in borderline with depression. Paper presented at the 141st annual meeting of the American Psychiatric Association, Montreal, May 1988

Silk KR, Lohr NE, Gold LJ, et al: Standard rating scales and depression in borderline personality disorder. Paper presented at the 143rd annual meeting of the American Psychiatric Association, New York, May 1990a

Silk KR, Lohr NE, Ogata S, et al: Borderline in patients with affective disorders: preliminary follow-up data. Journal of Personality Disorders 4:213–224, 1990b

Snyder S, Pitts WM, Goodpaster WA, et al: MMPI profile of DSM-III borderline personality disorder. Am J Psychiatry 139:1046–1048, 1982

Soloff PH, Millward JW: Psychiatric disorders in the families of borderline patients. Arch Gen Psychiatry 40:37–44, 1983

Soloff PH, George A, Nathan RS: The dexamethasone suppression test in patients with borderline personality disorders. Am J Psychiatry 139:1621–1623, 1982

Soloff PH, George A, Nathan RS, et al: Paradoxical effects of amitriptyline on borderline patients. Am J Psychiatry 143:1603–1605, 1986a

Soloff PH, George A, Nathan RS, et al: Progress in pharmacotherapy of borderline disorders: a double-blind study of amitriptyline, haloperidol, and placebo. Arch Gen Psychiatry 43:691–697, 1986b

Spitzer RL, Endicott J, Robins E: Research Diagnostic Criteria (RDC) for a Selected Group of Functional Disorders, 2nd Edition. New York, New York State Psychiatric Institute, Biometrics Research, 1975

Stangl D, Pfohl B, Zimmerman M, et al: A structured interview for the DSM-III personality disorders: a preliminary report. Arch Gen Psychiatry 42:591–596, 1985

Steele TE: Depression, borderline disorder, and the DST (letter). Am J Psychiatry 140:818, 1983

Sternbach HA, Fleming J, Extein I, et al: The dexamethasone suppression and thyrotropin-releasing hormone tests in depressed borderline patients. Psychoneuroendocrinology 8:459–462, 1983

Stone MH: Contemporary shift in the borderline concept from a subschizophrenic disorder to a subaffective disorder. Psychiatr Clin North Am 2:577–594, 1979

Val ER, Nasr SJ, Gaviria FM, et al: Depression, borderline disorder, and the DST (letter). Am J Psychiatry 140:819, 1983

Westen D, Moses JA, Lohr NE, et al: Quality of depressive experience in BPD and MDD. Paper presented at the 143rd annual meeting of the American Psychiatric Association, New York, May 1990

Widiger TA: The categorical distinction between personality and affective disorders. Journal of Personality Disorders 3:77–91, 1989

Widiger TA, Sanderson C, Warner L: The MMPI, prototypal typology, and borderline personality disorder. J Pers Assess 50:540–553, 1986

Zanarini MC, Frankenburg FR, Chauncey DL, et al: The Diagnostic Interview for Personality Disorders: interrater and test-retest reliability. Compr Psychiatry 28:467–480, 1987

CHAPTER 3

Borderline Personality Disorder as an Impulse Spectrum Disorder

Mary C. Zanarini, Ph.D.

TERN (1938) WAS THE FIRST AUTHOR TO USE THE TERM "borderline" to describe a specific pathological condition—a condition that he thought had both neurotic and psychotic features. Since that time, there have been four main conceptualizations of this term. The first of these conceptualizations is based on the work of Kernberg (1975), in which the term borderline is used to describe most serious forms of character pathology. The second conceptualization reflects the work of Gunderson (1984). In this view, the term borderline describes a specific form of personality disorder that can be distinguished from a substantial number of other Axis II disorders, particularly those in the "odd" and "anxious" clusters of DSM-III (American Psychiatric Association 1980) and DSM-III-R (American Psychiatric Association 1987). The third conceptualization, which flourished in the 1960s and 1970s, focused on the propensity of borderline patients to have transient psychotic or psychotic-like experiences. In this view, borderline personality was thought of as being a schizophrenia spectrum disorder (Wender 1977). The fourth of these conceptualizations, which organized much of clinical care and empirical research in the 1980s, focused on the chronic dysphoria and affective lability of borderline patients. In this view, borderline personality was thought of as being an affective spectrum disorder (Akiskal 1981; Stone 1980). In this chapter the alternative theory will be proposed that borderline personality disorder (BPD) is best conceptualized as an impulse spectrum disorder (i.e., a disorder related to substance use disorders, antisocial personality disorder, and perhaps eating disorders). In this view, BPD is not seen as an attenuated or atypical form of one of these impulse spectrum disorders. Rather, it is being proposed that BPD is a specific form of personality disorder that may share a propensity to action with these disorders of impulse control.

The empirical evidence from the realms of phenomenology and family history will first be reviewed to show the strength of the relationship between BPD and impulse spectrum disorders. Alternative ways of understanding the relationship between borderline psychopathology, substance use disorders, and antisocial personality disorder will then be described.

BORDERLINE PERSONALITY DISORDER AND AXIS I AND AXIS II PHENOMENOLOGY

To date, eight studies that have assessed a range of Axis I and Axis II disorders in the histories of criteria-defined borderline patients have been published (see Table 3–1 for details). In the first of these studies, Akiskal (1981) studied outpatients at two urban mental health centers in Tennessee who met at least five of the six Gunderson-Singer (Gunderson and Singer 1975) criteria for BPD. Each of these patients also met the DSM-III criteria for BPD. A semistructured interview was administered by a research psychiatrist to obtain phenomenological information according to DSM-III criteria. Using this information, Akiskal then made all Axis I and Axis II diagnoses that were applicable. He found that 66% of these borderline outpatients met criteria for some form of affective disorder: 45% had a primary affective disorder, while 21% had a secondary depression, usually of a chronic intermittent nature. Akiskal also found that 57% of the borderline cohort met criteria for a substance use disorder, 16% met criteria for schizotypal personality disorder, and 13% met criteria for antisocial personality disorder.

McGlashan (1983) studied the Axis I phenomenology of a retrospectively diagnosed sample of inpatients meeting Diagnostic Interview for Borderlines (DIB; Gunderson et al. 1981) and/or DSM-III criteria for BPD. A research team reviewed the charts of all patients discharged from the Chestnut Lodge between 1950 and 1975 who 1) were between 16 and 55 years of age on admission, 2) had a hospitalization of at least 90 days, and 3) did not have an organic brain syndrome. Each patient was rated as to the presence of DSM-III schizophrenia, bipolar disorder, and major depression as well as DIB and DSM III BPD. McGlashan found that 82 patients met DIB criteria for BPD and 97 patients met DSM-III criteria for this disorder. A surprising 10% of the DIB borderline patients met DSM-III criteria for schizophrenia, while 5% met DSM-III criteria for bipolar disorder and 30% met DSM-III criteria for major depression. However, an even more surprising 20% of DSM-III BPD patients met DSM-III criteria for schizophrenia, while 12% met DSM-III criteria for bipolar disorder and 31% met DSM-III criteria for major depression. In a related study of the same cohort, McGlashan (1987) found that 18.2% of 99 definite or probable DIB and/or DSM-III borderline patients met DSM-III criteria for schizotypal personality disorder.

Pope and colleagues (1983) studied the Axis I and Axis II phenomenology of a group of inpatients at McLean Hospital who met the DSM-III criteria for BPD. An investigator reviewed the charts of patients who had previously been given a clinical or DIB diagnosis of BPD and determined

Table 3–1. Comorbidity studies of borderline personality disorder and Axis I and Axis II phenomenology

Study	BPD (n)	Schizophrenia (%)	Affective disorder (%)	Substance abuse (%)	APD (%)	STPD (%)
Akiskal (1981)	100	0.0	66.0	57.0	13.0	16.0
McGlashan (1983)[a]	82	10.0	35.0			18.2
	97	20.0	42.0			
Pope et al. (1983)	33	0.0	48.0	67.0	9.0	0.0
Andrulonis and Vogel (1984)	106	0.0	66.0	69.0	69.0	
Frances et al. (1984)	26	0.0	38.0	23.0	0.0	27.0
Perry and Cooper (1985)[b,c]	23	0.0	87.0	43.0		
			35.0	87.0	25.5	
Links et al. (1988b)[b,c]	88	1.1	59.5	31.4	13.1	6.8
			3.6	22.9		
Zanarini et al. (1989a)[b,c,d]	50	0.0	78.0	66.0	60.0	68.0
			0.0	70.0		18.0

Note. BPD = borderline personality disorder; APD = antisocial personality disorder; STPD = schizotypal personality disorder.
[a]These percentages are based on a sample of 99 patients who met probable or definite Diagnostic Interview for Borderlines (DIB) (top row) and/or DSM-III (bottom row) criteria for BPD.
[b]The top row pertains to major depression and the bottom row to bipolar disorder.
[c]The top row pertains to alcohol abuse and the bottom row to drug abuse.
[d]The top row pertains to DSM-III and the bottom row to DSM-III-R schizotypal personality disorder.

which of them met DSM-III criteria for this disorder. Pope et al. found that 48% of the BPD patients had conditions diagnosed as either possible or probable major affective disorder (MAD) (i.e., bipolar disorder or major depression). They also found that 67% of the sample met criteria for some type of substance use disorder, and 85% met criteria for one of the other personality disorders in the "dramatic" cluster of DSM-III. More specifically, 73% met criteria for histrionic personality disorder, 9% met criteria for antisocial personality disorder, and 3% met criteria for narcissistic personality disorder. In addition, they found that none of their cohort met DSM-III criteria for either schizophrenia or schizotypal personality disorder.

Andrulonis and Vogel (1984) studied the phenomenology of three groups of inpatients at the Institute of Living who met DSM-III criteria for the following disorders: nonschizotypal BPD, schizophrenia, and affective disorder. These diagnoses were made by a research psychiatrist on the basis of a clinical interview and chart review. None of the borderline patients was currently suffering from MAD, and none of the control patients had a concurrent Axis II diagnosis. In addition, no patient had an IQ of less than 80 or a primary diagnosis other than BPD, schizophrenia, or an affective disorder. Phenomenological data, which was collected through a chart review, had to be well documented by past psychiatric or legal records. Andrulonis and Vogel found that 69% of their borderline cohort had engaged in antisocial acting out (i.e., violence toward property or others, criminal acts, promiscuity, and running away) or had a history of serious substance abuse. In addition, they found that 66% of the borderline patients had a history of depressive behavior (i.e., chronic withdrawal and isolating behavior, self-mutilation, and suicidal efforts). Andrulonis and Vogel also found that borderline patients were significantly more likely than those in either control group to have engaged in antisocial acting out and to have a history of substance abuse.

Frances and associates (1984) studied outpatients between the ages of 18 and 45 at the Payne Whitney Evaluation Service who met criteria for either BPD or other personality disorders; 38% of the borderline patients met criteria for an affective disorder (most often dysthymic disorder), and 23% met criteria for a substance use disorder. The authors found that 27% of the borderline patients met DSM-III criteria for schizotypal personality disorder and that none met DSM-III criteria for antisocial personality disorder. Only the high rate of comorbid schizotypal personality disorder significantly discriminated the borderline patients from non-borderline control subjects.

Perry and Cooper (1985) studied the syndromal phenomenology of a group of outpatients, symptomatic volunteers, and individuals who were on probation from the metropolitan Boston area. After a lengthy semi-structured diagnostic interview, the sample was divided into the following five groups: definite BPD, BPD trait, antisocial personality disorder, BPD and antisocial personality disorder, and bipolar II disorder. After the initial interview, trained research assistants administered the Diagnostic Interview Schedule (DIS) (Robins et al. 1981), a structured interview designed to assess the lifetime prevalence of various psychiatric disorders. Perry and Cooper found that 87% of their definite BPD group had a history of major depression, 100% had a history of dysthymic disorder, and 35% had a history of bipolar disorder. They also found that 43% of this group met DSM-III criteria for alcohol abuse/dependence and that 87% met DSM-III criteria for drug abuse/dependence. However, each of these Axis I disorders was also common among antisocial and bipolar II patients, and no significant between-group differences were found. In addition, 25.5% of the definite and trait borderline patients met DSM-III criteria for antisocial personality disorder.

Links and colleagues (1988b) screened consecutive inpatients who met three or more of the seven best indicators for BPD (Gunderson and Kolb 1978). The patients were interviewed with the DIB and the Schedule for Affective Disorders and Schizophrenia (SADS) (Endicott and Spitzer 1978), which assesses disorders according to Research Diagnostic Criteria (RDC) (Spitzer et al. 1978). In terms of lifetime diagnoses, 1.1% of the BPD patients met RDC criteria for schizophrenia, 3.6% met RDC criteria for bipolar disorder, 59.5% met RDC criteria for major depression, 31.4% met RDC criteria for alcoholism, 22.9% met RDC criteria for drug abuse, 13.1% met RDC criteria for antisocial personality disorder, and 6.8% met DSM-III criteria for schizotypal personality disorder. No significant differences emerged between the BPD patients and the BPD trait control subjects.

Zanarini and associates (1988a, 1989a) studied the lifetime Axis I and Axis II phenomenology of 50 borderline patients meeting both Revised Diagnostic Interview for Borderlines (DIB-R) (Zanarini et al. 1989b) criteria for BPD and DSM-III criteria for BPD using the Structured Clinical Interview for DSM-III Axis I Disorders (SCID-I) (Spitzer and Williams 1984) and the Diagnostic Interview for Personality Disorders (DIPD) (Zanarini et al. 1987). They also studied the lifetime syndromal phenomenology of antisocial control subjects and control subjects who met the DSM-III criteria for dysthymic disorder and the DSM-III criteria for a nonborderline and nonantisocial form of personality disorder. All patients met the following inclusion criteria: 1) age between 18 and 40, 2) average or better intelligence, and 3) no history or current symptomatology of a clear-cut organic condition or major psychotic disorder (i.e., schizophrenia or bipolar disorder).

Zanarini et al. found that 100% of the borderline patients met DSM-III criteria for dysthymic disorder, 78% met DSM-III criteria for major depression, 70% met DSM-III criteria for drug abuse/dependence, and 66% met DSM-III criteria for alcohol abuse/dependence, whereas none met DSM-III criteria for schizophrenia or bipolar disorder. In addition, Zanarini et al. found that 60% of their borderline cohort met DSM-III criteria for antisocial personality disorder and 68% met DSM-III criteria for schizotypal personality disorder (but only 18% met the DSM-III-R criteria for this disorder). When compared with control subjects, borderline patients were significantly more likely than those in either control group to have met the DSM-III criteria for schizotypal personality disorder. They were also significantly more likely than dysthymic outpatient control subjects and significantly less likely than antisocial control subjects to have met the DSM-III criteria for alcohol abuse/dependence, drug abuse/dependence, and antisocial personality disorder. In addition, borderline patients were significantly more likely than antisocial control subjects to have met the DSM-III criteria for dysthymic disorder.

Taken together, these studies suggest that BPD bears little relationship to schizophrenia spectrum disorders in the realm of phenomenology. The fact that only two studies found any comorbidity between BPD and schizophrenia (Links et al. 1988b; McGlashan 1983) despite the fact that only two of the eight explicitly excluded patients with psychotic disorders from their borderline cohorts (Frances et al. 1984; Zanarini et al. 1989a) lends weight to the argument that BPD is not a schizophrenia spectrum disorder. The low rate of DSM-III schizotypal personality disorder found in all but one of these studies lends additional weight to the argument that

BPD is not strongly linked to schizophrenia. Even the fact that the study of Zanarini et al. (1988a) found a high rate of DSM-III schizotypal comorbidity does not necessarily link BPD to the schizophrenia spectrum, as only 18% of the borderline patients in this study met the more stringent and narrowly focused DSM-III-R criteria for schizotypal personality disorder—a finding of decreased comorbidity that has been found in other studies that have assessed the comorbidity between BPD and both DSM-III and DSM-III-R schizotypal personality disorder (Morey 1988; Silk et al. 1990).

These studies also suggest that the relationship between BPD and affective spectrum disorders is strong but not specific, because most control groups also exhibited high rates of affective disorder. Particularly telling in this regard are the very high rates of affective disorder reported in control subjects with antisocial personality disorder (Perry and Cooper 1985; Zanarini et al. 1989a), the other "dramatic" cluster personality disorder with a very strong penchant for impulsivity.

These studies further suggest a strong phenomenological link between BPD and impulse spectrum disorders; the borderline patients in these studies exhibited rates of substance abuse and/or antisocial personality disorder that were comparable to their rates of affective disorder. In addition, the borderline patients in all five of the controlled studies described above reported higher rates of substance abuse and/or antisocial personality disorder than did a variety of near-neighbor control groups (Andrulonis and Vogel 1984; Frances et al. 1984; Links et al. 1988b; Perry and Cooper 1985; Zanarini et al. 1988a, 1989a).

BORDERLINE PERSONALITY DISORDER AND FAMILY HISTORY OF PSYCHIATRIC DISORDERS

To date, nine studies that have assessed a range of psychiatric disorders in the first-degree relatives of borderline patients meeting modern research criteria for BPD have been published (see Table 3–2; also see van Reekum et al., Chapter 1). In the first of these studies, Loranger and colleagues (1982) examined the family history of female borderline patients, female bipolar patients, and female schizophrenic patients who had been hospitalized at the Westchester Division of New York Hospital between 1976 and 1980. Two raters reviewed the charts of all female patients who had been given a DSM-II discharge diagnosis of "other personality disorder" (borderline), manic-depressive illness (circular type), and schizophrenia (exclusive of latent and schizoaffective types), and selected those patients who unequivocally met DSM-III criteria for their respective disorder. Two raters who were blind to proband diagnosis then reviewed the chart information on the parents, siblings, and children of patients who had been treated for some type of emotional disorder. Diagnoses of BPD, bipolar disorder, schizophrenia, and major depression were assigned. It should be noted that while the criteria sets for the Axis I disorders were

Table 3–2.   Family history studies of first-degree relatives of patients with borderline personality disorder

Study	BPD (n)	Schizophrenia (%)	Affective disorder (%)	Substance abuse (%)	BPD (%)	APD (%)	STPD (%)
Loranger et al. (1982)[a] Loranger and Tulis (1985)	83	0.0	7.0	18.4	11.7		
Pope et al. (1983)[b]	33	0.0	6.2	11.5		6.2	0.0
Soloff and Millward (1983)[b]	48	2.6	8.7	11.8 3.9		7.0	
Andrulonis and Vogel (1984)[c]	106	4.0	32.0	35.0			
Akiskal et al. (1985)[c]	97	3.0	35.0				
Baron et al. (1985)[d]	17		13.3	13.6	17.9		3.1
Links et al. (1988a)[a,e,f]	69	0.0	26.6 4.4	21.0 12.7	15.3	9.6	
Zanarini et al (1988b)[a,e,f]	48	0.0	31.2 0.7	24.3 10.7	24.9	13.6	
Schulz et al. (1989)[b,e,f]	26	4.6	15.3 0.0	15.3 1.5		7.5	

Note.   BPD = borderline personality disorder; APD = antisocial personality disorder; STPD = schizotypal personality disorder.
[a]These studies pertain to lifetime expectancy (morbid risk) rates.
[b]These studies pertain to unadjusted prevalence rates.
[c]These studies pertain to the percentage of patients with at least one first-degree relative with the disorder.
[d]Prevalence rates are provided for BPD and substance abuse, while morbid risk rates are provided for major depression and STPD.
[e]The top row pertains to major depression and the bottom row to bipolar disorder.
[f]The top row pertains to alcohol abuse and the bottom row to drug abuse.

somewhat less stringent than those found in DSM-III, the criteria set used to diagnose BPD in treated relatives was far more encompassing than that found in DSM-III (i.e., only two of the following criteria were required: emotional, dramatic, demanding, angry, sexually acting out, antisocial, physically self-damaging, abusing substances, physically violent). The lifetime expectancy (morbid risk) of these disorders was then calculated. Loranger et al. found that the first-degree relatives of these borderline probands had a morbid risk of 11.7% of being treated for BPD, a morbid risk of 6.4% of being treated for major depression, a morbid risk of 0.5% of being treated for bipolar disorder, and no morbid risk of being treated for schizophrenia. They also found that the morbid risk of being treated for BPD among the first-degree relatives of borderline probands was significantly higher than that found for the relatives of those in either control group. In addition, the first-degree relatives of these borderline probands had a significantly higher morbid risk of being treated for major depression than did the first-degree relatives of schizophrenic control subjects.

Loranger and Tulis (1985) later studied the family history of alcohol abuse/alcoholism in the sample described above. A rater who was not blind to proband diagnosis assigned a diagnosis of alcohol abuse/alcoholism if a parent or sibling was so described in the chart. Loranger and Tulis found that the first-degree relatives of these borderline probands had a morbid risk for alcohol abuse/alcoholism of 18.4%. They also found that this morbid risk rate was significantly higher than that found in either control group.

Pope and his McLean associates (1983) also studied the family histories of their sample of BPD patients. A research psychiatrist who was blind to all information about the proband reviewed the chart of each borderline patient and assigned DSM-III diagnoses, when appropriate, to all first-degree relatives. The charts of bipolar and schizophrenic control subjects were reviewed in a similar manner. Pope et al. found that 11.5% of the first-degree relatives of the borderline patients met criteria for some form of substance use disorder. They also found that 6.2% of these 130 first-degree relatives met criteria for MAD (i.e., major depression or bipolar disorder) and 7.7% met criteria for a "dramatic" cluster personality disorder (6.2% meeting criteria for antisocial personality disorder). None of these relatives, however, met criteria for schizophrenia or schizotypal personality disorder. Pope et al. also found that the borderline probands were significantly more likely than schizophrenic control subjects to have a family history of MAD and that they were significantly more likely than those in either control group to have a family history of a "dramatic" cluster personality disorder. No significant family history differences were found for substance abuse or schizophrenia.

Soloff and Millward (1983) studied the family histories of BPD patients, schizophrenic patients, and patients with unipolar depressions. Family histories were obtained by experienced social workers: 43% of the data was gathered through interviews with the patient and family members, while 57% was obtained through retrospective chart review. Soloff and Millward found that 8.7% of the first-degree relatives of the BPD patients had a history of depression, 11.8% had a history of alcoholism, 3.9% had a history of substance abuse, 2.6% had a history of schizophrenia, and 7.0% had a history of antisocial behavior. They also found that depressed control patients were significantly more likely than BPD patients to have a first-degree relative with a history of depression.

Andrulonis and Vogel (1984) also studied the family histories of their borderline and control patients. Raters who were not blind to the diagnosis of the index patient interviewed the patient and family members and reviewed chart material as well. Andrulonis and Vogel found that 35% of the borderline probands had a family history of severe substance abuse, 32% had a family history of clinically treated depression, and 4% had a family history of schizophrenia. They also found that the borderline patients were significantly less likely than the schizophrenic patients to have a family history of schizophrenia, while there was a tendency for depressed control subjects to be more likely than borderline patients to have a family history of treated depression.

Akiskal and colleagues (1985) also studied the family history of their borderline sample using a method that combined chart review, family informants, and direct interviews. They found that borderline subjects had first-degree relatives with bipolar disorder and that another 18% had first-degree relatives who met criteria for a major depression. However, only three borderline probands had first-degree or second-degree relatives with schizophrenia. When these results were compared with those found in the families of four groups of outpatient control subjects (schizophrenic patients, nondepressed patients with personality disorders, bipolar patients, and patients with recurrent major depressive episodes), Akiskal et al. found that a significantly higher percentage of the borderline probands had a family history of affective disorder (bipolar disorder or major depression) than did schizophrenic control subjects (35% vs. 9%, respectively) and those with other forms of personality disorder (35% vs. 12%, respectively). They also found that a significantly lower percentage of borderline patients had a family history of schizophrenia than did schizophrenic control subjects (3% vs. 21%, respectively). Borderline patients and those in the control groups did not differ significantly in terms of a family history of major depression. However, borderline patients were significantly more likely to have a family history of bipolar disorder than were those with other Axis II disorders or major depressive episodes.

Baron and associates (1985) interviewed college students and hospital employees with an abbreviated version of the SADS and the Schedule for Interviewing Borderlines (SIB) (Baron and Gruen 1980). Of the 310 volunteers, 2 were diagnosed as having definite BPD (met five or more DSM-III criteria), and 15 others were diagnosed as having probable BPD (met three or four DSM-III criteria). Thirteen other volunteers were diagnosed as having definite schizotypal personality disorder (met four or more DSM-III criteria), and 23 were diagnosed as having probable schizotypal personality disorder (met two or three DSM-III criteria). Of the 36 schizotypal probands, 20 also met criteria for BPD.

Ninety normal control subjects were also selected for study. The same rater who had diagnosed the proband assessed the subject's family history using the Family History Research Diagnostic Criteria (Endicott et al. 1978) and a family history version of the SIB. Prevalence rates for BPD and substance abuse, as well as morbid risk rates for schizotypal personality disorder and major depression, were then calculated. These rates were then adjusted for the lower sensitivity of the family history method when compared with the family study method (Thompson et al. 1982). Baron et al. (1985) found that 17.9% of the first-degree relatives of the borderline probands met criteria for either definite or probable BPD, 13.6% met criteria for substance abuse, 13.3% were at risk for major depression, and 3.1% were at risk for definite or probable schizotypal personality disorder. Baron et al. also found that the borderline probands had a significantly higher percentage of relatives with BPD (definite and probable categories combined) than either the subjects with definite schizotypal personality disorder or the normal control subjects. In addition, the borderline pro- bands had a significantly lower percentage of relatives at risk for schizo- typal personality disorder (definite and probable categories combined) than did the subjects with pure schizotypal personality disorder. How- ever, the rates of major depression and substance abuse did not signifi- cantly distinguish the borderline probands from any of the schizotypal groups or the normal control subjects.

Links and his colleagues (1988a) also collected family history data on their borderline cohort using RDC criteria. Information was obtained on 320 family members; 36% were interviewed directly and 64% were diag- nosed based on indirect data. Links et al. calculated morbid risks for seven disorders and found that no relatives were at risk for schizophrenia and that the morbid risk of bipolar disorder was low (4.4%). However, the authors found that 26.6% of the first-degree relatives of their borderline patients were at risk for major depression, 21.0% were at risk for alcohol- ism, 12.7% were at risk for drug abuse, 15.3% were at risk for BPD, and 9.6% were at risk for antisocial personality disorder.

Zanarini and her associates (1988b) also collected family history data on their cohort of 50 borderline patients, 29 antisocial control subjects, and 26 dysthymic OPD control subjects by interviewing the proband using a semistructured interview based on DSM-III criteria. Information was collected on a total of 488 first-degree relatives. Zanarini et al. then calculated morbid risk rates for eight disorders and found that none of the first-degree relatives of the 48 borderline patients (two of the sample of 50 were adopted and had no knowledge about their biological relatives) were at risk for schizophrenia and 0.7% were at risk for bipolar disorder. However, 31.2% were at risk for major depression, 13.6% were at risk for dysthymic disorder, 24.3% were at risk for alcohol abuse/alcoholism, 10.7% were at risk for drug abuse/dependence, 24.9% were at risk for BPD, and 13.6% were at risk for antisocial personality disorder. Zanarini et al. also found that a significantly higher percentage of the first-degree relatives of borderline probands were at risk for BPD than were the relatives of those in either control group. In addition, a significantly higher percentage of the first-degree relatives of the borderline probands were at risk for dysthymic disorder than were the relatives of antisocial control subjects.

Schulz and her colleagues (1989) studied the family histories of borderline inpatients who met both DIB and DSM-III criteria for BPD and compared them to the family histories of schizophrenic control subjects. Borderline probands who met all but one of the required number of criteria for any personality disorder other than BPD or schizotypal personality disorder as assessed by Pfohl's Structured Interview for DSM-III Personality Disorders (SIDP) (Stangl et al. 1985) were excluded. All borderline and schizophrenic probands were interviewed about their families using the family history version of the RDC criteria. In addition, at least one relative of each schizophrenic patient and at least one relative of 42.3% of the borderline probands were interviewed using the same criteria. Schulz et al. found that 4.6% of the first-degree relatives of the BPD patients met criteria for schizophrenia, while none met criteria for bipolar disorder. In addition, 15.3% met criteria for major depression and alcoholism, 1.5% met criteria for drug abuse, and 7.5% met criteria for antisocial personality disorder. The authors also found that relatives of BPD patients had significantly higher prevalence rates of major depression, alcoholism, and antisocial personality disorder than did the relatives of the schizophrenic control subjects.

Taken together, the results of these studies, which vary considerably in their methodology, are very consistent in indicating little if any familial link between BPD and schizophrenia and/or schizotypal personality disorder. Only four of the nine studies found any schizophrenia among the first-degree relatives of borderline subjects (Andrulonis and Vogel 1984; Akiskal et al. 1985; Schulz et al. 1989; Soloff and Millward 1983), and each of these four studies found a morbid risk rate of less than 5%. In addition, only Baron et al. (1985) found any morbid risk for schizotypal personality disorder among the first-degree relatives of borderline probands, and this rate (3.1%) was both low and significantly less than that found among the first-degree relatives of schizotypal probands.

The results of these studies are also very consistent in indicating that affective disorder, particularly unipolar affective disorder, is very common among the first-degree relatives of borderline probands. However, unipolar depression was also found to be common among the relatives of control subjects: about equally common among the relatives of personality-disordered control subjects (Akiskal et al. 1985; Baron et al. 1985; Zanarini et al. 1988b), significantly more common among the relatives of depressed control subjects than among borderline probands (Andrulonis and Vogel 1984; Soloff and Millward 1983), and significantly more common among the relatives of borderline probands than among the relatives of schizophrenic subjects (Loranger et al. 1982; Schulz et al. 1989).

Taken together, the results of these studies suggest a strong familial link between BPD, substance use disorders, and antisocial personality disorder. The results of these studies indicate that substance use disorders are somewhat more common than affective disorders among the first-degree relatives of borderline probands. They also indicate that alcoholism, in particular, is significantly more common among the relatives of borderline probands than among the relatives of schizophrenic and bipolar control subjects (Loranger and Tulis 1985; Schulz et al. 1989). Additionally, these studies indicate that about 1 out of every 11 first-degree relatives of borderline probands meets research criteria for antisocial personality disorder. This was the case even in Schulz et al.'s (1989) study, which specifically excluded borderline probands who met criteria for antisocial personality disorder. The rate of antisocial personality disorder found in the relatives of borderline probands was also higher than that found in the relatives of all control groups other than the antisocial patients themselves (Pope et al. 1983; Schulz et al. 1989; Soloff and Millward 1983; Zanarini et al. 1988b). Additionally, Loranger et al. (1982) found that BPD "breeds true" (i.e., is significantly more common among the first-degree relatives of borderline probands than among control subjects). However, unlike the other two controlled studies that have found the same result (Baron et al. 1985; Zanarini et al. 1988b), many of the borderline relatives in Loranger et al.'s study may well have had antisocial personality disorder rather than BPD, given the strong antisocial trend in their criteria set for familial BPD.

IMPULSIVITY AND BORDERLINE PSYCHOPATHOLOGY

The results of these studies of phenomenology and family history of psychiatric disorder are consistent in indicating that there is a strong relationship between BPD and impulse spectrum disorders and that this relationship is as strong and perhaps more specific than that between BPD and affective disorders. It could be argued that this relationship is primarily based on an inherited propensity for impulsivity. Alternatively, it could be argued that this relationship represents a way of dealing with emotional pain in a motoric fashion and that borderline patients use impulsivity as a means of self-soothing as well as a way to express their desperation, rage, and intense frustration. Ultimately, it may well turn out that both are true. However, it is not my intention in this chapter to suggest that BPD is a subimpulse disorder (i.e., simply an attenuated or atypical form of substance abuse or antisocial personality disorder). Clearly, all of the empirical research on the phenomenology (Widiger and Frances 1989), pathogenesis (Gunderson and Zanarini 1989), and course of BPD (Stone 1989) strongly supports the validity of the disorder. However, it is a disorder characterized by symptomatology in the spheres of cognition, affect, and impulsivity (as well as highly troubled interpersonal relationships).

Recent research would seem to indicate that the cognitive difficulties of borderline patients are very distinct from those of schizophrenic patients, patients with other forms of personality disorders, and normal control subjects (Zanarini et al. 1990a). Recent research also indicates that the affective symptomatology of borderline patients is somewhat unique (Snyder et al. 1982; Soloff et al. 1987). In the same vein, some of these patients' impulsive acts, such as deliberately self-mutilative acts and manipulative suicide efforts, have been found to be very specific, and perhaps even pathognomonic, to BPD, whereas others, such as the propensity to abuse substances and to engage in antisocial acts, have been found to be characteristic of, but not totally discriminating for, BPD (Zanarini et al. 1990b).

Taken together, these results suggest that BPD is a valid disorder characterized by a high degree of impulsivity, some of which is specific to BPD and some of which represents a strong relationship to a spectrum of impulsive disorders. This view has important implications for both prognosis and treatment. In terms of prognosis, the results of the long-term follow-back study of Stone (1990) suggest that having a comorbid impulse spectrum disorder is strongly related to outcome for borderline patients. More specifically, Stone has found that those borderline patients who have gained control of a serious substance abuse problem tend to have a good outcome, whereas those with a continuing pattern of serious antisocial acting out tend to have a poor outcome. In terms of treatment, clinical experience suggests that participation in self-help groups, vocational training, and maturation may well prove to be more efficacious forms of treatment for borderline patients with comorbid substance use disorders and/or antisocial personality disorder than intensive psychotherapy or pharmacotherapy.

Borderline patients subjectively experience themselves as being in tremendous pain—pain that is often associated with a childhood history of chronic abuse and/or neglect (Gunderson and Zanarini 1989). Many individuals handle this pain and/or signal others about their pain through impulsivity. The results of the studies reviewed above suggest a strong relationship between BPD and impulse spectrum disorders. However, further research is necessary to assess the strength and nature of this relationship as well as its clinical implications.

REFERENCES

Akiskal HS: Subaffective disorders: dysthymic, cyclothymic and bipolar II disorders in the "borderline" realm. Psychiatr Clin North Am 4:25–46, 1981

Akiskal HS, Chen SE, Davis GC, et al: Borderline: an adjective in search of a noun. J Clin Psychiatry 46:41–48, 1985

American Psychiatric Association: Diagnostic and Statistical Manual of Mental Disorders, 3rd Edition. Washington, DC, American Psychiatric Association, 1980

American Psychiatric Association: Diagnostic and Statistical Manual of Mental Disorders, 3rd Edition, Revised. Washington, DC, American Psychiatric Association, 1987

Andrulonis PA, Vogel NG: Comparison of borderline personality subcategories to schizophrenic and affective disorders. Br J Psychiatry 144:358–363, 1984

Baron M, Gruen R: The Schedule for Interviewing Borderlines. New York, New York State Psychiatric Institute, 1980

Baron M, Gruen R, Asnis L, et al: Familial transmission of schizotypal and borderline personality disorders. Am J Psychiatry 142:927–934, 1985

Endicott J, Spitzer RL: A diagnostic interview: the Schedule for Affective Disorders and Schizophrenia. Arch Gen Psychiatry 35:837–844, 1978

Endicott J, Andreasen N, Spitzer RL: Family History Research Diagnostic Criteria. New York, New York State Psychiatric Institute, 1978

Frances A, Clarkin JF, Gilmore M, et al: Reliability of criteria for borderline personality disorder: a comparison of DSM-III and the Diagnostic Interview for Borderline Patients. Am J Psychiatry 141:1080–1084, 1984

Gunderson JG: Borderline Personality Disorder. Washington, DC, American Psychiatric Press, 1984

Gunderson JG, Kolb JE: Discriminating features of borderline patients. Am J Psychiatry 135:792–796, 1978

Gunderson JG, Singer MT: Defining borderline patients: an overview. Am J Psychiatry 132:1–10, 1975

Gunderson JG, Zanarini MC: Pathogenesis of borderline personality, in American Psychiatric Press Review of Psychiatry, Vol 8. Edited by Tasman A, Hales RE, Frances AJ. Washington, DC, American Psychiatric Press, 1989, pp 25–48

Gunderson JG, Kolb JE, Austin V: The diagnostic interview for borderline patients. Am J Psychiatry 138:896–903, 1981

Kernberg O: Borderline Conditions and Pathological Narcissism. New York, Jason Aronson, 1975

Links PS, Steiner M, Huxley G: The occurrence of borderline personality disorder in the families of borderline patients. Journal of Personality Disorders 2:14–20, 1988a

Links PS, Steiner M, Offord DR, et al: Characteristics of borderline personality disorder: a Canadian study. Can J Psychiatry 33:336–340, 1988b

Loranger AW, Tulis EH: Family history of alcoholism in borderline personality disorder. Arch Gen Psychiatry 42:153–157, 1985

Loranger AW, Oldham JM, Tulis EH: Familial transmission of DSM-III borderline personality disorder. Arch Gen Psychiatry 39:795–799, 1982

McGlashan TH: The borderline syndrome, II: is it a variant of schizophrenia or affective disorder? Arch Gen Psychiatry 40:1319–1323, 1983

McGlashan TH: Testing DSM-III symptom criteria for schizotypal and borderline personality disorders. Arch Gen Psychiatry 44:143–148, 1987

Morey LC: Personality disorders in DSM-III and DSM-III-R: convergence, coverage, and internal consistency. Am J Psychiatry 145:573–577, 1988

Perry JC, Cooper SH: Psychodynamics, symptoms, and outcome in borderline and antisocial personality disorders and bipolar type II affective disorder, in The Borderline: Current Empirical Research. Edited by McGlashan TH. Washington, DC, American Psychiatric Press, 1985, pp 19–41

Pope HG Jr, Jonas JM, Hudson JI, et al: The validity of DSM-III borderline personality disorder: a phenomenologic, family history, treatment response, and long-term follow-up study. Arch Gen Psychiatry 40:23–30, 1983

Robins LN, Helzer JE, Croughan J, et al: National Institute of Mental Health Diagnostic Interview Schedule: its history, characteristics, and validity. Arch Gen Psychiatry 38:381–389, 1981

Schulz PM, Soloff PH, Kelly T, et al: A family history of borderline subtypes. Journal of Personality Disorders 3:217–229, 1989

Silk KR, Westen D, Lohr NE, et al: DSM-III and DSM-III-R schizotypal symptoms in borderline personality disorder. Compr Psychiatry 31:103–110, 1990

Snyder S, Sajadi C, Pitts WM Jr, et al: Identifying the depressive border of the borderline personality disorder. Am J Psychiatry 139:814–817, 1982

Soloff PH, Millward JW: Psychiatric disorders in the families of borderline patients. Arch Gen Psychiatry 40:37–44, 1983

Soloff PH, George A, Nathan RS, et al: Characterizing depression in borderline patients. J Clin Psychiatry 48:155–157, 1987

Spitzer RL, Williams JBW: Structured Clinical Interview for DSM-III Axis I Disorders. New York, New York State Psychiatric Institute, 1984

Spitzer RL, Endicott J, Robins E: Research Diagnostic Criteria: rationale and reliability. Arch Gen Psychiatry 35:773–782, 1978

Stangl D, Pfohl B, Zimmerman M, et al: A structured interview for the DSM-III personality disorders. Arch Gen Psychiatry 42:591–596, 1985

Stern A: Psychoanalytic investigation of and therapy in the borderline group of neuroses. Psychoanal Q 7:467–489, 1938

Stone MH: The Borderline Syndromes: Constitution, Personality, and Adaptation. New York, McGraw-Hill, 1980

Stone MH: The course of borderline personality disorder, in American Psychiatric Press Review of Psychiatry, Vol 8. Edited by Tasman A, Hales RE, Frances AJ. Washington, DC, American Psychiatric Press, 1989, pp 103–122

Stone MH: The Fate of Borderline Patients: Successful Outcome and Psychiatric Practice. New York, Guilford, 1990

Thompson WD, Orvaschel H, Prusoff BA, et al: An evaluation of the family history method for ascertaining psychiatric disorders. Arch Gen Psychiatry 39:53–58, 1982

Wender PH: The contribution of the adoption studies to an understanding of the phenomenology and etiology of borderline schizophrenia, in Borderline Personality Disorders: The Concept, the Syndrome, the Patient. Edited by Hartocollis P. New York, International Universities Press, 1977, pp 255–269

Widiger TA, Frances AJ: Epidemiology, diagnosis, and comorbidity of borderline personality disorder, in American Psychiatric Press Review of Psychiatry, Vol 8. Edited by Tasman A, Hales RE, Frances AJ. Washington, DC, American Psychiatric Press, 1989, pp 8–24

Zanarini MC, Frankenburg FR, Chauncey DL, et al: The Diagnostic Interview for Personality Disorders: interrater and test-retest reliability. Compr Psychiatry 28:467–480, 1987

Zanarini MC, Gunderson JG, Frankenburg FR: Axis II phenomenology of borderline personality disorder, in Proceedings of the World Psychiatric Association Regional Symposium. Washington, DC, 1988a

Zanarini MC, Gunderson JG, Marino MF, et al: DSM III disorders in the families of borderline outpatients. Journal of Personality Disorders 2:292–302, 1988b

Zanarini MC, Gunderson JG, Frankenburg FR: Axis I phenomenology of borderline personality disorder. Compr Psychiatry 30:149–156, 1989a

Zanarini MC, Gunderson JG, Frankenburg FR, et al: The revised Diagnostic Interview for Borderlines: discriminating BPD from other Axis II disorders. Journal of Personality Disorders 3:10–18, 1989b

Zanarini MC, Gunderson JG, Frankenburg FR: Cognitive features of borderline personality disorder. Am J Psychiatry 147:57–63, 1990a

Zanarini MC, Gunderson JG, Frankenburg FR, et al: Discriminating borderline personality disorder from other Axis II disorders. Am J Psychiatry 147:161–167, 1990b

Etiology of Borderline Personality Disorder: Psychobiological Factors Contributing to an Underlying Irritability

Michael H. Stone, M.D.

Etiologic Heterogeneity

The tendency was common a generation ago to view the factors leading to borderline personality disorder (BPD) purely from a narrow, psychological perspective. Masterson and Rinsley (1975), for example, ascribed the abnormalities of BPD to mothers who interfered with the needs of their offspring to become emotionally separate and to develop as distinct individuals. Masterson regarded many of the mothers of borderline patients as themselves having BPD, as though the disorder were "transmissible" psychologically. Others, noting that there is an excess (over the expectable number) of mothers with BPD among the relatives of identified BPD cases, have speculated that the condition is transmissible, to a certain extent, genetically (Loranger et al. 1982).

In an early reformulation concerning etiology, emphasis was placed on a familial predisposition to affective disorders (Akiskal 1981; Stone 1977). Although no claim was made that all BPD cases stemmed from this source, some investigators made a special point of demonstrating that familial affective illness was a factor in only a proportion of BPD patients and might, furthermore, be a "nonspecific" factor, inasmuch as affective illness was common in the families of index cases with other personality disorders (Barasch et al. 1985; Torgersen 1984).

In the last decade, formulations have taken yet another path: one in which much of the responsibility for BPD is assigned to intrafamilial abuse in all its various forms (sexual, physical, psychological). A number of investigators now consider an abusive family environment not only common in the histories of borderline (especially hospitalized borderline) patients, but fairly specific, in the sense that such abuse is not so common in the lives of patients with other personality disorders, with the exception of antisocial personality disorder (Byrne et al. 1990; also see Perry and Herman, Chapter 6). Many borderline and antisocial individuals share the tendency to accumulate, through their own behavior as adults, the kind of untoward life events that may, during childhood, have contributed to the abnormal personality development. Abused children may, for example, become chronically irritable and angry. As adults, they often undermine through their hostility what would otherwise have been sustaining work and love relationships. Broken marriages and lost jobs become "life events" further aggravating the clinical picture of these personality-disordered patients (Seivewright 1987).

Now that genes, constitution, maternal overcontrol, family neglect, and family abusiveness have all been implicated in BPD, one can rightfully claim that every etiologic base has already been touched. With no new factors to look for, what remains for us is to ascertain the relative weights of these factors in each particular BPD patient and to distinguish, if we can, whether some common element exists among the various factors that might provide BPD with a unifying framework. At this point it will be useful to survey the data concerning two broad categories of contributing factors: those related to psychological traumata and those related to our biological substrate.

THE TRAUMA FACTOR

Since the late 1970s an ever-growing number of investigators have been impressed by the frequency of severe psychological traumata in the early lives of many of their BPD patients. The frequency of a history of incest is particularly high among hospitalized females with BPD (Stone 1990; Stone et al. 1988; Zanarini et al. 1989). In many carefully studied recent samples, this frequency will be in the range of 33% to 70%—that is, two to four times the frequency noted in the best epidemiologic study from the general population (Russell 1986). There is some evidence (Stone 1990) that, of the personality disorders outlined in DSM-III-R, the incest frequency is higher in hospitalized BPD females than in women with other personality disorders (apart from antisocial personality disorder). If this connection is borne out in further, larger-scale studies, the hypothesis of a causative relationship would be bolstered—that is, that incest, especially between father/stepfather and daughter, may induce, in effect, a chronic posttraumatic stress disorder whose symptoms and personality traits happen to include those we now associate with BPD.

Repeated physical assault by a parent can induce a similar clinical picture, one in which chronic irascibility and inordinate anger are especially prominent (Goodwin 1982; Stone 1990). Abusiveness toward children appears to be directed more toward boys than toward girls. But whereas incest engenders both rage and guilt, violence engenders intense rage but guilt only occasionally. The borderline picture, if it emerges in this context, may thus be slanted toward violence more than toward self-mutilation or other forms of self-destructiveness.

Physically abused males in particular, if they later develop the BPD syndrome, will often show an admixture of antisociality. This combination is common in the annals of forensic psychiatry. Among the recent biographies of notorious serial and multiple murderers, some make specific mention of consulting psychiatrists who diagnosed an underlying BPD, usually with concomitant antisocial features (Cahill 1986, writing on John Gacy; Kaplan et al. 1990, on Laurie Dann).

Cultural and hereditary influences, though perhaps separable for heuristic purposes, are intermixed in complicated ways. In certain cultures (e.g., Islamic culture) incest is quite rare (Stone 1989). Cultures vary as to the extent to which impulsive and aggressive behavior is tolerated. BPD might be proportionally less common, for example, in certain Islamic or Asian societies where such behavior is strongly discouraged. Etiologically speaking, over many generations, breeding advantages may accrue to those with milder temperaments, whose children are in turn also less violent on average—partly for genetic reasons and partly for not having been maltreated by their parents. And those who do have risk factors enough to predispose to BPD, were they to have been reared in our culture, might have developed along different lines in their culture—perhaps in the direction of anxiety states or psychosomatic disorders. To test whether the hypotheses concerning cultural factors adumbrated here prove correct will require considerable epidemiological work in a number of different countries.

CONTEMPORARY RESEARCH

Affective Illness

As reviewed by Gold and Silk in Chapter 2, a number of recent papers address the complicated issue of affective illness in relation to BPD. The area of conjunction between BPD and major affective disorder (MAD) is very great, raising the question of whether BPD is a forme fruste of MAD. Rippetoe and her colleagues (1986) noted that BPD inpatients with dysthymia showed more splitting, suicidality, clinging dependency, and feelings of emptiness than did BPD patients who did not show dysthymia concomitantly. Concluding that BPD is etiologically "amorphous" (i.e., heterogeneous), Rippetoe et al. included several varieties of depressive and personality disorders that are associated with different levels of function and different outcomes.

A balanced view of the question concerning BPD and its relation to affective illness requires our taking into consideration not only etiologic heterogeneity but also sample variation (Stone 1990, p. 74). The BPD patients who formed the basis of the PI500 follow-up study showed, for example, only a modest degree of abuse history. Affective illness in close relatives was fairly prominent (32 of 395 biological parents); 10 to 25 years after discharge, 8.5% of the borderline patients had themselves gone on to develop unipolar or bipolar illness. In a sample from Brisbane, Australia, in contrast, a history of incest was present in half the female BPD inpatients. If one included physical abuse or extreme verbal humiliation by caretakers as well, the "abuse" factor rose to 90% (Stone et al. 1988). Serious affective illness was present only in a scant few of the first-degree relatives. In the case of depressive disorders, biological factors could not easily be separated out from the harsh life circumstances and traumatic histories of these patients. Differing from either of these groups of borderline patients, those encountered in Japan often involve suicide gestures precipitated either by leaving close family ties (e.g., upon entering universities far from home) or by rejection in a love relationship (K. Okonogi, Y. Ono, personal communication, 1990). A history of sexual or physical abuse in the childhood of BPD patients is rare in Japan; nor is a family history of MAD a prominent accompaniment.

These examples illustrate how different are the weights an investigator would assign to the various factors relevant to the etiology of BPD depending upon sample and culture. Each investigator, so long as he or she remained within his or her solipsistic universe, would elaborate a different—and "convincing"—theory about the causative picture in BPD, until such time as he or she broke out of the narrower universe and made contact with other samples from around the world.

Aggression

One of the most salient characteristics of BPD is inordinate anger. This may take many forms, such as chronic hostility, intermittent rage outbursts, or extreme touchiness. As discussed in Chapter 1 by van Reekum et al., this aggression may have a neurological basis. As Gardner and Cowdry (1989) point out, this is a difficult phenomenon to capture in the laboratory, which does better with stable traits than it does with episodic traits. Positron-emission tomography or regional cerebral blood flow studies of BPD patients who are actually engulfed in a rage outburst have not been done and for obvious ethical reasons cannot be provoked in a laboratory setting. But the recent literature on aggression is often pertinent to a discussion of BPD even though directed originally toward other conditions. Merikangas (1981), in a study of 128 violent prisoners, underlined three important factors: 1) drive level, 2) stimulus threshold, and 3) response inhibition. High drive level, low threshold, and impaired ability to inhibit aggressive responses were all associated with the highest degrees of violence proneness. Hair-trigger sensitivity was often coupled with a tendency to respond maximally even to minimal threats. Epilepsy, abnormal EEG, and other evidence of brain damage were common. Similar abnormalities have been mentioned by Andrulonis et al. (1981) in their group of (mostly) young males with BPD and "episodic dyscontrol" (i.e., impulsive aggressivity). Huesman (1988), in connection with his information-processing model of aggression, speaks of aggressive "scripts," acquired during childhood, which then become resistant to change. Some persons, once made aggressive through either experiencing or witnessing abuse, tend to provoke aggressive responses in others (via taunts, menacing gestures, selection of abusive partners, etc.), heightening in the process their convictions concerning the "dangerousness" of other people in general (van der Kolk 1989).

If undampened, this cumulative learning can build enduring mental schemata for aggressive behavior. Many BPD patients, especially those who have been abused physically or sexually, behave as though their brains had been programmed for this type of "shoot first and then ask questions" responsivity. Under certain circumstances this hair-trigger responsivity can lead to assault or murder. It is of interest to note, in this connection, that among the 285 traced "borderlines" of the PI500 series, four (all males) had murdered one or more persons by the time of follow-up.

As Valzelli (1981) points out, aggression is an umbrella concept comprising many different forms: territorial, competitive, predatory, maternal-protective, irritative, and others. The behavioral programs within each of these forms can often be related to particular brain pathways— some specific to the particular variety of aggression, some overlapping with several varieties. The irritative form of aggression is of special relevance to BPD. This is the form of aggression unleashed by an opponent's attack (or, in laboratory animals, by aversive stimuli). In man, irritable aggression is associated with disproportionate intensity (the "inordinate anger" of BPD) as well as with the tendency to counterattack not the actual "offender" but often mere symbols of the offender.

In BPD patients, physical abuse during childhood, even more than sexual abuse, is often associated with an "enkindled" nervous system, poised and ready to overreact instantaneously in the face of real or perceived threats. The pathological alterations in patterns of central nervous system (CNS) arousal and reactivity appear to correlate with certain neurological abnormalities, whose attributes have come under intense study during the past decade. In the section that follows, we turn our attention to several of these lines of investigation.

Neurological Abnormalities

The role of neurological abnormalities in BPD has been discussed by van Reekum et al. in Chapter 1. Gardner et al. (1987) found neurologic soft signs in BPD that could relate to behavioral abnormalities. The finding of an abnormal auditory P300 in BPD (Blackwood et al. 1986) is particularly relevant to the impulsive aggressiveness seen in BPD. P300 is related to the evaluation of stimuli (Boddy 1978). It remains to be tested whether this technic will prove useful in discriminating BPD patients from patients with other personality disorders or noncomorbid affective illness. More work needs to be done to determine whether the P300 abnormality is an episode rather than a vulnerability marker (Zubin 1980, p. 283). Prolonged P300 latency is suggestive of impairment in the ability to form conditioned responses to a given stimulus. What the implications of such an abnormality might be for BPD is as yet unclear, though the abnormality may be related to the phenomenon of sensation seeking (Raine 1989; Raine and Venables 1988), a feature observable in many patients with BPD, especially those who show an admixture of sociopathic features.

Hegerl et al. (1989), in their study of evoked potentials in high and low sensation-seeking subjects among a normal population, found that high sensation-seekers showed steeper slopes in the amplitude/stimulus intensity function of the auditory evoked N^1/P^2 component. This phenomenon might be related to the "need for new and exciting sensations" (p. 186), as well as to the rapid loss of interest and high susceptibility to boredom. Hegerl et al.'s approach, if applied to a population of patients with personality disorders, would probably yield comparable neurophysiological results in many cyclothymic and Axis II Cluster-B patients, given their shared attribute of sensation seeking.

One peculiarity of memory in BPD patients is that they remain at the mercy of the latest sensory impression within personal relationships (Stone 1988). Thus, a mostly loving attitude on the part of a spouse known over many years can be erased from the screen of memory in a moment if the spouse's last interaction was interpreted (correctly or incorrectly) as annoying. A rage outburst may follow, accompanied by vituperations such as, "You never loved me," or "You've always been a no-good . . ." The person with BPD behaves as though the links between short- and long-term memory are severed. Yet the next day, given enough reassurance and soothing, the attitudinal pointer may swing to the opposite extreme. Are there neurophysiological correlates to this phenomenon, and if so, of what do they consist? Here again, there are major obstacles to research, owing to the difficulties inherent in testing BPD patients during moments of interpersonal crisis. Studies of memory storage and neural systems (Alkon 1989) are still conceptually remote from the particularities of the borderline personality. The work of McGaugh et al. (1989) may nonetheless be relevant. These investigators note that memory storage is modulated by a variety of hormones released under the impact of aversive experience that activate, for example, noradrenergic receptors within the amygdaloid complex. It may be that past traumatic experiences may become so "italicized" within the stored memory of certain BPD patients as to give undue weight to subsequent inputs of even a faintly similar nature, in the meantime trivializing the significance of later positive experiences, no matter how intense and consistent these may be.

Possible disturbances in amygdala-mediated memory point to the limbic system in general as a region that may be implicated in various manifestations of BPD. Kellner et al. (1987) were able to compare the effects of intravenous procaine in BPD patients with those in either affectively ill patients or normal control subjects. Procaine appeared to activate temporal lobe and limbic system structures in the patients as well as in the control subjects, leading to cognitive and sensory distortions, increased cortisol secretion, and heightened EEG fast activity over the temporal lobes. Preliminary results with subsequent use of carbamazepine in the BPD group showed no correlation between degree of procaine-induced EEG activation and degree of improvement on carbamazepine. Procaine may in future studies emerge as a useful pharmacological probe of limbic system function, especially if it turns out that identifiable subgroups of BPD patients could be distinguished, in their responsivity, from patients with other personality disorders.

As for such temporal lobe disorders as partial complex seizures, the diagnostic overlap was once thought to be fairly common. Similarly, cases of multiple personality often receive a diagnosis of BPD and at times have been considered a manifestation of partial complex seizures. Using the Dissociative Disorders Interview Schedule, Ross et al. (1989) were able to discriminate effectively between multiple personality and partial complex seizures, suggesting that the former is not simply a type of temporal lobe disorder. Occasionally, patients with partial complex seizures also satisfy criteria for BPD, raising the question of whether the temporal lobe disorder is of etiologic significance in a subset of BPD, as some have argued, or whether the connection is spurious (Andrulonis et al. 1981). While BPD, multiple personality, and partial complex seizures may share certain clinical features in common, it seems prudent not to regard multiple personality as a special variety of, or model for, BPD—in the same way that LSD-induced psychosis is not a reliable copy of idiopathic schizophrenia. Multiple personality stems from severe abuse and represents the extreme of "splitting" (hence the confusion with BPD). Partial complex seizures are only occasionally associated with head trauma. A connection between BPD and anatomically identifiable (as opposed to functional) temporal lobe disorders is in all likelihood neither typical nor spurious, but simply uncommon.

The limbic system can also be viewed as an element in the more complex limbic-hypothalamic-pituitary-adrenocortical system. Excessive secretory activity of this neuroendocrine system is, as Holsboer (1989) mentions, part of an acute stress response or depressive symptom pattern. The steroids and peptides involved in this system, given the stress overload and maladaptive stress reactions in BPD, may in future studies show characteristic deviations in various groups of borderline patients.

Though it has not been studied in relation to BPD, another memory system has been outlined in recent years by Mishkin et al. (1984). This so-called "habit" or procedural memory system is subserved not by limbic structures but by the basal ganglia (namely, the caudate and putamen). These structures are central to the mechanism for storage of nonverbal habit patterns, apparently including the ineradicable beliefs and identifications formed in the first few years of life. There is growing evidence that obsessive-compulsive disorder (OCD) is related to the function of this memory system (Hantouche et al. 1990; Rapoport et al. 1981). Some BPD patients are comorbid for OCD or for other disorders in which irrational beliefs exercise dominion over rational thought processes. The body-image distortions in anorexic and bulimic patients and the terror mobilized by any attempts to change their eating habits offer a compelling example of this phenomenon. BPD patients who were abused sexually, physically, and verbally during the formative years also tend to form patterns of reaction and thought consonant with the original victimization but highly skewed with respect to the more benign persons they will encounter later in life. Their distortions are clung to tenaciously and acquire a life-or-death quality, seldom yielding to the most accurate and oft-repeated psychodynamic interpretations. Attempts to overwhelm the habit-memory system of such patients and to reprogram them along more adaptive lines have spawned many new treatment approaches in the last decade, ranging from serotonergic drugs to special forms of cognitive and group therapy. The latter includes the whole gamut of special groups oriented toward control of specific impulses (Alcoholics Anonymous, Overeaters Anonymous, Narcotics Anonymous, Gamblers Anonymous, etc.).

In the area of neurotransmitter research, much attention has focused recently on serotonin, once it was ascertained that suicide, and, later, aggressivity, were often correlated with low CNS levels of serotonin. Serotonin serves in the CNS as a neurotransmitter mediating inhibitory pathways; its deficiency is associated with dis-inhibition (Coccaro 1989). The ability of serotonergic drugs like clomipramine and fluoxetine to ameliorate some cases of OCD has also heightened interest in this neurotransmitter (Murphy et al. 1989). Bulimic-anorexic patients often show concomitantly the features of OCD, and both these syndromes are common in patients with BPD. Impulsive aggression, including multiple suicide attempts, is characteristic of BPD patients, some of whom have already shown a reduction in such aggressivity when administered drugs that augment serotonin levels in key CNS regions either in a more specific manner (e.g., clomipramine) or in a nonspecific manner (e.g., carbamazepine; cf. Cowdry and Gardner 1988). In females with BPD, emotional dysregulation, with heightened tendencies to depression and irritability, commonly occurs in the paramenstrual phase of the menstrual cycle; those individuals with eating disorders may exhibit intensification of bulimic or anorectic symptoms during this phase. Further study of serotonin, along with other transmitter metabolites, throughout the cycle might well yield interesting results concerning possible neurophysiological correlates of this phenomenon, especially in women with BPD.

CONCLUSIONS

Among the most striking features of BPD are emotional instability, over-reaction (going to extremes, "all-or-none" responses), irascibility, and unreasonableness. The latter often expresses itself in the patient's rigid adherence to maladaptive patterns or else in overvalued ideas to which the patient clings with a tenacity reminiscent of delusion and despite awareness of the indefensibility of his or her assertions. These phenomena may be seen as various facets of a general tendency toward unmodulated responses and are accompanied by spasmodic, unstable behavior—much as one witnesses in a child's first day on ice skates or a bicycle.

Irritability may be the red thread running through all the major manifestations of BPD, with this irritability either causing or accompanying the characteristic disturbances in modulation (Stone 1988). BPD appears to be the final common pathway of many influences: hereditary, constitutional, organic-traumatic, neurologic (including attention-deficit disorder), and environmental, the latter usually in the form of parental cruelty, extreme neglect, or incest. While certain prenatal factors seem able to destabilize the CNS in ways predisposing to BPD, chronic abuse may leave quite similar traces within the nervous system via "kindling" effects (especially following parental violence or erotization), the imprints of which within the CNS appear to be just as deeply etched and just as resistant to conventional therapies as are the abnormalities stemming from constitutional sources. As Steiner et al. (1988) suggest, the symptomatology of some personality-disordered patients seems unrelated to Axis I conditions, whereas that of others is genetically related to the major mental disorders. Figure 4–1 outlines the various factors that may contribute, initially, to abnormal levels of CNS irritability and, then, to the formation of the clinical syndrome we now identify as BPD.

The faulty modulation in BPD appears to correlate, in part, with malfunction of the limbic system, which under normal circumstances operates as an "amplifier or filter through which stimuli and responses pass" (Zarr 1984, p. 220). Specifically, an "irritable" (i.e., overreactive) limbic system would set the thermostat of reactivity too high—too near an emotional "boiling point"—such that minor stresses are experienced as major threats prompting "kill or be killed" responses. Psychodynamic explanations by themselves cannot account for these drastic reactions, although they may be accurate in delineating interactional patterns that trigger the catastrophic response. Being alone on Saturday, being rejected, being yelled at by a parent are all unpleasant experiences that by themselves do not lead to mayhem or suicidal acts. A trigger in an unloaded gun makes only a click. What loads the gun in BPD is the abnormal neurophysiological substrate. As alluded to earlier, malfunction of the habit memory system often appears as a component of this substrate, mediating the all-or-none responses that help define those who exhibit these exaggerated responses as examples of "borderline personality disorder." Further research in the areas adumbrated above, both the psychological and the biological, should lead to improved subtyping of conditions within the domain of BPD, and thus to better and more integrated treatment that is drawn from psychological, sociocultural, and biological sources.

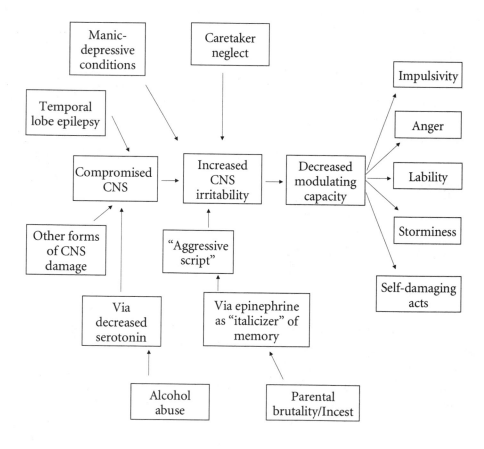

Figure 4–1. Etiologic factors in borderline personality disorder

REFERENCES

Akiskal HS: Subaffective disorders dysthymic, cyclothymic, and bipolar II disorders in the "borderline" realm." Psychiatr Clin North Am 4:25–46, 1981

Alkon DL: Memory storage and neural systems. Sci Am, July 1989, pp 42–5O

Andrulonis PA, Glueck BC, Stroebel CF, et al: Organic brain dysfunction and the borderline syndromes. Psychiatr Clin North Am 4:47–66, 1981

Barasch A, Frances A, Hurt S, et al: Stability and distinctness of borderline personality disorder. Am J Psychiatry 142:1484–1486, 1985

Blackwood DHR, St Clair DM Kutcher SP: P-300–event related potential abnormalities in borderline personality disorder. Biol Psychiatry 21:560–564, 1986

Boddy J: Brain Systems and Psychological Concepts. New York, Wiley, 1978

Byrne CP, Velamoor VR, Cernovsky ZZ, et al: A comparison of borderline and schizophrenic patients for childhood life events and parent-child relationships. Can J Psychiatry 35:590–595, 1990

Cahill T: Buried Dreams. New York, Bantam, 1986

Coccaro EF: Central serotonin and impulsive aggression. Br J Psychiatry 155 (suppl 8):52–62, 1989

Cowdry RW, Gardner DL: Pharmacotherapy of borderline personality disorder: alprazolam, carbamazepine, trifluoperazine and tranylcypromine. Arch Gen Psychiatry 45:111–119, 1988

Gardner DL, Cowdry RW: Borderline personality disorder: a research challenge. Biol Psychiatry 26:655–658, 1989

Gardner D, Lucas PB, Cowdry RW: Soft sign neurological abnormalities in borderline personality disorder and normal control subjects. J Nerv Ment Dis 175:177–180, 1987

Goodwin J: Sexual Abuse: Incest Victims and Their Families. Littleton, MA, PSG Publishing, 1982

Hantouche E, Gueguen B, Martinot JL, et al: Arguments en faveur d'un dysfonctionnement cerebral dans le trouble obsessionel-compulsif. L'Encephale 16:23–30, 1990

Hegerl U, Prochno I, Ulrich G, et al: Sensation-seeking and auditory evoked potentials. Biol Psychiatry 25:179–190, 1989

Holsboer F: Psychiatric implications of altered limbic hypothalamic-pituitary-adrenocortical activity. Eur Arch Psychiatr Neurol Sci 238:302–322, 1989

Huesman LR: An information processing model for the development of aggression. Aggressive Behavior 14:13–24, 1988

Kaplan J, Papajohn G, Zorn E: Murder of Innocence: The Tragic Life and Final Rampage of Laurie Dann. New York, Warner Books, 1990

Kellner CH, Post RM, Putnam F, et al: Intravenous procaine as a probe of limbic system activity in psychiatric patients and normal controls. Biol Psychiatry 22:1107–1126, 1987

Loranger AW, Oldham JM, Tulis EH: Familial transmission of DSM-III borderline personality disorder. Arch Gen Psychiatry 39:795–799, 1982

Masterson JF, Rinsley DB: The borderline syndrome: the role of the mother in the genesis and psychic structure of the borderline personality. Int J Psychoanal 56:163–177, 1975

McGaugh JL, Introini-Collinson LB, Nagahara AH, et al: Involvement of the amygdala in hormonal and neurotransmitter interactions in the modulation of memory storage, in Aversion, Avoidance, and Anxiety. Edited by Archer T, Nilsson LG. Hillsdale, NJ, Erlbaum, 1989, pp 231–248

Merikangas JR: The neurology of violence, in Brain Behavior Relationships. Edited by Merikangas JR. Lexington, MA, Lexington Books, 1981, pp 155–185

Mishkin M, Malamut B, Bachevalier J: Memories and habits: two neural systems, in Neurobiology of Learning and Memory. Edited by Lynch J, McGaugh J, Weinberger NM. New York, Guilford, 1984, pp 65–77

Murphy DL, Zohar J, Benkelfat C, et al: Obsessive-compulsive disorder as a 5-HT subsystem-related behavioural disorder. Br J Psychiatry 155 (suppl 8):15–24, 1989

Raine A: Evoked potentials and psychopathology. Int J Psychophysiol 8:1–16, 1989

Raine A, Venables PH: Enhanced P-3 evoked potentials and longer P-3 recovery time in psychopaths. Psychophysiology 25:30–38, 1988

Rapoport JL, Elkins R, Langer DH: Childhood obsessive-compulsive disorder. Am J Psychiatry 138:1545–1554, 1981

Rippetoe PA, Alarcon RD, Walter-Ryan WG: Interactions between depression and borderline personality. Psychopathology 19:340–346, 1986

Ross CA, Heber S, Anderson G, et al: Differentiating multiple personality disorder and complex partial seizures. Gen Hosp Psychiatry 11:54–58, 1989

Russell D: The Secret Trauma. New York, Basic Books, 1986

Seivewright N: Relationship between life-events and personality in psychiatric disorder. Stress Medicine 3:163–168, 1987

Steiner M, Links PS, Korzekwa M: Biological markers in borderline personality disorders: an overview. Can J Psychiatry 33:350–354, 1988

Stone MH: The borderline syndrome: evolution of the term, genetic aspects, and prognosis. Am J Psychother 31:345–365, 1977

Stone MH: Toward a psychobiological theory of borderline personality disorder: is irritability the red thread that runs through borderline conditions? Dissociation 1:2–15, 1988

Stone MH: Incest, Freud's seduction theory, and borderline personality. Paper presented at the annual meeting of the American Academy of Psychoanalysis, San Francisco, CA, May 1909

Stone MH: The Fate of Borderline Patients: Successful Outcome and Psychiatric Practice. New York, Guilford, 1990

Stone MH, Unwin A, Beacham B, et al: Incest in female borderlines: its frequency and impact. International Journal of Family Psychiatry 9:277–293, 1988

Torgersen S: Genetic and nosological aspects of schizotypal and borderline personality disorders: a twin study. Arch Gen Psychiatry 41:546–554, 1984

Valzelli L: Psychobiology of Aggression. New York, Raven, 1981

van der Kolk BA: The compulsion to repeat the trauma: attachment, reenactment, and masochism. Psychiatr Clin North Am 12:389–411, 1989

Zanarini MC, Gunderson JG, Marino MF, et al: Childhood experiences of borderline patients. Compr Psychiatry 30:18–25, 1989

Zarr ML: Psychobiology of the borderline disorders—a heuristic approach. Psychiatr Q 56:215–228, 1984

Zubin J: Chronic schizophrenia from the standpoint of vulnerability, in Perspectives in Schizophrenia Research. Edited by Baxter CF, Melnechuk T. New York, Raven, 1980, pp 269–294

A Behavioral Theory of Borderline Personality Disorder

Marsha M. Linehan, Ph.D.
Kelly Koerner, B.A.

B EHAVIORISTS HAVE HISTORICALLY PAID LITTLE ATTENTION to personality disorders in general and to borderline personality disorder (BPD) in particular. The limited attention to BPD by behaviorists is not surprising given the fact that the borderline construct itself was initially developed within the psychoanalytic community. More recently, behavioral and cognitive theories of BPD have emerged (Turner 1984, 1987). In the following chapter we will present Linehan's (1987a, 1987b, 1989) biosocial-behavioral theory of BPD. The biosocial-behavioral theory of BPD is based on transactional and learning models in its hypothesis that emotion regulation dysfunction is the primary underlying mechanism for the disorder. The theory proposes a model of the pathogenesis of the disorder, specifying how particular developmental environments influence and are influenced by the dysfunction of emotional dysregulation to produce a developmental course that leads to BPD. Further, the theory specifies the patterns of adult borderline behavior one would predict as sequelae of the interaction of emotion regulation dysfunction with certain developmental circumstances. Linehan's theory is the basis of her treatment method, *dialectical behavior therapy* (DBT), described in further detail in Chapter 14 (see also Linehan 1987b, 1989; Linehan and Wasson 1990; Linehan et al. 1989, 1991).

We begin with an overview of the assumptions inherent in the theory and then present the biosocial-behavioral theory of the core pathology of BPD and its pathogenesis. We then present the behavioral characteristics and dialectical dilemmas that are predicted from this hypothesis. We close with a summary and recommendations for future research.

BASIC ASSUMPTIONS

The basic assumptions inherent in Linehan's theory are dialectical. First, the theory implicitly assumes that psychological disorders are best conceptualized as systemic dysfunctions. Hollandsworth (1990) argues that rather than modeling psychological disorders after infectious disease, in which an identifiable pathogen is present, psychological disorders are better thought of as analogous to systemic disease or systemic dysfunction. Systemic dysfunction is characterized by 1) defining disorder with respect to normal functioning, 2) assuming continuity between health and disorder, and 3) assuming that disorder results from multiple rather than single causes.

Hollandsworth presents essential hypertension as a good example of systemic dysfunction:

> It is defined in terms of a deviation from normal rather than by the presence of some pathogen. Also there is a continuity between normal and high blood pressure so that the decision regarding diagnosis and treatment is often a matter of judgment rather than some absolute standard. And finally the development of essential hypertension appears to result from a number of factors, some inherited by the person and some found in his or her interaction with the environment. The "disease" aspect of hypertension comes into play when, as a result of this dysfunctional state, a cardiovascular crisis (e.g., stroke, heart failure) eventually occurs. (pp. 20–21)

Similarly, the theory assumes that BPD represents a breakdown in normal functioning and that this disorder is best conceptualized as a systemic dysfunction of the emotion regulation system. The biosocial theory proposes that the pathogenesis of BPD results from numerous factors, some inherited biological predispositions that create individual differences in susceptibility to emotion dysregulation, others resulting from the individual's interaction with the environment. Making the assumption of a systemic view has the advantage of compelling the theorist to integrate work from a variety of fields and disciplines.

A second assumption that underlies the biosocial theory presented here is that the relationship between the individual and the environment constitutes a process of reciprocal influence and that the outcome at any given moment is due to the transaction between the person and the environment.

A further assumption here, which comes from behavior genetics, is that people make their own environments (Scarr and McCartney 1983). Scarr and McCartney propose three effects through which genes influence what we experience: passive, reactive, and active genotypic effects. The *passive genotypic effect* is influential primarily during infancy and represents those gene-environment interactions that are independent of the individual—that is, those gene environment effects that are due solely to individuals' genetic makeup and to their parents in the sense that individuals do not determine their own genetic makeup or their own parental environment in the beginning. The second effect—the *reactive effect*—occurs when the genotype elicits particular responses from the social and physical environment. The example of cooperative and attentive preschoolers receiving more pleasant and instructional attention from adults than do uncooperative and easily distracted preschoolers is an example of a reactive genotypic effect. The third way that genes influence what we experience is by an *active genotypic effect,* which occurs when the individual seeks out environments that support his or her genetic potential. An example here is an individual with high genetic potential for athletics or for intellectual pursuits who seeks out these opportunities. From the perspective of a biosocial-behavioral theory, much of the pathogenesis of BPD represents exactly these sorts of genotypic influences on the environment, such that individuals who are predisposed to emotion regulation dysfunctions influence their environments in ways that make the full systemic dysfunction become apparent. A transactional, or *dialectical,* account of psychopathology may allow greater compassion because it is incompatible with the assignment of blame. This is particularly relevant with a label as stigmatizing among mental health professionals as "borderline" (Reiser and Levenson 1984).

CORE PATHOLOGY OF BORDERLINE PERSONALITY DISORDER: THE EMOTION DYSREGULATION HYPOTHESIS

A main tenet in Linehan's biosocial theory is that the core pathology in BPD is emotion dysregulation. Although affective instability, particularly the control and expression of anger, is an important defining characteristic of BPD in most diagnostic schemes (American Psychiatric Association 1987; Gunderson et al. 1981; Kernberg 1984), and although affective regulation has been related to mood disorder (Gunderson and Elliott 1985), Linehan's theory conceptualizes the relationship of emotion dysregulation to BPD as the primary dysfunction in the disorder rather than as simply symptomatic or definitional. The theory here is that individuals with BPD have emotion dysregulation across several, if not all, emotions. From our perspective, this systemic dysregulation is produced by emotional vulnerability and maladaptive and inadequate emotion regulation.

Emotional vulnerability is characterized by 1) high sensitivity to emotional stimuli, 2) intense response to emotional stimuli, and 3) slow return to baseline. Emotion regulation is the ability to a) inhibit inappropriate behavior related to strong negative or positive affect, b) self-soothe any physiological arousal that the strong affect has induced, c) refocus attention, and d) organize oneself for coordinated action in the service of an external goal (Gottman and Katz 1990, p. 373). Emotion dysregulation in BPD individuals, then, is a product of an oversensitive and overreactive emotional response system and an inadequate emotion regulation system—that is, the core pathology is a combination of emotion vulnerability and the inability to adequately regulate affect. The premise of excessive emotional vulnerability fits empirical descriptions of both parasuicidal and borderline populations. Individuals with histories of chronic parasuicide tend to react to emotional stimulation with extreme expressions of anger, hostility, irritability, depression, anxiety, and social discomfort (Linehan 1981). By definition, a wide spectrum of difficulties regulating emotion are part of the borderline syndrome, including emotional lability, problems with anger, fear of abandonment (related possibly to intense sadness and or emptiness consequent to loss), and boredom. Individuals who meet criteria for BPD often experience depressive disorders as well, including dysphoria, atypical depression, and major affective disorders

(MADs) (Barasch et al. 1985; Perry 1985; Plakun et al. 1985; Pope et al. 1983; Widiger and Frances 1989).

The mechanisms of this emotion dysregulation among individuals with BPD are unclear. Given the complexity of the emotion regulation system, there is no a priori reason to expect that the dysfunction will be due to a common factor in all borderline individuals. Biological contributions to emotion dysregulation may enter the causal pathway at any time in development, ranging from genetic influences to disadvantageous intrauterine events, to early childhood environmental effects on development of the brain and nervous system. As discussed by van Reekum et al. in Chapter 1, some empirical evidence suggests that difficulties in limbic system reactivity and attention control may contribute to emotion dysregulation in BPD (Cowdry et al. 1985; Gardner and Cowdry 1986; Snyder and Pitts 1984). Especially relevant here would be research linking BPD to temperamental characteristics already suspected to be related to emotion regulation difficulties. This type of prospective research would allow more sophisticated analyses of genotype-environment influences.

THE PATHOGENESIS OF EMOTION DYSREGULATION IN BORDERLINE PERSONALITY DISORDER

As mentioned above, the biosocial theory argues that the main pathology of BPD is emotion dysregulation and that this dysregulation is due to emotional vulnerability and inadequate emotion regulation. Emotion dysregulation represents a systemic dysfunction that results from the confluence of particular developmental circumstances, both genetic-biological and environmental, which in turn set the stage for later adult pathology. The development of emotion dysregulation can best be understood in terms of a dysfunction of normal emotion regulation.

Emotions are innate, hard-wired responses consisting of feeling-experiencing, cognitive, and motor components selected over the course of evolution as a result of their functional value. Emotions can be thought of as complex behavioral responses, as sensations of bodily change, as biology, and as cognition. In other words, emotions are often analyzed as different components or at different levels of analysis: the neurobiological component, the behavioral component, and the experiencing-feeling component. These divisions are based on conventions that are thought to be useful rather than on any certainty regarding the nature of emotion. In fact, it is well recognized by researchers of emotion that the different aspects of emotions—the behavioral, the cognitive-experiential, the somatic and visceral-physiological—are not perfectly or even highly correlated. For example, there is a growing body of research that suggests that affect and cognition are partially independent systems such that information can be encoded emotionally without conscious cognitive activity (Derryberry and Rothbart 1984).

Maccoby (1980) has argued that the inhibition of action is the basis for the organization of all behavior. The development of self-regulatory repertoires, especially the ability to inhibit and control affect, is one of the most important self-regulatory repertoires a child develops. The ability to regulate the experience of affect and control the expression of emotion is crucial because the failure to regulate and modulate strong emotion leads to the disruption of behavior, especially goal-directed and other prosocial behavior. Alternatively, strong emotion reorganizes or redirects behavior, preparing the individual for alternative actions that compete with the first nonemotional or less emotional behavioral repertoire.

Research on the development of emotion regulation indicates the importance of genotypic environmental influences. For example, Porges (1984) has suggested that there is a physiological basis for the development of emotion regulation ability related to the activation of the parasympathetic branch of the autonomic nervous system. There is also some evidence to suggest that individuals with reactive physiologies tend to prefer passive stimulus regulation strategies (Eliasz 1985). These sorts of findings highlight the importance of continued investigation of genotypic influences on the environment. The nature of emotional responding activates all response systems (cognitive, physiological, expressive, and phenomenological), and it is this whole response system that is difficult to regulate. Emotional arousal and mood states affect diverse phenomena such as concepts of self, self attributions, perceptions of control, learning and performance on various tasks, patterns of self-reward, and delay of gratification (Izard et al. 1984). Therefore, difficulties regulating emotion affect functioning across a wide range of areas. It is exactly this sort of disruption across response systems under conditions of high arousal that one sees in patients with BPD.

BEHAVIORAL CHARACTERISTICS OF PATIENTS WITH BORDERLINE PERSONALITY DISORDER

Reviews of the research on the effects of emotional states on various cognitive processes (Bower 1981; Gilligan and Bower 1984) indicate that emotional states selectively bias recall of affectively toned material, enhance the learning of mood-congruent material, and can bias interpretation, fantasies, projections, free associations, personal forecasts, and social judgments so that they are congruent with current mood. Intense negative affect also seems to interfere with learning. Additionally, there is evidence that increasing emotional arousal is associated with increasingly narrowed attention such that emotion-relevant stimuli become more salient and more attention is given to them (Bahrick et al. 1952; Bursill 1958; Callaway and Stone 1960; Cornsweet 1969; Easterbrook 1959; McNamara and Fisch 1964). This restricted attention, or cognitive rigidity, is a preoccupation with mood-congruent material during emotional reactivity. Other forms of altered attentional and cognitive processes, such as dissociation and brief psychotic symptoms, may be more extreme, "automatic" strategies for regulating emotion.

Impulsive behavior, and especially parasuicide, can also be thought of as maladaptive but highly effective emotion regulation strategies. For example, overdosing usually leads to long periods of sleep, which in turn reduces one's susceptibility to emotion dysregulation. Although the mechanism by which self-mutilation exerts affect-regulating properties is unknown, it is very common for borderline patients to report substantial relief from anxiety and other intense, negative affective states following such acts. Suicidal behavior is also very effective in eliciting helping behaviors from the environment, help which may be effective in avoiding or changing situations that elicit emotional pain. For example, suicidal behavior is generally the most effective way for a nonpsychotic individual to be admitted on an inpatient psychiatric unit.

The inability to consistently regulate arousal of emotions also interferes with the development and maintenance of a sense of self. Generally, one's sense of self is formed by one's own observations of oneself and observation of others' reactions to one's actions. Emotional consistency and predictability, across time and similar situations, are prerequisites of identity development. Unpredictable emotional lability leads to unpredictable behavior and cognitive inconsistency and, consequently, interferes with identity development. The tendency of borderline individuals to inhibit or attempt to inhibit emotional responses may also contribute to an absence of a strong sense of identity. The numbness associated with inhibited affect is often experienced as emptiness, further contributing to an inadequate, and at times completely absent, sense of self. Similarly, if an individual's sense of events is never "correct" or is unpredictably "correct"—the situation in an invalidating environment—then one would expect the individual to develop an overdependence on others.

Effective interpersonal relationships depend on both a stable sense of self and a capacity for spontaneity in emotional expression. Successful relationships also require a capacity to self-regulate emotions in appropriate ways and to tolerate some emotionally painful stimuli. Emotion regulation difficulties interfere with a stable sense of self and with normal emotional expression. Without such capabilities, it is understandable that individuals with BPD develop chaotic relationships. These individuals have difficulty controlling impulsive behaviors and expressions of extreme negative emotions, which often wreaks havoc on their relationships. Difficulties with anger and anger expression preclude the maintenance of stable relationships. The inability to control affect expression contributes in many ways to chaotic interpersonal relationships.

THE ROLE OF THE INVALIDATING ENVIRONMENT IN EMOTION DYSREGULATION

The emotion dysregulation proposed here as the core pathology of BPD is a joint outcome of temperamental emotional vulnerability and certain developmental circumstances. The crucial developmental circumstance is the *invalidating environment,* by which Linehan (1987b, 1989) means those aspects of the social and physical environment that are particularly likely to generate and exacerbate emotional vulnerability and difficulties regulating emotions.

A defining characteristic of the invalidating environment is the tendency of the family to respond erratically and inappropriately to private experience and, in particular, to be insensitive (i.e., nonresponsive) to private experience that does not have public accompaniments. These families also tend to respond extremely (i.e., over- or underrespond) to private experience that does have public accompaniments. Phenomenological, physiological, and cognitive components of emotions are prototypic private experiences that lead to invalidation in these families. Here again it is important to define disorder with respect to more normal functioning. To understand the invalidating environment's contribution to BPD, one can contrast it to environments that foster more adaptive emotion regulation skills.

For example, in more optimal environments, public validation of private experience is important because successful communication of one's private experience is followed by changes in other people's behavior that increase the probability that one's needs will be met and that decrease the probability of negative consequences. Parental responding that is attuned and nonaversive results in children who are better able to discriminate their own and others' emotions. Invalidating environments are problematic because people in the social environment respond to the communication of emotions with abnormal responses, specifically with either nonresponsiveness or more extreme consequences than in more normal, validating social environments. This leads to an intensification of the differences between the individual's private experience and the experience the social environment actually supports and responds to. Persistent discrepancies between private experience and what others in one's environment describe as one's experience provide the fundamental learning environment necessary for many of the behavioral problems associated with BPD.

In addition to early failures to respond optimally, those families that provide invalidating environments more generally emphasize controlling emotional expressiveness and especially disapprove of the expression of negative affect. Painful experiences are trivialized and attributed to negative traits such as lack of motivation, lack of discipline, and failure to adopt a positive attitude. Other characteristics of the invalidating environment include restricting the demands the child may make upon the environment. Also, individuals in an invalidating environment tend to use punishment (from criticism to abuse) to control behavior.

Invalidating environments contribute to emotion dysregulation by 1) failing to teach the child to label and modulate arousal, 2) failing to teach the child to tolerate distress, 3) failing to teach the child to trust his or her own emotional responses as valid interpretations of events, and 4) actively teaching the child to invalidate his or her own experiences by making it necessary for the child to scan the environment for cues about how to act and feel. By oversimplifying the ease of solving life's problems, the child fails to learn to form realistic goals. By punishing the expression of negative emotion and responding erratically to emotional communication only after escalation by the child, the family shapes an emotional expression style that vacillates between extreme inhibition and suppression of emotional experience and extreme emotion styles, as the family's usual response cuts off the communicative function of emotion to elicit helping responses.

Such parental responding probably differentially affects different children. The emotion control strategies used in these families may have little negative impact or may even be useful to some children who are physiologically well equipped to regulate their emotions. One example here is the different effects parental strategies have on one child who has attention-deficit disorder versus another who does not. If a parent comes into a room where the two children are playing around with each other rather than doing their homework, the parent might tell the children to pay attention and get to work or else lose future play time. This may be sufficient to allow the child without attention-deficit disorder to regulate his or her behavior and get to the homework. However, for the child with attention-deficit disorder, parental admonishment alone will be insufficient because the child lacks the ability to comply.

One of the most traumatic invalidating experiences is childhood sexual abuse. This is particularly relevant to BPD, given the research reporting high prevalence of sexual abuse in this population. Reported prevalence rates of childhood sexual abuse (incest and other forms of child sexual abuse, including exposure to genitals, fondling, and penetration) among BPD patients range from 37% to 86% (Briere and Zaidi 1989; Bryer et al. 1987; Herman et al. 1989). Histories of childhood sexual abuse seem to distinguish BPD clients from other outpatient diagnostic groups (Herman et al. 1989; Westen et al. 1990; Zanarini et al. 1989). This research strongly indicates that childhood sexual abuse is an important factor in the development of BPD. It is unclear, however, whether the abuse in and of itself facilitates the development of BPD or whether the abuse and the development of BPD both result from the extent of the familial dysfunction and invalidation. In other words, the history of victimization and the emotion regulation problems seen in BPD patients may both arise from the same set of developmental circumstances. Nevertheless, the high incidence of sexual abuse in BPD patients points to the possibility that this is a distinguishing precursor to the disorder.

There is some research and clinical evidence that parasuicide may be a particular coping response developed among survivors of childhood sexual abuse (Briere 1989; Briere and Runtz 1986; Herman and Hirschman 1981). Clinically, there are many examples of the functional value that self-harm and parasuicide have had in these patients' lives. For example, one client in our clinic made her first suicide attempt after her attempts to tell school counselors, the Child Protection Service, and even a court-appointed psychologist failed to stop her stepfather's sexual abuse of her. Her suicide attempt finally did stop the abuse: she was hospitalized. Another client in our clinic found that the care she received at the hospital was the only source of care she received as a child, and describes getting to go to the doctor as a major reinforcer in her family.

THE PHENOMENOLOGICAL EXPERIENCE OF BORDERLINE PERSONALITY DISORDER: DIALECTICAL DILEMMAS

The interplay between an emotionally vulnerable temperament on the one hand, and a developmental environment characterized by emotional invalidation on the other, should have a number of interesting theoretical consequences for adult BPD behavior patterns. Linehan (1987b), on the basis of clinical observations, has proposed three bipolar dimensions, representing dialectical dilemmas, that characterize the behavior of BPD patients in therapy. According to Linehan's theory, BPD patients oscillate along each dimension, usually alternating between the extremes at each pole.

Emotional Vulnerability Versus Self-Invalidation

Emotional vulnerability, as discussed earlier, refers to high sensitivity to emotional stimuli, intense responses to even low-level stimuli, the inability to consistently regulate emotional responses, and a slow return to emotional baseline. High emotional vulnerability has two important consequences: intensely painful feelings and equally intense experiences of helplessness and being out of control. In some senses, emotional vulnerability can be thought of as the psychological equivalent of third-degree burns; even the slightest touch or movement can create immense suffering. The inability to consistently regulate emotional arousal leads to disruptions across entire behavioral repertoires. The subsequent subjective experience of being unable to regulate one's emotions and behavior despite one's best efforts creates the sense of being out of control and involves intense feelings of frustration and disillusionment with oneself.

Borderline individuals learn to respond to their own emotional experiences as their environments have modeled, that is, with shame, criticism, and punishment. Invalidation of one's own emotions (i.e., *self-invalidation*) leads to attempts to inhibit both the experience and the expression of emotion. Doubting and criticizing one's own perceptions prohibits developing a sense of identity or confidence in one's self. Oversimplification of life's difficulties leads inevitably to self-hate following failure to achieve goals.

Therefore, the dilemma for patients is that they vacillate between these two poles. At one pole they adopt an emotionally invalidating attitude toward themselves, thereby oversimplifying the ease of achieving behavioral and emotional regulation. The inevitable failure associated with such excessive aspirations is met with shame, extreme self-criticism, and self-punishment, including parasuicide and suicide. At the other pole, borderline individuals at times are keenly aware of their emotional and behavioral lack of control. Recognition of the discrepancy between their own capacities for emotional and behavioral control and excessive demands and criticism by themselves and from the environment can lead to anger and attempts to prove to significant others the error of their ways.

Active Passivity Versus Apparent Competence

Active passivity refers to a tendency to approach problems passively and helplessly as well as a corresponding tendency under extreme distress to demand from the environment solutions to life's problems. Active passivity is similar to Lazarus and Folkman's (1984) emotion-focused coping.

This style of coping consists of efforts to reduce negative emotional reactions to stress, for example, by distracting or seeking comfort from others. This is in contrast to problem-focused coping, in which the individual takes action directly to solve the problem. The tendency to actively seek help from the environment, combined with an absence of active problem solving, defines the active passivity pattern. The attempt to elicit or expect help from the environment differentiates active passivity from learned helplessness. This type of passive self-regulation style probably results from both temperamental disposition and the individual's history of failed attempts to independently control emotional arousal and associated maladaptive behaviors. Interesting research by Eliasz (1974) suggests that people with high autonomic reactivity, independent of other considerations, will prefer passive self-regulation styles, i.e., those that involve minimal active efforts to improve one's own abilities and one's environment.

Active passivity is associated with *apparent competence*. Apparent competence refers to the tendency to appear competent, in control emotionally, and able to cope with everyday life at some times, and at other times to unexpectedly behave as if the observed competencies did not exist. Two factors can account for the discrepancy. First, a consequence of emotion dysregulation is that cognitive, emotional, and behavioral competencies become extremely variable. The variability is due to variability in emotional arousal, but the observed effect is that competencies one would ordinarily expect to generalize across apparently similar situations do not generalize. This failure to generalize may be a function of both mood-dependent learning and situation-specific learning, both of which may be particularly influential in BPD clients.

A second factor, one that is due to the influence of invalidating environments, is that individuals with BPD may also learn communication styles that foster the perception of apparent competence. Frequently, borderline individuals communicate in a manner that appears competent and in control and that fails to communicate actual vulnerability to others. This may be a function of having learned to suppress emotional expression, resulting in communications that convey distress verbally but in which nonverbal cues do not support such a message. The effect is that inner emotional chaos is experienced but not expressed, a hypothesis in line with a finding recently reported by Edell et al. (1990).

The dilemma for individuals with BPD is that, on the one hand, they have tremendous difficulties regulating their emotions and subsequent behavioral competence. They frequently but unpredictably need a great deal of assistance. Without the ability to predict and control their own well-being, they depend on the social environment to regulate affect and behavior. On the other hand, they experience intense shame at behaving dependently, especially given our society's intolerance of dependency, and have learned to inhibit expressions of negative affect and helplessness whenever they can. Observing the unpredictability and tenuousness of one's competence may lead to the experience of intense guilt about presumed lack of motivation when one falls short of objectives. At other times, this can lead to the experience of extreme anger at others for their lack of understanding and unrealistic expectations. For the apparently competent person, suicidal behavior is sometimes the only means to communicate to others that one really cannot cope and needs help. Suicidal behavior also may change others' unrealistic expectations and in some way "prove" to them that one really cannot do what is expected.

Unrelenting Crisis Versus Inhibited Grieving

Many individuals who meet the criteria for BPD are in a state of perpetual, *unrelenting crisis*. This state of chronic, unrelenting crisis is debilitating not necessarily because of the magnitude of any one stressful event but rather because of the individual's high reactivity as well as the chronic nature of the stressful events. For example, the simultaneous loss of job, spouse, children, and concomitant serious illness would theoretically be easier to cope with than the same set of events experienced sequentially. Repetitive stressful events coupled with an inability to ever recover fully from any one stressful event result in, as Berent (1981) suggests, a "weakening of the spirit" and subsequent suicidal or other "emergency" behaviors. In a sense, the patient never returns to an emotional baseline before the next blow hits.

The inability to return to baseline may be a result of several factors. Many borderline individuals both create and are controlled by aversive environments. Temperamental factors exacerbate the individual's initial emotional response and rate of return to baseline after each stressor. An inability to tolerate or reduce short-term stress without emitting dysfunctional escape behaviors brings about further stressors. Inadequate interpersonal skills create interpersonal stress and preclude solving many of life's problems. Equally inadequate social support networks may contribute to the inability to control negative environmental events. In turn, an absence of positive, supportive individuals in the environment further weakens the ability to develop needed capabilities. Seemingly incomprehensible overreactions to apparently minor events such as criticism become understandable when viewed against the backdrop of the unrelenting nature of the chronic crises experienced by these patients.

The corresponding countertendency here is to avoid or inhibit the experience or expression of extreme, painful emotional reactions. The result is *inhibited grieving* and a pattern of repetitive, significant trauma and loss, together with an inability to fully experience and personally integrate or resolve these events. Crises of any type entail loss—whether of a job or a relationship; psychological loss of ever having nurturing parents; or loss of interpersonal acceptance. We can only stay with very painful emotions if we are confident that someday, sometime, they will end. It is not uncommon to hear borderline patients say they feel that if they ever do cry they will never stop. Indeed, their experience is that of being unable to consistently control, modulate, or titrate their own emotional experience. This avoidance of feeling painful emotions leads to the avoidance of cues associated with painful emotions.

The dilemma for the patient is that the inhibition of grief reactions and the consequent avoidance of exposure to cues are extraordinarily difficult when at the same time one is in a perpetual state of crisis. Although inhibition of affective responses associated with grief may be effective in the short term, it does not in the long term facilitate social support for one's crises, nor does it lead to successful "working through" of grief. Indeed, the escape behaviors associated with inhibited grieving (impulsive behaviors such as drinking, driving fast, spending money, having unprotected sex, and leaving situations) are often instrumental in creating new crises.

SUMMARY AND FUTURE DIRECTIONS

Linehan has proposed a biosocial-behavioral theory of the development of BPD. The theory, which is based on a set of dialectical philosophical assumptions, proposes that BPD is an outcome of temperamental factors in transaction with an invalidating developmental environment. The resulting disorder is, at core, a dysfunction of the emotion regulation system. Although the ideas presented in this chapter are extensions of basic psychological research that seem to fit the available data on BPD, there is not yet a body of prospective empirical evidence to support the particular hypotheses put forward here. Nevertheless, there are at least three reasons that Linehan's theory should be given consideration. First, it has been heuristic in developing one of the few empirically supported treatments of BPD (Linehan 1987a, 1989; Linehan et al. 1991). Second, it fosters integration between biological and psychological variables and may foster integration across a variety of knowledge domains in psychology. Third, its propositions are testable for the most part and therefore should generate empirical research by both proponents and opponents of the theory.

Two lines of research are needed to support Linehan's theory. First, a body of programmatic research is needed to demonstrate the pervasiveness and parameters of emotional vulnerability and emotion dysregulation among individuals meeting criteria for BPD. In particular, temperamental mapping, using well-regarded measures and methodologies, is essential. Second, longitudinal research is needed to demonstrate the relationship of invalidating environments to the development of BPD. Although cross-sectional designs at the adult level might have some use, the fallibility of retrospective reports makes such approaches tenuous at best. The notion of dialectical dilemmas, proposed by Linehan, has not yet been subjected to prospective empirical testing. Such research is needed if the theory is to be developed and modified further.

REFERENCES

American Psychiatric Association: Diagnostic and Statistical Manual of Mental Disorders, 3rd Edition, Revised. Washington, DC, American Psychiatric Association, 1987

Bahrick HP, Fitts PM, Rankin RE: Effect of incentives upon reactions to peripheral stimuli. Journal of Experimental Psychology 44:400–406, 1952

Barasch A, Frances A, Hurt S, et al: Stability and distinctness of borderline personality disorder. Am J Psychiatry 142:1484–1486, 1985

Berent I: The Algebra of Suicide. New York, Human Sciences Press, 1981

Bower GH: Mood and memory. Am Psychol 36:129–148, 1981

Briere J: Therapy for Adults Molested as Children. New York, Springer, 1989

Briere J, Runtz M: Suicidal thoughts and behaviors in former sexual abuse victims. Canadian Journal of Behavioral Sciences 18:413–423, 1986

Briere J, Zaidi LY: Sexual abuse histories and sequelae in female psychiatric emergency room patients. Am J Psychiatry 146:1602–1606, 1989

Bryer JB, Nelson BA, Miller JB, et al: Childhood sexual and physical abuse as factors in adult psychiatric illness. Am J Psychiatry 144:1426–1430, 1987

Bursill AE: The restriction of peripheral vision during exposure to hot and humid conditions. Quarterly Journal of Experimental Psychology 10:123–129, 1958

Callaway E, Stone G: Re-evaluating the focus of attention, in Drugs and Behavior. Edited by Uhr L, Miller JG. New York, Wiley, 1960

Cornsweet DJ: Use of cues in the visual periphery under conditions of arousal. Journal of Experimental Psychology 80:14–18, 1969

Cowdry RW, Pickar D, Davies R: Symptoms and EEG findings in the borderline syndrome. Int J Psychiatry Med 15:201–211, 1985

Derryberry D, Rothbart M: Emotion, attention, and temperament, in Emotions, Cognition and Behavior. Edited by Izard CE, Kagan J, Zajonc RB. Cambridge, UK, Cambridge University Press, 1984, pp 132–166

Easterbrook JA: The effect of emotion on cue utilization and the organization of behavior. Psychol Rev 66:183–201, 1959

Edell WS, Joy SB, Yehuda R: Discordance between self-report and observer-rated psychopathology in borderline patients. Journal of Personality Disorders 4:381–390, 1990

Eliasz A: Temperament a osobowosc. Wroclaw-Warsaw: Ossolineum, 1974

Eliasz A: Mechanisms of temperament: basic functions, in The Biological Bases of Personality and Behavior: Theories, Measurement Techniques, and Development. Edited by Strelau J, Farley FH, Gale A. Washington, DC, Hemisphere, 1985, pp 45–49

Gardner DL, Cowdry RW: Positive effects of carbamazepine on behavioral dyscontrol in borderline personality disorder. J Pers Soc Psychol 143:519–522, 1986

Gilligan SG, Bower GH: Cognitive consequences of emotional arousal, in Emotions, Cognition, and Behavior. Edited by Izard CE, Kagan J, Zajonc RB. Cambridge, UK, Cambridge University Press, 1984, pp 547–588

Gottman JM, Katz LF: Effects of marital discord on young children's peer interaction and health. Developmental Psychology 25:373–381, 1990

Gunderson JG, Elliott GR: The interface between borderline personality disorder and affective disorder. J Pers Soc Psychol 142:277–288, 1985

Gunderson JG, Kolb JE, Austin V: The diagnostic interview for borderline patients. Am J Psychiatry 138:896–903, 1981

Herman J, Hirschman L: Families at risk for father-daughter incest. Am J Psychiatry 138:967–970, 1981

Herman JL, Perry JC, van der Kolk BA: Childhood trauma in borderline personality disorder. Am J Psychiatry 146:490–495, 1989

Hollandsworth JG Jr: The Physiology of Psychological Disorders. New York, Plenum, 1990

Izard CE, Kagan J, Zajonc RB (eds): Emotions, Cognition, and Behavior. Cambridge, UK, Cambridge University Press, 1984

Kernberg OF: Severe Personality Disorders: Psychotherapeutic Strategies. New Haven, CT, Yale University Press, 1984

Lazarus RS, Folkman S: Stress, Coping, and Adaptation. New York, Springer, 1984

Linehan MM: A social-behavior analysis of suicide and parasuicide: implications for clinical assessment and treatment, in Depression: Behavioral and Directive Intervention Strategies. Edited by Clarkin JF, Glazer HI. New York, Garland STPM Press, 1981, pp 229–294

Linehan MM: Dialectical behavior therapy: a cognitive behavioral approach to parasuicide. Journal of Personality Disorders 1:328–333, 1987a

Linehan MM: Dialectical behavior therapy for borderline personality disorder: theory and method. Bull Menninger Clin 51:261–276, 1987b

Linehan MM: Cognitive and behavior therapy for borderline personality disorder, in American Psychiatric Press Review of Psychiatry. Edited by Tasman A, Hales RE, Frances AJ. Washington, DC, American Psychiatric Press, 1989, pp 84–102

Linehan MM, Armstrong HE, Suarez A, et al: Cognitive-behavioral treatment of chronically parasuicidal borderline patients. Arch Gen Psychiatry 48:1060–1064, 1991

Linehan MM, Wasson EJ: Behavior therapy, in Comparative Handbook of Treatment for Adult Disorders. Edited by Hersen M, Bellack A. New York, Wiley, 1990, pp 420–435

Linehan MM, Miller ML, Addis ME: Dialectical behavior therapy for borderline personality disorder: practical guidelines, in Innovations in Clinical Practice: A Source Book. Edited by Keller PA, Heyman SR. Sarasota, FL, Professional Resource Exchange, 1989, pp 43–54

Maccoby EE: Social Development. New York, Harcourt, Brace, and Jovanovich, 1980

McNamara H, Fisch R: Effect of high and low motivation on two aspects of attention. Percept Mot Skills 19:571–578, 1964

Perry JC: Depression in borderline personality disorder: lifetime prevalence at interview and longitudinal course of symptoms. Am J Psychiatry 142:15–21, 1985

Plakun E, Burkhardt P, Muller J: Fourteen-year follow-up of borderline and schizotypal personality disorders. Compr Psychiatry 26:448–455, 1985

Pope HG Jr, Jonas JM, Hudson JI, et al: The validity of DSM-III borderline personality disorder: a phenomenologic, family history, treatment response, and long-term follow-up study. Arch Gen Psychiatry 40:23–30, 1983

Porges SW: Heart rate oscillation: an index of neural mediation, in Psychophysiological Perspectives: Festschrift for Beatrice and John Lacey. Edited by Coles GH, Jennings JR, Stern JA. New York, Van Nostrand Reinhold, 1984, pp 229–241

Reiser DE, Levenson H: Abuses of the borderline diagnosis: a clinical problem with teaching opportunities. Am J Psychiatry 141:1528–1532, 1984

Scarr S, McCartney K: How people make their own environments: a theory of genotype-environmental effects. Child Dev 54:424–435, 1983

Snyder S, Pitts WM Jr : Electroencephalography of DSM-III borderline personality disorder. Acta Psychiatr Scand 69:129–134, 1984

Turner RM: Assessment and treatment of borderline personality disorder. Paper presented at the 18th meeting of the Association for the Advancement of Behavior Therapy, Philadelphia, PA, November 1984

Turner RM: A bio-social learning approach to borderline personality disorder. Paper presented at the Association for the Advancement of Behavior Therapy. Boston, MA, 1987

Westen D, Ludolph P, Misle B, et al: Physical and sexual abuse in adolescent girls with borderline personality disorder. Am J Orthopsychiatry 60:55–66, 1990

Widiger TA, Frances AJ: Epidemiology, diagnosis, and comorbidity of borderline personality disorder, in American Psychiatric Press Review of Psychiatry. Edited by Tasman A, Hales RE, Frances AJ. Washington, DC, American Psychiatric Press, 1989, pp 8–24

Zanarini MC, Gunderson JG, Marino MF, et al: Childhood experiences of borderline patients. Compr Psychiatry 30:18–25, 1989

Trauma and Defense in the Etiology of Borderline Personality Disorder

J. Christopher Perry, M.D., M.P.H.
Judith L. Herman, M.D.

W HEN ADOLPH STERN (1938) FIRST DESCRIBED THE "borderline group of neuroses" he offered his observations about the etiologic factors to which these patients were exposed as children. He noted that the following factors were present in at least three-quarters of cases, operating "more or less constantly over many years from earliest childhood . . . not single experiences": lack of spontaneous maternal affection; many parental quarrels, including temper outbursts directed at the child, early divorce and separation, or desertion; and actual cruelty, neglect, and brutality by the parents of many years duration.

Because the subsequent literature on borderline personality disorder (BPD) focused largely on diagnostic confusion and difficulties in the treatment, it lost touch with the import of Stern's initial observations. However, recent empirical studies have taken up where Stern left off, validating his observations and thereby yielding a quantum leap in understanding the etiology of BPD. In this chapter we review the evidence for the role of childhood trauma in the genesis of BPD and for the function of certain learned defense mechanisms in maintaining borderline psychopathology. Our conclusion is that, while multiple etiologic factors clearly operate, childhood trauma is the most significant known contributor in the majority of cases.

Clinicians and researchers vary somewhat in their views of what constitutes trauma. The narrow view encompasses gross or objective trauma, consisting of those events that would be expected to have traumatic consequences for anyone. This includes gross physical abuse resulting in bodily injury and fear of death, dismemberment, or severe pain; sexual abuse, including incest and rape, nonconsensual fondling, or other physical sexual contact; and witnessing violence resulting in physical injury or the reasonable expectation of injury to others. A broader definition of trauma includes events that are traumatic partially because of subjective traumatic meaning, that is, the conscious or unconscious meaning that the events have for the individual. This might include death of a loved one, witnessing parental sexual behavior (primal scene), or being inadvertently hurt in an accident caused by a parent. This review generally follows the narrow definition, that of gross trauma, that has been employed in a number of research studies.

The lifetime population prevalence of childhood trauma has been estimated by several authors. Finkelhor (1984) estimated that a history of incest can be found in approximately 5% of women in the United States. Russell (1986) found that 16% of women surveyed reported some history of incest. Furthermore, the incidence of sexual abuse is thought to be much higher than that of incest alone. While boys and girls are believed to be at equal risk for physical abuse, girls are at two to three times greater risk for sexual abuse, and sexual abuse may be more prevalent and occur over a more prolonged period of time than physical abuse (Pagelow 1984). The gender differences in sexual abuse find a parallel in the gender ratio of BPD. Although the population prevalence of BPD is unknown, it is unlikely to be as high as 5% to 16% of the female population, underlining that BPD is not a necessary consequence of trauma and that other etiologic factors may also operate. However, we believe the high prevalence of childhood trauma in BPD has important treatment implications that link the therapeutic process directly to etiologic factors (Perry et al. 1990; van der Kolk 1989).

EMPIRICAL RESEARCH ON TRAUMA AND BORDERLINE PERSONALITY DISORDER: A REVIEW

The studies on trauma and BPD are reviewed below in order of their appearance in the literature. Table 6–1 displays a summary of the childhood prevalence of physical and sexual abuse from each study. Comparison of the figures must be carried out with caution, given that each study used different definitions and different methods of ascertainment of diagnosis and childhood trauma. Also, some studies conditioned their samples on diagnoses, whereas others conditioned on abuse histories, yielding figures with different interpretations.

Bryer et al. (1987) examined consecutive female inpatients by ques-

Table 6–1. Summary of studies of the childhood prevalence of physical and sexual abuse

Study	Sample	Methods	Physical abuse	Sexual abuse
More rigorous				
Herman et al. (1989)	55 subjects; naturalistic follow-up	Blind systematic interviews	BPD: 71% non-BPD: 39%	BPD: 67% non-BPD: 26%
Zanarini et al. (1989)	50 BPD, 29 ASP, 26 other PD, outpatients	Blind systematic interviews	BPD: 46% ASP: 28% Other PD: 35%	BPD: 26% ASP: 7% Other PD: 4%
Ogata et al. (1990)	Adult inpatient: 24 BPD, 18 depression	Blind systematic interviews	BPD: 42% Depressed: 33%	BPD: 71% Depressed: 22%
Less rigorous				
Bryer et al. (1987)	66 female inpatients	Questionnaire		BPD: 86%
Briere and Zaidi (1989)	50 women: 35 sexually abused, 15 not	Chart review: sex abuse data systematic		Abused v. nonabused: 37% v. 7% given diagnosis of BPD
Goodwin et al. (1990)	20 women, hospitalized, incest histories	Questionnaires, chart reviews, treatment	All patients reported physical abuse	Among abused, 95% had BPD
Ludolph et al. (1990)	Adolescent girls, inpatients: 27 BPD, 23 non-BPD	Diagnostic interview, chart reviews	BPD: 52% Non-BPD: 26%	BPD: 52% Non-BPD: 19%
Swett et al. (1990)	125 adult male outpatients	Questionnaires; contact with therapist: $n = 34$		16 abused v. 18 nonabused: BPD: 25% v. 6%
Stone (1990)	181 borderline, 104 other former female inpatients	Retrospective chart review, clinicians' recollections	Parental brutality: BPD: 11% Others: 14%	Incest only: BPD: 19% Others: 14%

Note. BDP = borderline personality disorder; ASP = antisocial personality disorder; PD = personality disorders (other than BPD).

tionnaire and other self-report instruments. Fifty-nine percent experienced abuse before age 16: specifically 21% sexual abuse only, 15% physical abuse only, and 23% both types of early abuse. Fifty-eight percent of the women also reported abuse occurring after age 16. Of the 29 women reporting early sexual abuse, 52% also reported later sexual abuse, while of the 25 women reporting early physical abuse, 80% also reported later physical abuse. Family members were the perpetrators in 52% of the cases reporting early sexual abuse, with fathers and brothers mentioned most often. Of those women reporting early physical abuse, the perpetrators most often reported were (in descending order) fathers, siblings, and mothers. On the SCL-90-R (Derogatis 1983), women reporting both early sexual and physical abuse generally scored higher than those reporting either type of abuse alone, who in turn scored higher than women without abuse histories. These findings were based on scales reflecting global severity, psychoticism, anxiety, phobic anxiety, paranoid ideology, interpersonal sensitivity, depression, and somatization. On the Millon Clinical Multiaxial Inventory (MCMI) (Millon 1983), a self-report measure of Axis II and other pathology, sexual abuse and combined sexual and physical abuse were strongly associated with the borderline personality scale ($P = .002$); trends were evident for the passive-aggressive scale, and there was a negative trend for the compulsive personality scale. Of 14 patients given chart diagnoses of BPD, 12 (86%) had experienced early sexual abuse, with or without physical abuse ($P = .009$).

Herman et al. (1989) interviewed a sample of individuals with personality and/or affective disorders participating in a prospective, naturalistic, longitudinal study. Histories of childhood trauma were obtained by direct interview in which the interviewers were blind to initial diagnostic and other data. Fifty-three percent of the subjects were female. Of 21 definite BPD subjects, 81% gave a history of significant childhood trauma, including physical abuse (71%), sexual abuse (67%), and witnessing domestic violence (62%). Any form of abuse was less common among those subjects with borderline traits (73%) and least common among nonborderline subjects (52%). When quantitative assessment about the number of perpetrators and the duration of trauma was analyzed, the differences were even more pronounced. The cumulative score of childhood trauma was significantly correlated with borderline pathology ($r = .53$, $P < .001$) but not antisocial or schizotypal pathology. The occurrence of trauma especially before age 6 was found significantly more often in BPD than in non-BPD subjects (57% v. 13%, $P < .001$). While BPD patients generally scored higher on the Dissociative Experiences Scale (Bernstein and Putnam 1986), a measure of dissociative symptoms, cumulative childhood trauma scores predicted dissociation scores even after controlling for BPD pathology. This suggests that dissociation has an ongoing functional role in BPD, apart from sharing traumatic origins with BPD.

Zanarini et al. (1989) studied a group of outpatients with either borderline, antisocial, or other personality disorders with dysthymia. Childhood histories were obtained independently of diagnostic data. Eighty percent of BPD subjects reported some type of abuse, compared with 38% of the antisocial subjects and 50% of the subjects with other personality disorders. BPD patients reported significantly more verbal abuse (72%) and sexual abuse (26%) than did patients with the other disorders and reported (nonsignificantly) more physical abuse. Abuse was found in early childhood in 60% of BPD patients, compared with 21% to 31% of patients with the other diagnoses, and remained significantly higher throughout latency and adolescence. The authors also examined histories of physical and emotional neglect, and separations from caretakers of more than 1 month. The incidence of any form of neglect was higher in BPD patients (76%) than in antisocial patients (47%), but not compared to patients with other personality disorders (77%). Among subjects with BPD, emotional withdrawal (56%) and inconsistency (48%) were more prevalent than physical neglect (24%). Significant periods of separation from caretakers were found in BPD patients in 46% to 58% of cases over early, middle, and late childhood; however, other diagnoses obtained similar figures with the exception that patients with other personality disorders reported fewer separations during early childhood (19%). The authors concluded that their findings underscored the importance of abuse in the etiology of BPD, while giving minor support for the role of neglect, and even less for the role of separations. Nevertheless, many BPD subjects underwent all three forms of childhood adverse experiences, suggesting that the effects may be additive.

Briere and Zaidi (1989) conducted a chart review study of female patients seen by clinicians in a psychiatric emergency room. Among the first 50 subjects, the chart revealed a history of sexual abuse in 6% of cases. The next 50 subjects were specifically interviewed about histories of sexual abuse, yielding positive responses in 70% of cases. This highly significant difference underscores the serious possibility of underreporting of sexual abuse unless systematic efforts are made to obtain information. When the authors examined chart diagnoses they found that a diagnosis of any personality disorder was given more often in the sexually abused (63%) than in the nonabused (20%) women, most particularly in the case of BPD (37% v. 7%, $P < .03$). The sexually abused women also showed evidence reported in the chart for current or past suicidal ideation (77%), history of suicide attempts (66%), drug use (57%), sexual problems or inappropriateness (31%), trends toward self-mutilation (17%), and legal problems (17%). Among the sexually abused women, BPD subjects reported a significantly greater number of perpetrators ($P = .44$). Women with the greatest severity and number of perpetrators also tended to be given a greater number of psychiatric diagnoses. The authors noted that the lack of systematic procedures for making diagnoses and obtaining other data affected the interpretation of their findings.

Goodwin et al. (1990) reported a sample of female incest survivors with recent hospitalizations. Data was gathered from questionnaires, chart review, and ongoing treatment. In this sample, 95% of the women had been diagnosed with BPD, while 90% had mood disorders, and all had one or more major dissociative symptoms. Sequelae of posttraumatic stress disorder were found in all subjects and included nightmares and pronounced startle reactions, as well as flashbacks to abusive events accompanied by hearing the perpetrator's voice (60%). Multiple symptoms and syndromes were prevalent, including eating disorders (75%), antisocial behavior toward children (40%), alcohol and other substance abuse (80%), and somatization (95%). All 20 patients had made two or more suicide attempts, and 60% were self-mutilators. Multiple abusers were found in 95% of the patients, with the father the most common perpetrator, and all had an age of onset for first abuse by 8 years of age. All had been physically abused, had witnessed violence, and had reported emotional abuse as well. Adult reenactments of abuse were common: 90% of the subjects had been raped and 55% had been battered. The authors suggest that severe incest histories are accompanied by other childhood adversity and lead both to BPD and to multiple severe symptoms.

Shearer et al. (1990) studied female inpatients given BPD diagnoses. Childhood abuse histories were obtained by semistructured interviews:

40% of the patients gave histories of sexual abuse, while 25% reported having been physically abused. BPD patients with histories of sexual abuse were significantly more likely to have suspected complex partial seizure disorder or an eating or drug abuse disorder. Incest in particular was associated with greater lethality of self-destructive behavior. BPD patients with histories of physical abuse were more likely to have been concomitantly diagnosed with antisocial personality disorder and showed trends toward having more psychotic symptoms and somatization. The authors suggested that complex partial seizure phenomena were not likely to have been due to physical abuse, because they were associated only with sexual abuse. Whether these are dissociative phenomena or subsequent manifestations of a kindling effect of the original trauma affecting levels of arousal remains an open question.

Ogata et al. (1990) studied inpatients with either BPD, diagnosed by the Diagnostic Interview for Borderlines (DIB) (Gunderson et al. 1982), or major depression, diagnosed according to Research Diagnostic Criteria (RDC) (Spitzer et al. 1975). Childhood antecedents were gathered systematically and blindly by a specific interview with explicit criteria for abuse, neglect, etc. Sexual abuse, which included exposure to genitals as well as fondling and penetration, was significantly more common in patients with BPD (71%) than in depressed (22%) subjects. Most abuse began before age 12, with the mean age of onset earliest when perpetrated by fathers (7.4 years) and siblings (8 years). In descending order, the most frequent perpetrators were nonrelatives, siblings, other relatives, and fathers. Four of the seven BPD patients without sexual abuse histories were men. Sixty-five percent of the sexually abused BPD patients also reported physical abuse. Although BPD patients reported more physical abuse (42% v. 33%) and physical neglect (17% v. 6%) than depressed patients, the differences were not significant. When the authors entered all abuse and neglect variables in a stepwise regression, sexual abuse alone predicted the BPD diagnosis; no other variable significantly added unique variance. A history of sexual abuse itself was predicted by the following DIB symptoms: derealization, promiscuity, unstable close relationships, chronic dysphoria (i.e., loneliness, emptiness), and depersonalization. The authors suggested that the high prevalence of multiple forms of abuse indicates that BPD patients come from highly disturbed families that do not protect them and fail to attend to their needs.

Ludolph et al. (1990) retrospectively examined the charts from a sample of adolescent girls for abuse data. Based on the DIB, subjects were diagnosed as having BPD or other nonborderline diagnoses (exclusive of psychosis). The BPD group had a higher frequency of disrupted attachments, including early parental divorce, adoption, expulsion from home, and multiple foster placements and surrogate parents. Adverse childhood experiences were more common among the BPD subjects than among the nonborderline adolescents: sexual abuse (52% v. 19%), physical abuse (52% v. 26%), neglect by primary caretaker (44% v. 17%), expulsion from home by primary caretaker (41% v. 9%), and involvement with protective services (37% v. 13%). BPD subjects were also more likely to have been the recipient of grossly inappropriate parental behavior (44% v. 9%). The authors noted several examples, including a girl "double-dating with her father and his girlfriend and watching each other's sexual behavior; parents threatening to maim family pets; and a mother giving her borderline daughter a loaded gun, saying 'Shoot me if you hate me that much'" (p. 473). Interestingly, psychiatric illness diagnosed in the fathers was equally high (about two-thirds) in the two groups, although there was a trend for mothers of the BPD group to have more borderline and other personality pathology and histories of physical abuse themselves. The authors concluded that BPD adolescents have been subjected to multiple traumas, neglect, disruptions, and chaos that generally begin early in life and have a cumulative effect. While the chart reviews were retrospective, the fact that parents were often interviewed as part of the adolescents' hospitalizations adds an external source of data to that provided by the patients.

Swett et al. (1990) obtained self-report data from a series of consecutive males seeking outpatient treatment. Information about early traumas was attained from questionnaires, while Axis II data was obtained from the treating therapists in a subsample of 34 patients. Forty-eight percent of the entire sample reported some form of abuse, including physical abuse only (35%), sexual abuse only (7%), and both types of abuse (6%). Similar to the findings of Bryer et al. (1987), in descending order, reports of sexual abuse only, both types of abuse, and physical abuse only were highly related to elevations of all scales of the SCL-90. Half of the abused sample reported multiple perpetrators, most frequently family members, especially among the physically abused. In the limited subsample with

Axis II data, BPD was diagnosed more frequently among the abused than among the nonabused men (25% v. 6%), yielding a relative risk of 4.5 for BPD among the abused. The authors did note the methodological limitations of using self-report data.

Stone (1990) conducted a long-term follow-up study (mean length = 16 years) of former inpatients. Diagnoses and data on childhood antecedents were obtained by retrospective chart review with explicit criteria. The patients were generally from middle- and upper-socioeconomic-class family backgrounds. Histories of incest were noted in 19% of borderline cases, compared with 5% of schizophrenic cases. However, the author noted that active inquiry about incest was not common in the psychiatric hospital setting of the time, thereby ensuring underestimates of the true prevalence. Stone noted that incest tended to be most pathogenic when it occurred across generations (e.g., father, uncle), involved force, and occurred repetitively and well within the victims' memory. These factors tended to lead to personality characteristics such as compulsive sexuality, impulsivity, a propensity toward relationships that involve boundary violations (e.g., sexual involvement with helping professionals), sadomasochism, extreme jealousy, substance abuse, and a sense of being a pariah. In some cases, incest with extreme sadism led to psychotic symptoms. The frequency of nonincestuous, early sexual abuse was not reported. Parental brutality was found in 11% of borderline subjects, compared with 6% of psychotic individuals. The frequency of physical abuse by others was not reported. Although only five cases were noted to have overlapping incest and parental brutality, this group was the most severely impaired.

Studies of multiple personality disorder have also examined traumatic antecedents. Ross et al. (1990) gathered 102 cases of multiple personality from four sites and administered a structured interview, the Dissociative Disorders Interview Schedule (Ross et al. 1989), which includes data on borderline personality criteria and trauma. Multiple personality was highly associated with histories of sexual abuse (90%), physical abuse (82%), or either or both types of abuse (95%). In addition, 91% and 64% of the subjects met criteria for major depressive disorder and BPD, respectively. The sample as a whole had a mean of 5.2 positive criteria for BPD and a mean score of 41.4 on the Dissociative Experiences Scale. The frequency of sexual and/or physical abuse was not reported separately for those subjects with concurrent BPD; however, given the high base rate of abuse in the sample as a whole, it could not be much lower than the mean for the sample. The authors also reviewed four other studies of multiple personality, noting that abuse rates ranged from 68% to 90% for sexual abuse, 60% to 82% for physical abuse, and over 88% for either or both forms of abuse. This study in particular demonstrated that there is a relationship between childhood abuse and adult BPD and multiple personality disorder. Cases of multiple personality disorder show a very high degree of dissociation and have a high rate of concurrent BPD, but what differentiates the two disorders is not yet known, although severity of abuse and higher degrees of dissociation may be likely factors.

The above studies are divided into two groups in Table 6–1.[1] The first group includes three studies that had adequate attention to independent and blind ascertainment of diagnoses and abuse histories, and minimization of sample biases that affect interpretation. By and large these studies demonstrate the highest frequencies of sexual and physical abuse. The remaining studies have more methodological limitations, such as using chart review rather than direct patient ascertainment for diagnosis or abuse histories. Although as a group they obtained somewhat lower frequencies of abuse, their findings are remarkably consistent in direction with the first three studies. Furthermore, those studies that used quantitative measures of abuse (Briere and Zaidi 1989; Herman et al. 1989) found the most highly specific relationships between abuse and BPD psychopathology. As a whole, these findings are highly suggestive that childhood abuse, particularly that beginning in early childhood, is a major etiologic factor in the adult development of BPD.

However, abuse does not occur in a vacuum. There are other childhood factors that are associated with BPD for which scientific evidence exists. In the schema presented in Table 6–2, childhood trauma, especially recurrent and multiple forms of abuse, is a major cause, facilitated by other factors listed in the second column. The fact that some cases of BPD have no demonstrable histories of abuse suggests that in a minority of cases, these facilitating factors may sometimes be sufficient to cause BPD. Most of these facilitating factors were noted in the above studies. The one exception is what we have termed "noninvulnerable" temperament. Some

---

[1]The study by Ross et al. is not summarized in Table 6–1 because selection was conditioned on multiple personality disorder.

Table 6–2. Schema for the development of borderline personality disorder

Major factors	Facilitating factors
Sexual abuse	Physical and emotional neglect
Physical abuse	Separations from caretakers
Witnessing violence	Verbal abuse
	Noninvulnerable temperament
	Parental psychopathology
	Lack of protective, confiding relationships
	Ability to dissociate
	Chaotic home environment
	Grossly inappropriate parental behavior

children who have grown up in very adverse circumstances have entered adulthood with little evidence of psychopathology and have been termed "resilient" or "invulnerable." We do not see these temperamental characteristics in BPD subjects, although adequate characterization of these temperamental features remains to be done. While it is possible that there is a specific temperamental vulnerability to developing BPD, studies to date (e.g., Soloff and Millward 1983) have found little evidence for this. Perhaps most children have temperaments that are not invulnerable enough to mitigate the effects of abuse, while a few have temperaments that render them relatively invulnerable. This certainly warrants further study.

THE ROLE OF DEFENSES

Studies examining dissociative experiences in BPD have found high degrees of dissociation, although perhaps not as high as those found in multiple personality (Herman et al. 1989; Ross et al. 1990). Both dissociative symptoms and BPD result from traumatic experiences, but dissociation appears to help maintain borderline pathology, as noted by Herman et al. (1989). Furthermore, dissociation adds to the prediction of self-mutilation in BPD subjects who have been prospectively followed (van der Kolk et al. 1991). Dissociation appears to keep both the ideational memories and attendant affects associated with trauma out of consciousness at a price. Memories are reenacted rather than recalled, and the inhibition of intolerable affects is accompanied by high levels of anxiety leading to clouding of conscious experience. Periodically, the dissociative symptoms become intolerable themselves, and the BPD patient relieves the underlying affects by self-destructive behaviors, such as cutting himself or herself, simultaneously enacting the role of abuser and victim. Any successful treatment for BPD must help the individual to overcome dissociation, recall the unconscious traumatic memories when they are activated by events, and handle the attendant affects with healthier defenses, such as self-assertion, affiliation, and suppression.

Studies that have examined major image-distorting defenses (splitting of self and others' images, projective identification) have found these defenses to be more prevalent in BPD than in comparison disorders, whether measured by clinical observers (Bond 1990; Perry and Cooper 1986) or by projective testing (Cooper et al. 1988; Lerner et al. 1987). Certain defenses—denial, devaluation, idealization, and omnipotence—originally proposed by Kernberg (1975) to cohere at a borderline level of defensive functioning, are not as specifically associated with BPD as are the major image-distorting defenses noted above (Perry and Cooper 1986). The major image-distorting defenses also predicted higher rates of psychotic and psychotic-like symptoms and depression on follow-up (Perry 1988; Perry and Cooper 1989).

Splitting and projective identification may be understood best clinically when their adaptive value for the physically or sexually abused child is considered. The abused child must continue to depend on caretakers who are all powerful, for better or worse, whether in taking care of the child's basic needs or in threatening or carrying out a painful or injurious assault. When abuse begins in early childhood (especially before 6 years of age), the child has not yet learned to reach out to other more protective surrogate caregivers. Instead, he or she must coexist with one or more unpredictably malevolent persons who either ignore or actively punish and suppress the child's protest.

Learning to split off bad self image and others' images minimizes awareness of the ever-constant threat from which the child cannot escape. While adaptive in such horrible childhood circumstances, these defenses are not adaptive later in adulthood in other contexts. Instead, splitting and projective identification are triggered by situations that remind the subject unconsciously of earlier abuse situations, leading to reenactments of traumatic relationships. Ambiguous cues trigger anxiety that abuse might be impending; splitting resolves ambiguous roles into all good or all bad, the scripts or outlines of which are readily retrieved from memory. Furthermore, because BPD patients also use other defenses such as acting out, passive-aggression, and help-rejecting complaining (i.e., hypochondriasis) (Perry and Cooper 1986), reenactments of traumatic relationships adversely affect others as well. This may paradoxically lead others to retraumatize the subject, thereby reinforcing splitting and maintaining borderline psychopathology. Examples of this include being battered by a sexual partner or being sexually victimized by a health care professional. Thus, defenses protect the individual against anxiety but at the price of continuing to perceive the world as it existed in childhood, even to the extent of reenacting abusive scenarios. To the degree that others unwittingly play the scripted role in the reenactment, splitting is reinforced, and borderline psychopathology along with it.

DISCUSSION

Many of the most troubling and difficult features of BPD become more comprehensible in the light of a history of early, prolonged, severe childhood trauma. The psychopathology becomes an understandable adaptation to an environment of fear, secrecy, and betrayal rather than an innate defect in the self. Chronic childhood abuse takes place in a familial climate of pervasive terror. The abused child cannot turn to a parent for protection, either because the parent is himself the abuser, or because the abuser has succeeded in alienating the child from his or her primary caretaker. Father-daughter incest, for example, often occurs in conjunction with battering (Bowker et al. 1988; Herman 1981). The abused child who sees her mother being beaten dares not disclose the incest secret, while the intimidated mother dares not ask too many questions, even if her suspicions are aroused. Thus, the mother-child relationship is seriously undermined, and the child often feels abandoned to the abuser.

When ordinary caregiving relationships are disrupted, the abused child faces formidable developmental tasks in isolation. He or she must find a way to form primary attachments to caretakers who are either dangerous or incapable of protecting him or her. The capacity to trust must develop in an environment where trust is not warranted. The capacity for bodily self-regulation must develop in an environment in which the child's body is periodically attacked. The capacity to experience and modulate affect must develop in an environment that provokes extreme feelings of terror and rage and that does not provide reliable soothing.

The characteristic borderline defense of splitting may be understood as an adaptive attempt to maintain some positive image of an idealized, nurturing parent as a figure for attachment while segregating the image of the abusive or neglectful parent. The twin fears of abandonment and domination, which the borderline patient carries into subsequent relationships, and which result in unstable, oscillating attachments (Melges and Swartz 1989), accurately reflect the reality of the abusive childhood environment. The child's developing capacity to regulate affective states is repeatedly disrupted by traumatic experiences that evoke overwhelming terror, rage, and grief. These emotional states ultimately coalesce in a chronic posttraumatic syndrome. While intrusive posttraumatic symptoms such as nightmares may be present only intermittently, the hyperarousal and numbing components of the posttraumatic syndrome become most pronounced, resulting in a dysphoric state that victims find almost impossible to describe. It is a state of emotional confusion, agitation, emptiness, and utter aloneness. The emotional state of the chronically abused child ranges from a baseline of uneasiness, through intermediate states of anxiety and dysphoria, to extremes of panic, fury, and despair (Herman et al. 1986). Not surprisingly, a great many survivors develop chronic anxiety and mood disorders that persist into adulthood (Chu and Dill 1990; Krystal 1978).

In an environment of neglect as well as abuse, the child victim cannot turn to a safe and reliable caregiver for comfort. Indeed, the only source of solace may be the abusive caretaker. This is particularly true in incestuous relationships, where the sexual abuse may offer some degree of pleasure or soothing to the child, at the price of utter humiliation and helplessness. Thus, relational methods of self-soothing are profoundly compromised, and the abused child is forced to develop alternative methods in isolation. Most commonly, the child does this by learning to self-induce altered states of consciousness. The capacity for trance or dissociative states, normally high in school-age children, is apparently developed to a fine art in children who have been severely punished or abused (Spiegel 1990). In our own study (Herman et al. 1989), the degree of familiarity with dissociative states closely paralleled the severity of reported childhood abuse.

Dissociation, however, is not a fully adaptive defense, either because it fails at crucial moments or because it becomes too effective, resulting in a frightening sense of numbness, detachment, or inner deadness. Later elaborations of self-destructive behavior, including self-mutilation, binge eating and purging, substance abuse, and risk taking, may represent additional attempts to regulate affective states or terminate dissociative states by producing intense bodily crises.

Finally, the literature on treating BPD patients is fraught with descriptions of regression partially induced by treatment that can become a reenactment of traumatic experiences and relationships. Regression is often stimulated or exacerbated by the therapist's failure to recognize the validity of the patient's perceptions in light of past traumas (Perry et al. 1990). The therapist may inadvertently repeat the trauma of blaming, thus misunderstanding and invalidating the kernels of truth in the patient's perceptions. These kernels of truth must be nurtured in order for more adaptive adult defenses and behaviors to develop.

REFERENCES

Bernstein EM, Putnam FW: Development, reliability and validity of a dissociation scale. J Nerv Ment Dis 174:727–735, 1986

Bond M: Are "borderline defenses" specific for borderline personality disorders? Journal of Personality Disorders 4:251–256, 1990

Bowker L, Arbitel M, McFerron JR: On the relationship between wife-beating and child abuse, in Feminist Perspectives on Wife Abuse. Edited by Yllo K, Bograd M. Beverly Hills, CA, Sage, 1988, pp 158–174

Briere J, Zaidi LY: Sexual abuse histories and sequelae in female psychiatric emergency room patients. Am J Psychiatry 146:1602–1606, 1989

Bryer JB, Nelson BA, Miller JB, et al: Childhood sexual and physical abuse as factors in adult psychiatric illness. Am J Psychiatry 144:1426–1430, 1987

Chu JA, Dill DL: Dissociative symptoms in relation to childhood physical and sexual abuse. Am J Psychiatry 147:887–892, 1990

Cooper SH, Perry JC, Arnow D: An empirical approach to the study of defense mechanism, I: reliability and preliminary validity of the Rorschach defense scales. J Pers Assess 52:187–203, 1988

Derogatis LR: SCL-90-R Administration, Scoring, and Procedures Manual, II. Towson, MD, Clinical Psychometric Research, 1983

Finkelhor D: Child Sexual Abuse. New York, Free Press, 1984

Goodwin JM, Cheeves K, Connell V: Borderline and other severe symptoms in adult survivors of incestuous abuse. Psychiatric Annals 20:22–32, 1990

Gunderson JG, Kolb JE, Austin V: The Diagnostic Interview for Borderline Patients. Am J Psychiatry 138:896–903, 1982

Herman JL: Father-Daughter Incest. Cambridge, MA, Harvard University Press, 1981

Herman J, Russell D, Trocki K: Long-term effects of incestuous abuse in childhood. Am J Psychiatry 143:1293–1296, 1986

Herman JL, Perry JC, van der Kolk BA: Childhood trauma in borderline personality disorder. Am J Psychiatry 146:490–495, 1989

Kernberg OF: Borderline Conditions and Pathological Narcissism. New York, Jason Aronson, 1975

Krystal H: Trauma and affects. Psychoanal Study Child 33:81–116, 1978

Lerner H, Albert C, Walsh M: The Rorschach assessment of borderline defense: a concurrent validity study. J Pers Assess 51:334–338, 1987

Ludolph PS, Westen D, Misle B, et al: The borderline diagnosis in adolescents: symptoms and developmental history. Am J Psychiatry 147:470–476, 1990

Melges FT, Swartz MS: Oscillations of attachment in borderline personality disorder. Am J Psychiatry 146:1115–1120, 1989

Millon T: Millon Clinical Multiaxial Inventory, 3rd Edition. Minneapolis, MN, Interpretive Scoring Systems, 1983

Ogata SN, Silk KR, Goodrich S, et al: Childhood sexual and physical abuse in adult patients with borderline personality disorder. Am J Psychiatry 147:1008–1013, 1990

Pagelow M: Family Violence. New York, Praeger, 1984

Perry JC: A prospective study of life stress, defenses, psychotic symptoms, and depression in borderline and antisocial personality disorders and bipolar type II affective disorder. Journal of Personality Disorders 2:49–59, 1988

Perry JC, Cooper SH: A preliminary report on defenses and conflicts associated with borderline personality disorder. J Am Psychoanal Assoc 34:863–893, 1986

Perry JC, Cooper SH: An empirical study of defense mechanisms, I: clinical interview and life vignette ratings. Arch Gen Psychiatry 46:444–452, 1989

Perry JC, Lavori PW, Hoke L: A Markov model for predicting levels of psychiatric service use in borderline and antisocial personality disorders and bipolar type II affective disorder. J Psychiatr Res 21:215–232, 1987

Perry JC, Herman JL, van der Kolk BA, et al: Psychotherapy and psychological trauma in borderline personality disorder. Psychiatric Annals 20:33–43, 1990

Ross CA, Heberf S, Norton GR, et al: The Dissociative Disorders Interview Schedule: a structured interview. Dissociation 2(3):169–189, 1989

Ross CA, Miller SD, Reagor P, et al: Structured interview data on 102 cases of multiple personality disorder from four centers. Am J Psychiatry 147:596–601, 1990

Russell DE: The Secret Trauma. New York, Basic Books, 1986

Shearer SL, Peters CP, Quaytman MS, et al: Frequency and correlates of childhood sexual and physical abuse histories in adult female borderline inpatients. Am J Psychiatry 147:214–216, 1990

Soloff PH, Millward JW: Developmental histories of borderline patients. Compr Psychiatry 24:574–588, 1983

Spiegel D: Trauma, dissociation, and hypnosis, in Incest-Related Syndromes of Adult Psychopathology. Edited by Kluft R. Washington, DC, American Psychiatric Press, 1990, pp 247–262

Spitzer RL, Endicott HJ, Robins E: Research Diagnostic Criteria (RDC) for a Selected Group of Functional Disorders, 2nd Edition. New York, New York State Psychiatric Institute, Biometrics Research, 1975

Stern A: Psychoanalytic investigation of and therapy in the borderline group of neuroses. Psychoanal Q 7:467–489, 1938

Stone M: The Fate of Borderline Patients: Successful Outcome and Psychiatric Practice. New York, Guilford, 1990

Swett C Jr, Surrey J, Cohen C: Sexual and physical abuse histories and psychiatric symptoms among male psychiatric outpatients. Am J Psychiatry 147:632–636, 1990

van der Kolk BA: The compulsion to repeat the trauma: attachment, reenactment, and masochism. Psychiatr Clin North Am 12:389–411, 1989

van der Kolk BA, Perry JC, Herman JL: Childhood origins of self-destructive behaviors. Am J Psychiatry 148:1665–1671, 1991

Zanarini MC, Gunderson JG, Marino MF, et al: Childhood experiences of borderline patients. Compr Psychiatry 30:18–25, 1989

CHAPTER 7

Parental Bonding in Borderline Personality Disorder

Joel Paris, M.D.
Hallie Zweig-Frank, Ph.D.

THE DIMENSIONS OF PARENTING

Developmental psychology has described two factors that determine the quality of parenting: *affection* and *control* (Rowe 1981). Ideal parenting in this model would consist of providing sufficient emotional support and affection to promote bonding and allowing sufficient autonomy to promote separation.

The importance of bonding and secure attachment to parents has been developed in theoretical detail by Bowlby (1969, 1973, 1980). Bowlby has shown that failure to provide secure attachment leads to a number of psychopathological consequences, and he has collected a great deal of empirical evidence to support his views. The consequences of failing to encourage autonomy in children have been described by Levy (1943). There is significant clinical and empirical literature supporting the idea that overprotection of children can lead to psychopathology (Parker 1983).

As reviewed by Parker (1983), the dimensions of affection and control appear in a number of studies in which inventories of parental behavior were subjected to factor analysis. Schaefer (1959) has described the two factors of this theory of parenting as constituting a *circumplex model,* paralleling the circumplex theory of personality developed by Leary (1957), Kiesler (1983), and Wiggins (1982), in which dimensions of affiliation and control are seen as being basic to interpersonal behavior.

The Role of Parenting
in Borderline Personality Disorder:
Clinical Theories

Psychotherapists working with patients with borderline personality disorder (BPD) have frequently reported that their patients' experiences with their parents during childhood are abnormal (Gunderson 1984). Virtually every clinical report drawn from psychodynamic exploration is rich with interpretation of adult pathology as related to problems in parental bonding. Some theoretical formulations have attempted to relate the symptoms of BPD to such experiences.

Adler (1985) has suggested that the borderline syndrome can be explained as a failure of parental affection and bonding. Adler argues that borderline individuals experience unresponsiveness in their parents to their needs, which leads to a failure of the holding environment. Adler describes "borderline aloneness," the absence of good parental introjects to buffer emotions that creates the dysphoria and affective instability characteristic of the borderline syndrome.

One could further speculate that when negative affects are elicited in borderline individuals, rather than being buffered by an internal "good parent," these affects cycle out of control and flood the patient. Unresponsiveness also creates severe deficiencies in self-esteem that interfere with finding substitute objects to replace the missing parental images. In fact, the interpersonal relationships of the borderline individual are characterized by sensitivity to rejection, which recapitulates the experience of having unresponsive parents. The repeated dissolution of such relationships creates more affective dysphoria, which rises to intolerable levels. In an attempt to control the dysphoria, the borderline individual then acts out. Substance use reduces dysphoric affects. Self-mutilation is described by some borderline individuals as a relief from painful feelings of depersonalization (Gunderson 1984), and suicide attempts are an ultimate strategy for escaping from psychological pain.

A theory of emotional neglect could explain many of the symptoms of BPD. This theory has the further advantage of concordance with the clinical reports on borderline patients. However, like any theory, it requires empirical verification. In addition, the etiologic effects of emotional neglect lack specificity. As with other psychodynamic theories, the same factor can be used to explain a wide range of psychopathological outcomes. Not only do patients with entirely different pathology present similar histories, but only a proportion of those with poor parental bonding end up as "borderline."

There are several ways of accounting for this discrepancy. One possibility is that although borderline patients have problems in parental bonding similar to those of other patients, their difficulties are more severe, and it is the extent of the failure to provide secure attachment that accounts for the syndrome. This idea could be tested by comparing in a systematic way the reports of BPD patients with those of non-BPD patients. A second possibility is that there is a phase-specific factor in borderline development, such that parental failure affects the child either at an earlier stage of development or at a stage during which the child is particularly sensitive. Such formulations are not generally amenable to empirical testing. They seem to rely on traditions in psychoanalysis that emphasize epigenesis and assume that the deeper the pathology, the earlier the "fixation."

A third possibility is that there is an interaction between constitutional vulnerability and childhood experience. The child who becomes "borderline" could 1) be more vulnerable to parental failure because of increased sensitivity, 2) have an unusual need for parental affection that cannot be met by neglectful parents, or 3) receive less affection because of low sociability (Rowe 1981). Constitutional vulnerability could produce a pathological response to neglect such as affective instability and/or impulsivity (see van Reekum et al., Chapter 1). These theories would be empirically verifiable if we could identify biological markers of constitutional vulnerability that either relate specifically to BPD or relate to impulse spectrum disorders as a group (Gunderson and Zanarini 1989).

Finally, it is possible that failure of parental bonding in BPD patients interacts with other specific trauma in childhood, as suggested by Perry and Herman (see Chapter 6). The interaction could work in two ways: 1) physical and sexual abuse produces problems in attachment, or 2) abuse is an outgrowth of a failure of attachment. Multivariate studies of neglect and trauma in the childhood of BPD patients could help sort out this complex issue.

Adler's theory of emotional neglect in the childhood of BPD patients suggests parental failure on the dimension of affection. Could there also be failure on the dimension of parental control? Masterson (1981) suggested that borderline individuals grow up with a mother who may herself be "borderline" and who interferes with separation so as to keep the child near her, particularly during the separation-individuation phase. The phase-specific aspect of the theory is not really testable empirically. Moreover, it has been shown that most borderline individuals do not have a borderline parent (Links et al. 1988), although there may be a subgroup of patients who do (Feldman and Guttman 1984). However, the behavior of parents preventing autonomous development in children could be sufficiently pervasive throughout childhood so as to correspond to Levy's (1943) description of parental overprotection, an aspect of Masterson's theory that is open to empirical investigation.

Methodological Approaches to Childhood Experience and Parental Bonding

Ideally, prospective studies could test clinical hypotheses about the relationship of childhood experience to borderline pathology. However, there are difficulties with such research. A large cohort would be required to obtain a significant number of BPD cases in a community sample, given that preliminary estimates of prevalence of the disorder are not greater than 2% (Swartz et al. 1990). Prospective studies suffer from attrition, and from what we know of the families of borderline patients, these cases might be particularly vulnerable to loss during follow-up. Finally, a study with a 20-year follow-up might suffer from using baseline measures that prove to be anachronistic by the time data are collected.

Another possibility, suggested by Gunderson and Zanarini (1989), is to study high-risk populations that are more likely to develop BPD. These could include children from disturbed families, children who have suffered abuse, or children with borderline parents. These studies will no doubt be carried out in the near future, but the choice of measures of developmental factors in BPD will be informed by retrospective research.

Retrospective studies quantify the histories we get from our patients, which have been the source of hypotheses for empirical research on the childhood of borderline individuals. Most investigations of childhood experience have used a retrospective approach in which patients are asked to describe their earlier life through self-report scales or structured interviews. The assumption of the retrospective method is that most patients can recall their childhood and their parents with reasonable accuracy. The validity of such measures can be established in a number of ways. For example, concordance with sibling ratings is of particular value (Robins et al. 1985). Validity is also provided when such ratings can differentiate psychopathology from normality.

Retrospective studies have been criticized on a number of grounds. The memory of parenting experiences may be falsified in an attempt to blame the parents for one's problems, or else a discrepancy between the abnormal needs of the child and the ability of the parents to meet such needs may be reported as inadequate parenting. In the case of borderline patients, who tend to distort their perceptions of interpersonal relationships, retrospective falsification is a particular problem.

In order to validate retrospective measures we require instruments that have been shown to correlate with other measures of childhood experience. Most data from semistructured interviews, even if relatively factual, lack such validation. Scales designed to measure the dimensions of parental behavior during childhood, and which have been used in a number of other studies of clinical and nonclinical populations, would be ideal.

Such a measure was developed by the Australian psychiatrist Gordon Parker (1983), who specifically designed an instrument to score the two basic parental dimensions of affection and control. The Parental Bonding Index (PBI) consists of 25 items, 12 of which are a care scale, and 13 of which are a control scale. Each item is scored on a 4-point Likert scale. The PBI is filled out by the subject on mother and father separately and represents an overview of experience with parents in the first 16 years of life. The scales have good test-retest, as well as split-half, reliability. Scores are not influenced by the age, sex, or socioeconomic class of subjects. There are community norms drawn from three sites and from a large number of studies on psychiatric patients. The findings for depression (in which care is low and control high) have been the most striking.

Validity of the PBI has been established by showing that scores correlate highly with reports of siblings, with parental self-reports, and with data drawn from interviews. In addition, its ability to discriminate both

Axis I (Parker 1983) and Axis II (Paris et al. 1991) disorders so that those with more severe pathology have more abnormal scores provides support for its validity.

PREVIOUS STUDIES OF THE CHILDHOOD EXPERIENCES OF PATIENTS WITH BORDERLINE PERSONALITY DISORDER

Over the last decade a number of investigators, using different methodologies, have examined how BPD patients remember their childhoods. Although the results vary somewhat, there are a number of important convergences that, in spite of differing methodological approaches, suggest some degree of consistency.

A large group of studies, summarized in Table 7–1, provide evidence for failure of parental bonding in BPD patients. The first to appear, by Gunderson et al. (1980), used data from family interviews of borderline, depressed, and schizophrenic patients of both sexes admitted to a hospital. The transcripts were rated blind to diagnosis. The findings suggested that borderline patients suffer emotional neglect from both parents and that they are scapegoated by a parental coalition against them. This study is the only one to use direct family observation as data, and it strengthens the findings of all the other studies that are based on retrospective self-report. Its primary limitation is that the data can also be interpreted as parental reactions to the behavioral disturbance of their borderline children. The sample, drawn from a private hospital, was limited to intact families, which could be unrepresentative.

Frank and Paris (1981) administered a semistructured interview to groups of borderline patients, nonborderline patients, and a nonpsychiatric control group in a female university student population. The questions were designed to test hypotheses that borderline patients remember their parents as neglectful or overprotective. The findings showed that the borderline patients differed from the nonborderline patients in their recollections of their fathers as neglectful, while both the borderline and the nonborderline patients differed from the control subjects in reporting more maternal neglect. There were no differences on measures of overprotection. These somewhat surprising results suggest that, contrary to the emphasis in the psychodynamic literature on the role of the mother,

Table 7–1. Studies of the childhood experiences of patients with borderline personality disorder

Author	Sex	Source of sample	Comparison group	Instrument	Emotional neglect	Over-protection	Separation and loss
Gunderson et al. (1980)	Both	Inpatients	Depression, schizophrenia	Rating of family interviews	Biparental	—	—
Frank and Paris (1981)	Female	University student clinic	Non-BPD outpatients, normal subjects	Semistructured interviews	Father	No	—
Frank and Hoffman (1986)	Female	University student clinic	Non-BPD outpatients	Parental activity inventory	Biparental	No	—
Soloff and Millward (1983)	Both	Inpatients	Depression, schizophrenia	Semistructured interviews	Biparental	No	Increased
Zanarini et al. (1989)	Both	Outpatients	Dysthymia, antisocial personality disorder	Semistructured interviews	Biparental	—	Increased
Links et al. (1988)	Both	Inpatients	Borderline traits only	Semistructured interview; diagnostic interview of parents	Biparental	—	Increased
Paris et al. (1988)	Both	Mostly inpatients	Depression	Chart review	Mother	—	Increased
Goldberg et al. (1985)	Both	Inpatients	Non-BPD, normal subjects	Parental Bonding Index[a]	Biparental	Biparental	—
Byrne et al. (1990)	Both	Inpatients	Schizophrenia	Parental Bonding Index	Biparental	Biparental	Increased
Paris and Frank	Female	University student clinic	Non-BPD outpatients	Parental Bonding Index	Mother	—	—

[a]See Parker 1983.

both parents are involved in producing borderline pathology, supporting the findings of Gunderson et al. (1980). The explanation could be that borderline individuals suffer biparental failure, such that they are unable to buffer the neglect of one parent with the affection of the other (Feldman and Guttman 1984). The primary limitation of the study was the use of a nonstandardized instrument with only face validity.

In a second study on a population of female university students, Frank and Hoffman (1986, 1987) used another instrument, Bronfenbenner's Parent Activity Inventory, which, although not well standardized, had been used in a number of other research studies. The significant differences between borderline and nonborderline patients were all on scales that reflected emotional neglect from both parents, again supporting the idea of biparental failure in BPD. There were no differences on scales reflecting overprotection. In this study, borderline and nonborderline patients were also given the Profile of Nonverbal Sensitivity (PONS), which measures nonverbal sensitivity through the use of brief videotaped emotional states. The borderline patients scored significantly higher on the PONS, showing that they are particularly sensitive to the emotional states of others (Hoffman and Frank 1986), a possible factor in their response to parental psychopathology.

Soloff and Millward (1983) reported on family pathology in borderline, depressive, and schizophrenic patients of both sexes admitted to a hospital. The findings, based on data from interviews, suggest that borderline patients remember both parents as being emotionally neglectful. Although the authors interpreted these findings as also suggesting that there was maternal overprotection in borderline patients, those differences were not in fact statistically significant. Finally, Soloff and Millward (1983) found an increased frequency of histories of early separation and loss in borderline patients. This finding may have been missed in earlier studies using subjects from higher socioeconomic backgrounds.

In a study of male and female borderline outpatients as compared to dysthymic and antisocial control subjects, Zanarini et al. (1989) found that BPD patients were significantly more likely than antisocial subjects to report parental emotional withdrawal and significantly more likely than dysthymic subjects to report early separation experiences. Data were obtained with a semistructured interview, and the results were similar to Soloff and Millward's (1983) findings in a hospitalized population.

In a study using both semistructured interviews of male and female borderline inpatients and diagnostic interviews of their immediate relatives, Links et al. (1988, 1990) showed that 28% of the BPD patients in their sample had parents who both had a psychiatric diagnosis (mostly depression, but also a number of personality disorders). They described this group of borderline probands as suffering from biparental failure. Although the requirements of the operational definition of biparental failure were stringent (overt diagnosis as opposed to parental failure without a diagnosis), the findings support the idea that BPD patients have troubled parents.

Two of the long-term outcome studies of BPD have used data scored from charts to examine the frequency of negative events in the childhood of BPD patients as compared with non-BPD patients. Paris et al. (1988) used an index to score early separation or loss, mother problems, and father problems. The rater was blind to diagnosis. The BPD patients (males and females) had more mother problems and separation or loss than did a comparison group with major depression. The histories were given additional validity by the fact that mother problems correlated negatively with ultimate outcome. Stone (1990) found a high frequency of early loss in his long-term follow-up of male and female BPD patients: in the absence of a control group, he compared his frequency with population means but did not find a difference from the non-BPD patients in his cohort.

Three studies have examined childhood experiences in BPD patients using the PBI. As described above, the PBI is a well-standardized instrument with good reliability and reasonable validity, and is superior to other measures of parental emotional neglect and overprotection. Goldberg et al. (1985) administered the PBI to groups of BPD patients, non-BPD patients, and normal control subjects of both sexes. The BPD patients perceived both their parents to be both less caring and more overprotective than did the other two groups. Byrne et al. (1990) administered the PBI to a group of hospitalized BPD patients of both sexes, using schizophrenic and community norms developed on the instrument for comparison. The authors' findings were the same as those of Goldberg et al. These two studies provided support for the construct of biparental failure in BPD but found evidence for overprotection in parents as well. By contrast, Paris and Frank (1989), administering the PBI to a group of female university students, found evidence for low care from both parents in BPD but failed to find differences in overprotection.

The discrepancies between the studies reviewed might be partly accounted for by the use of different populations of BPD patients. Some studies used hospitalized subjects, some used outpatients, and some used university students. Another possible source for differences between studies was whether male BPD patients were included. BPD is a predominantly female disorder (Gunderson 1984), and it is not clear whether the developmental pathway to borderline pathology for males and females is the same.

In summary, there seems to be a reasonable concordance among studies of childhood experience in BPD patients that the degree of parental emotional neglect is greater than that in non-BPD patients. The evidence as a whole supports the theoretical position of Adler (1985). The evidence for early separation or loss in these patients (Paris et al. 1988; Soloff and Millward 1983; Zanarini et al. 1989) can be seen either as another developmental variable increasing the risk for BPD or as a factor contributing to the failure of parental affection.

Although earlier studies did not identify overprotection as a factor in BPD, more recent evidence supports this idea (Byrne et al. 1990; Goldberg et al. 1985). If it could be shown that BPD patients remember both low care and overprotection from their parents, one could derive a theoretical position that integrates both findings. Melges and Swartz (1989) have suggested that if one examines the object relations of patients with BPD, one sees that they fear abandonment, but also engulfment, and are in continuous conflict about closeness and distance. If adult relationships recapitulate those with parents during childhood, one would in fact expect BPD patients to have been both neglected and overprotected.

PARENTAL BONDING INDEX SCORES IN MALE AND FEMALE PATIENTS WITH BORDERLINE PERSONALITY DISORDER FROM TWO SITES

To clear up the contradictions in earlier studies of parental bonding in patients with BPD, we studied PBI scores in a large sample of BPD and non-BPD patients (Zweig-Frank and Paris 1991). In order to examine possible sex differences among BPD patients, males and females were studied separately. Because previous studies had been done on varying populations of borderline patients, we included two groups of subjects, one from an urban general hospital outpatient clinic and one from a university mental health service.

Diagnoses were established using the retrospective version of the Diagnostic Interview for Borderlines (DIB) (Armelius et al. 1985). The chart review was carried out on all subjects by a senior psychiatrist blind to other measures. (The same psychiatrist was also present at the initial evaluations of the majority of subjects.) Those subjects who scored 7 or more out of 10 on the DIB were diagnosed as borderline ($n = 62$). Those who received a score of 4 or less on the DIB were assigned to the nonborderline group ($n = 99$). (Patients scoring 5 or 6 on the DIB were excluded to ensure that we had two discrete groups.) The mean ages for the borderline and nonborderline samples were 29.6 and 29.3 years, respectively ($F = .03$, df $= 1$, NS). The subjects were subgrouped according to their sex and site.

The PBI scores for care and control are presented in Table 7–2. Two four-way mixed analyses of variance were carried out for both the care and the control scores, with diagnostic group, sex of patient, and site as the three between-subjects factors and sex of parent as the within-subjects factor.

The ANOVA for care yielded a highly significant main effect for diagnostic group, with BPD patients remembering their parents as being less caring than did non-BPD subjects ($F = 15.53$, df $= 1$, $P = .0001$). (Neither the main effect of sex of patient nor the main effect of site was significant.) The main effect of sex of parent was also significant, with mothers perceived as more caring than fathers ($F = 16.63$, df $= 1$, $P = .0001$).

The ANOVA for control also yielded a significant main effect of diagnosis, with BPD patients remembering their parents as more overprotective than did non-BPD subjects ($F = 8.69$, df $= 1$, $P = .0037$). Once again, neither the main effect of sex of patient nor the main effect of site reached significance.

The findings on the care scale are unequivocal in showing that patients with BPD remember both their parents as uncaring, a finding that supports the theories that view biparental emotional neglect as important in the development of BPD. Because the number of subjects was large, and because the findings applied to both male and female BPD patients, as well as to outpatients in a general hospital and university students, the results seem generalizable to borderline patients as a whole, and not just to any particular population.

The results on the control scale are also clear and support the idea that patients with BPD experienced overprotection as well as emotional neglect in childhood. These results, based on a larger and more widely representative sample of BPD patients, support the findings of Goldberg et al. (1985) and Byrne et al. (1990).

The picture of parental bonding in the PBI scores of BPD patients is of low care and high overprotection. Parker (1983) has called this pattern "affectionless control," and it is strongly related to depression. BPD patients who show dysthymic symptoms present a similar picture. The overlap between depressive and borderline subjects suggests that either a

Table 7–2.   Parental Bonding Index scores in male and female patients with borderline personality disorder from two sites

	BPD ($n = 62$)							
	Males ($n = 28$)				Females ($n = 34$)			
	University ($n = 10$)		Hospital ($n = 18$)		University ($n = 18$)		Hospital ($n = 16$)	
	Mean	SD	Mean	SD	Mean	SD	Mean	SD
Care[*]								
Mother	21.7	10.3	22.8	6.5	19.2	9.9	18.3	6.3
Father	16.2	5.3	15.3	7.3	18.1	8.3	20.2	8.6
Protection[**]								
Mother	17.8	10.3	19.6	9.5	15.4	10.6	18.3	10.0
Father	17.8	7.5	18.8	9.8	13.6	7.2	16.9	7.9

	Non-BPD (n = 99)							
	Males (n = 45)				Females (n = 54)			
	University ($n = 20$)		Hospital ($n = 25$)		University ($n = 29$)		Hospital ($n = 25$)	
	Mean	SD	Mean	SD	Mean	SD	Mean	SD
Care[*]								
Mother	28.0	7.3	25.2	6.6	25.2	9.7	23.5	8.5
Father	24.2	9.4	17.4	7.8	22.1	9.1	21.6	11.9
Protection[**]								
Mother	14.8	6.6	17.4	7.3	15.1	7.7	12.9	8.0
Father	10.5	6.2	14.4	7.8	15.0	8.8	12.6	7.6

Note. For discussion of the development of Parental Bonding Index, see Parker 1983.
[*]Four-way ANOVA: $F = 15.53$, $P = .0001$.
[**]Four-way ANOVA: $F = 8.69$, $P = .0037$.

relation exists between BPD and depression or the two disorders have common etiologic factors. Emotional neglect and biparental failure may produce a variety of psychopathological consequences in different individuals.

THE RELATIONSHIP BETWEEN TRAUMA AND EMOTIONAL NEGLECT

Recently, the focus of research on childhood experience in patients with BPD has shifted from emotional neglect to trauma. The high frequency of histories of sexual and physical abuse in their families of origin has been shown in a number of studies (Herman et al. 1989; Ogata et al. 1990; Stone 1990; Zanarini et al. 1989) to differentiate borderline patients from nonborderline patients. (This research is reviewed by Perry and Herman in Chapter 6.) However, the interaction of trauma and emotional neglect is an important issue that remains to be properly examined in empirical research.

In the first place, although the increased history of sexual and physical abuse in BPD patients has been shown statistically and confirmed with several different populations, abuse is by no means universal among these patients. Second, there is an important difference between *extrafamilial* and *intrafamilial* sexual abuse. Herman et al. (1989), in the report that found the highest rate of sexual abuse in BPD patients, obscured this difference. The rate of childhood sexual abuse by caretakers was only 26% in the studies of borderline populations by Zanarini et al. (1989) and Links et al. (1990). Research on the long-term effects of sexual abuse in nonclinical populations has shown that the effects of intrafamilial abuse are much more severe than molestation by noncaretakers (Browne and Finkelhor 1986; Russell 1986). Given the well-established long-term effects of incest, there seems to be a significant subpopulation in whom abuse plays a major role in producing the borderline syndrome. However, it is unreasonable to lump together all such experiences.

Research on childhood sexual abuse in community populations (Browne and Finkelhor 1986) has shown that the parameters of abuse (duration, severity, and relation to the perpetrator) are more predictive of later psychological disturbance than the mere fact of abuse alone. In fact, a large percentage of abuse involves single episodes (Peters 1988). We consider it as an oversimplification to view BPD as a posttraumatic stress disorder resulting exclusively from childhood sexual and physical abuse.

Sexual abuse tends to occur in disturbed families (Peters 1988), and these families have an atmosphere of emotional neglect that could be as significant for the development of BPD as the abuse itself. It would be important to examine the effects of abuse and neglect in the same study and to do a multivariate analysis of their interaction. In fact, in studies of sexual abuse in the community in which this has been done, general measures of family environment accounted for most of the variance (Fromuth 1986). If this is also the case for BPD in particular, then abuse may effect BPD through its association with dysfunctional families rather than via a posttraumatic mechanism. This would be true to some extent even with incest, and might be even more true for cases of extrafamilial molestation, where parents may fail to protect children, making them more vulnerable to the approach of strangers by denying them emotional security within the family and by not providing a setting for disclosure and appropriate action when molestation occurs. In fact, Peters (1988) showed that sexual abuse by nonfamily members in a community population was highly correlated with maternal neglect and did not have psychopathological effects independent of such neglect. It would therefore be crucial to determine whether sexual abuse in BPD has an effect independent of problems in parental bonding.

DEVELOPMENTAL SUBGROUPING OF BORDERLINE PERSONALITY DISORDER

One way of reconciling the contributions of trauma, emotional neglect, and other childhood experiences in the etiology of BPD would be to determine if there are subgroups within the heterogeneous population of borderline patients with different developmental pathways to the syndrome. For example, some of the symptoms of BPD are more clearly related to trauma than others. In particular, dissociation and self-mutilation have been shown to be related to childhood experiences of abuse (Ogata et al. 1990). Those patients who do not have these symptoms could have a greater contribution of emotional neglect to their psychopathology. It is also possible that constitutional factors could be weighted more heavily in some cases of BPD than in others (see Chapter 1), in parallel with the concept of process versus reactive schizophrenia.

Another possible way of subdividing BPD patients developmentally could be by age of onset, as has been done for the functional psychoses. Earlier onset suggests the possibility of either increased biological vulnerability or more severe environmental trauma. There is no research on this question, but we do know that the disorder is most frequently first recognizable in adolescence (Gunderson 1984). Although patients with BPD often describe an unhappy childhood, overt symptomatology such as suicide attempts or other impulsive behavior is associated with the biological changes of the adolescent years.

Recently, Petti and Vela (1990) have reviewed the literature on borderline disorders in childhood. It is unclear whether the concept of the borderline child overlaps with that of the borderline adolescent and adult; one possibility is that the concept confounds those who are schizotypal and those who are truly "borderline." Thus far, follow-up studies of children diagnosed as "borderline" have been contradictory. But if there is a subpopulation of children who either show the full syndrome prior to puberty or go on to develop the syndrome later after presenting clinically during childhood, this group is worthy of separate study to see if the developmental factors leading to borderline symptoms differ from those of individuals who fall ill in late adolescence or young adulthood.

EMOTIONAL NEGLECT AND CONSTITUTION IN BORDERLINE PERSONALITY DISORDER

It is our view that BPD is unlikely to develop in the absence of an abnormal constitution. As discussed by van Reekum et al. in Chapter 1, the nature of this constitutional abnormality has thus far proved elusive and may in fact involve multiple factors in a final common pathway. However, we speculate that emotional neglect could be a factor in phenotypic expression of constitutional vulnerability. For example, Klein's (1977) theory of affective dysregulation in BPD would suggest that children who later develop a borderline syndrome have the potential to respond with strong and unmodulated affective dysphoria to environmental insults.

This affective instability could be exacerbated by failed parental bonding.

Emotional neglect could also interact with constitutional impulsivity. Coccaro et al. (1989) found that impulsivity (and BPD specifically) is associated with decreased central serotonergic activity. A biological tendency to impulsive action would be exacerbated by neglectful parents who failed to provide the interest and affection that helps to prevent and contain acting-out behavior. The increased interpersonal sensitivity in BPD found by Frank and Hoffman (1986) could also represent a constitutional factor.

It is possible that defense mechanisms in general, which have been shown by Vaillant and Vaillant (1990) to be powerful predictors of lifetime psychopathology independently of childhood experience, represent constitutional vulnerability (or invulnerability) to environmental trauma. Given the evidence from such studies as Kauffman et al. (1979) that children with even the worst parents can become reasonably functioning adults, it is clear that there is no simple causal link between bad parenting and adult psychopathology. As reviewed by Rutter (1980), the pathway from risk factors in childhood to adult outcome is enormously complex. It is probable that any comprehensive theory of the causes of BPD will have to be multivariate and that borderline pathology is best considered a final common pathway for many etiologic factors.

SUMMARY

There is reasonably strong evidence that borderline individuals remember their parenting as abnormal on the parental dimensions of affection and control. There is fairly good reason to believe these reports, which make theoretical sense of much of the pathology seen in this population. Abnormal parental bonding does not by itself lead to BPD, but it is a likely risk factor for severe personality disorder.

REFERENCES

Adler G: Borderline Psychopathology and Its Treatment. New York, Jason Aronson, 1985

Armelius B-A, Kullgren G, Renberg F: Borderline diagnosis from hospital records: reliability and validity of Gunderson's Diagnostic Interview for Borderlines (DIB). J Nerv Ment Dis 173:32–34, 1985

Bowlby J: Attachment and Loss, Vol 1: Attachment. New York, Basic Books, 1969

Bowlby J: Attachment and Loss, Vol 2: Separation: Anxiety and Anger. New York, Basic Books, 1973

Bowlby J: Attachment and Loss, Vol 3: Loss: Sadness and Depression. New York, Basic Books, 1980

Browne A, Finkelhor D: Impact of child sexual abuse: a review of the literature. Psychol Bull 99:66–77, 1986

Byrne CP, Velamoor VR, Cernovsky ZZ, et al: A comparison of borderline and schizophrenic patients for childhood life events and parent-child relationships. Can J Psychiatry 35:590–595, 1990

Coccaro EF, Siever LJ, Klar HM, et al: Serotonergic studies in patients with affective and personality disorders: correlates with suicidal and impulsive aggressive behavior. Arch Gen Psychiatry 46:587–599, 1989

Feldman RB, Guttman HA: Families of borderline patients: literal-minded parents, borderline parents, and parental protectiveness. Am J Psychiatry 141:1392–1396, 1984

Frank H, Hoffman N: Borderline empathy: an empirical investigation. Compr Psychiatry 27:387–395, 1986

Frank H, Hoffman N: Borderline empathy: constitutional considerations. Compr Psychiatry 28:412–415, 1987

Frank H, Paris J: Recollections of family experience in borderline patients. Arch Gen Psychiatry 38:1031–1034, 1981

Fromuth ME: The relationship of childhood sexual abuse with later psychological and sexual adjustment in a sample of college women. Child Abuse Negl 10:5–15, 1986

Goldberg RL, Mann LS, Wise TN, et al: Parental qualities as perceived by borderline personality disorders. Hillside J Clin Psychiatry 7:134–140, 1985

Gunderson JG: Borderline Personality Disorder. Washington, DC, American Psychiatric Press, 1984

Gunderson JG, Zanarini ME: Pathogenesis of borderline personality, in American Psychiatric Press Review of Psychiatry, Vol 8. Edited by Tasman A, Hales RE, Frances AJ. Washington, DC, American Psychiatric Press, 1989, pp 25–49

Gunderson JG, Kerr J, Englund DW: The families of borderlines: a comparative study. Arch Gen Psychiatry 37:27–33, 1980

Herman JL, Perry JC, van der Kolk BA: Childhood trauma in borderline personality disorder. Am J Psychiatry 146:490–495, 1989

Hoffman N, Frank H: Borderline empathy and borderline pathology: an empirical investigation. Compr Psychiatry 27:387–395, 1986

Kauffman C, Grunebaum H, Cohler B, et al: Superkids: competent children of psychotic mothers. Am J Psychiatry 136:1398–1402, 1979

Kiesler DJ: The 1982 interpersonal circle: a taxonomy for complementarity in interpersonal transactions. Psychol Rev 90:185–214, 1983

Klein DF: Psychopharmacological treatment and delineation of borderline disorders, in Borderline Personality Disorders: The Concept, the Syndrome, the Patients. Edited by Hartocollis P. New York, International Universities Press, 1977, pp 365–383

Leary T: Interpersonal Diagnosis of Personality. New York, Guilford, 1957

Levy D: Maternal Overprotection. New York, Columbia University Press, 1943

Links PS, Steiner M, Huxley G: The occurrence of borderline personality disorder in the families of borderline patients. Journal of Personality Disorders 2:14–20, 1988

Links P, Boiago I, Huxley G, et al: Sexual abuse and biparental failure as etiologic models in borderline personality disorder, in Family Environment and Borderline Personality Disorder. Edited by Links P. Washington, DC, American Psychiatric Press, 1990, pp 105–120

Masterson J: Borderline and Narcissistic Disorders. New York, Brunner/Mazel, 1981

Melges FT, Swartz MS: Oscillations of attachment in borderline personality disorder. Am J Psychiatry 146:1115–1120, 1989

Ogata SN, Silk KR, Goodrich S, et al: Childhood sexual and physical abuse in adult patients with borderline personality disorder. Am J Psychiatry 147:1008–1013, 1990

Paris J, Nowlis D, Brown R: Developmental factors in the outcome of borderline personality disorder. Compr Psychiatry 29:147–150, 1988

Paris J, Frank H: Perceptions of parental bonding in borderline patients. Am J Psychiatry 146:1498–1499, 1989

Paris J, Frank H, Buonvino M, et al: Recollections of parental behavior and Axis II cluster diagnosis. Journal of Personality Disorders 5:102–106, 1991

Parker G: Parental Overprotection: A Risk Factor in Psychosocial Development. New York, Grune & Stratton, 1983

Peters SD: Child abuse and later psychological problems, in Lasting Effects of Child Sexual Abuse. Edited by Wyatt GE, Powell GJ, Peters SD. New York, Sage, 1988, pp 101–118

Petti TA, Vela RM: Borderline disorders of childhood: an overview. J Am Acad Child Adolesc Psychiatry 29:327–337, 1990

Robins LN, Schoenberg SP, Holmes SJ, et al: Early home environment and retrospective recall: a test for concordance between siblings with and without psychiatric disorders. Am J Orthopsychiatry 55:27–41, 1985

Rowe DC: Environmental and genetic influences on dimensions of perceived parenting. Developmental Psychology 17:203–208, 1981

Russell DEH: The Secret Trauma: Incest in the Lives of Girls and Women. New York, Basic Books, 1986

Rutter M: Scientific Foundations of Developmental Psychiatry. London, Heinemann, 1980

Schaefer ES: A circumplex model for maternal behavior. J Abnorm Soc Psychol 59:226–235, 1959

Soloff PH, Millward JW: Developmental histories of borderline patients. Compr Psychiatry 23:574–588, 1983

Stone MH: The Fate of Borderline Patients: Successful Outcome and Psychiatric Practice. New York, Guilford, 1990

Swartz M, Blazer D, George L, et al: Estimating the prevalence of borderline personality disorder in the community. Journal of Personality Disorders 4:257–272, 1990

Vaillant GE, Vaillant CO: Natural history of male psychological health, XII: a 45-year study of predictors of successful aging at age 65. Am J Psychiatry 147:31–37, 1990

Wiggins JS: Circumplex models of interpersonal behavior in clinical psychology, in Handbook of Research Methods in Clinical Psychology. Edited by Kendall PC, Butcher JN. New York, Wiley, 1982, pp 183–221

Zanarini MC, Gunderson JG, Marino MF, et al: Childhood experiences of borderline patients. Compr Psychiatry 30:18–25, 1989

Zweig-Frank H, Paris J: Parents' emotional neglect and overprotection according to the recollections of patients with borderline personality disorder. Am J Psychiatry 148:648–651, 1991

Developmental Factors in Borderline Personality Disorder and Borderline Personality Organization

John F. Clarkin, Ph.D.
Otto F. Kernberg, M.D.

I N THIS CHAPTER WE CONSIDER IN DETAIL BOTH THE PHE-
nomenological description (Axis II) and the struc-
tural diagnosis (borderline personality organization) of the borderline
patient. Subsequently, we examine the psychodynamic hypotheses and
related empirical data on the etiology of these conditions. A central thesis
here is that DSM-III-R Axis II borderline personality disorder (BPD) is
inadequate in its definitional criteria and in the way it is separated from
other Axis II disorders, which are conceived as distinct and unrelated.
Empirical studies of the overlap of BPD with other Axis II disorders and
family studies of BPD both are congruent with the theoretical articulation
of borderline personality organization (BPO), which is a broader concept
than BPD and one with an explicated theoretical conceptualization. A
combination of Axis II behaviors and structural diagnosis is most useful.

Axis II Borderline Personality Disorder Criteria

Theoretical Background

The initial formulation of the Axis II BPD in DSM-III (American Psychiatric Association 1980) was characterized by a concern to distinguish it
from schizotypal personality disorder (Spitzer et al. 1979). The highly
touted atheoretical orientation of DSM-III was not atheoretical at all. The

BPD criteria are, in fact, a mixture of behaviors and traits from various clinical orientations (Stone 1988), doing justice to none of them. In selecting a few criteria from each system, and in selecting only criteria that could be reliably assessed across clinicians with different theoretical orientations and training, the resulting eight criteria are too few in number to cover the salient issues and are stated at a concrete level of abstraction that becomes simplistic at times (e.g., criteria for identity diffusion), missing the heart of the clinical matter. This short set of criteria from several theoretical orientations is hardly adequate for research and clinical practice.

Criteria

The eight DSM-III-R (American Psychiatric Association 1987) criteria cover five different content areas: *identity diffusion* (one criterion); *dysfunctional affects* such as labile moods, intense and uncontrolled anger, and feelings of emptiness and boredom (three criteria); *disturbed interpersonal relations* (such as intense interpersonal relations characterized by idealization and devaluation) and *fear of real or imagined abandonment* (two criteria); *impulsive behavior* in two or more areas (one criterion); and *self-destructive and suicidal behavior* (one criterion). According to Stone (1988), the source of these criteria are the writings of Kernberg (identity, impulsivity, emptiness, boredom) and Gunderson (unstable intense relations, impulsivity, anger, self-damaging acts, affective instability, problems being alone).

CLUSTERS OF BORDERLINE PERSONALITY DISORDER

Lists of isolated criteria selected from various theoretical orientations are not adequate for research or treatment planning. A set of criteria with empirical interrelationships is more theoretically satisfying and more useful for further research. For example, to research the origins of borderline pathology in the family environment and family genetics, clusters of symptoms with construct validity are needed. To plan treatment interventions such as pharmacological targets, traits (not diagnostic categories) that have behaviors that form a coherent structure are the target of specific drugs (e.g., Cowdry 1987). In an attempt to obtain some conceptual coherence using the DSM-III BPD criteria, we clustered the eight criteria in a sample of 465 borderline patients (Hurt et al. 1990). The assumption of this work was that the interrelationships between the criteria might indicate possible underlying causal relationships and hence possible treatment foci (Hurt and Clarkin 1990).

Using this methodology, we isolated three clusters of BPD symptoms (see Figure 8–1). The first cluster, the *identity cluster*, is composed of Axis II criteria concerning identity diffusion, feelings of emptiness and boredom, and intolerance of being alone. The second cluster, the *affective cluster*, is composed of criteria for labile moods, uncontrolled and inappropriate anger, and unstable interpersonal relationships characterized by idealization and devaluation. The third cluster, the *impulse cluster*, is composed of impulsivity in two or more areas and self-destructive behavior.

Not only are the clusters empirically derived, but they also seem to have face validity. As expected from theory, identity diffusion correlates with feelings of emptiness. Intolerance of being alone is easily conceived as a need for others, furthering self-definition. The affect cluster contains anger, labile moods, and the interpersonal expression of anger (i.e., shifting relationships in which extremes of idealization and devaluation occur). Finally, it seems reasonable that impulsive acts (concerning food,

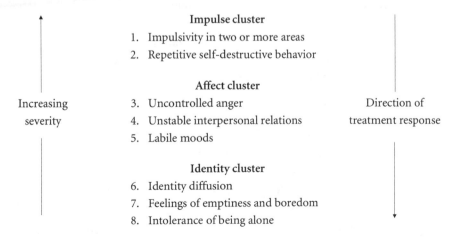

Figure 8–1. Clusters of symptomatology in borderline personality disorder

alcohol and drugs, promiscuous sex, etc.) might correlate with suicidal and self-destructive actions.

The impulsivity cluster is composed of actual behaviors (not personality traits), behaviors that come and go depending upon the condition of the patient and the stability of current object relations. In contrast, the affective cluster reflects a more trait-like condition of poor affect regulation and modulation, and the identity cluster relates to a more enduring aspect of identity formation. As we will see later, in the structural analysis of the borderline patient (and related narcissistic, antisocial, and histrionic personality disorders), the impulsive behaviors are not part of the personality structure but rather are resulting symptomatic behaviors that fluctuate with time.

Because a patient needs five of the eight criteria to meet the DSM-III-R BPD categorization, the patient may be borderline having none, one, two, or all three of the complete clusters. In our samples, the most commonly diagnosed BPD patient is one who meets criteria for the affect and impulse clusters. The most severely disturbed BPD patients are those with all three clusters (see Figure 8–1). These patients have disturbances in all three areas of human functioning: behavior (impulse cluster), affect (affective instability cluster), and cognition (identity cluster). The less disturbed borderline patients have the affect and/or the identity cluster. In reverse order to the severity of the disorder, the treatment response over time tends to involve, first, some change in the impulsive behavior, followed by some control of affect modulation and gradual change in identity formation. This order of change has been noted in our own psychotherapy research project (Clarkin et al. 1992). We also see this progression of change in the five successfully treated BPD patients documented by Waldinger and Gunderson (1984).

Etiology: Family Environment and Family History Studies

Given the behavioral and phenomenological criteria that can be reliably assessed, BPD (as opposed to BPO [see below]) can and has guided research concerning the family environment and family history of these patients. We will ask a number of questions from these studies:

1. What are the salient characteristics of the family environment that impacted on the BPD patient in the developmental years? Are those data consistent with the psychodynamic formulation of BPO, described later in this chapter? [To be consistent with the dynamic formulation, such a history would include early expression of anger by the patient, aggression in the family environment, events in the family environment that might stimulate aggression, and difficulty handling that aggression.]

2. What are the characteristics of the relatives of BPD patients, characteristics that could relate to both the heredity and the environment of the patient? [To be consistent with the dynamic formulation of BPO, such a family history would include the incidence of behaviors and conditions consistent with poor modulation and integration of intense anger and hostility.]

Family Environment

Family environment studies are relatively consistent in suggesting that the BPD patient is likely to experience early separation and loss of parental figures, and family disturbance including conflict, physical abuse, and sexual abuse (see Chapters 6 and 7).

Research suggests that the relationship between child and parents is disrupted in samples of borderline patients. Disruption takes the form of early physical separations and attitudes of parents toward children. In one sample of borderline outpatients (Zanarini et al. 1989) nearly one-half of the patients experienced a significant separation before age 6, and a majority experienced such a separation before age 18. This finding was not different from that seen in patients with antisocial personality disorder, but it did differ from what was seen in patients with other personality disorders. Likewise, in another sample (Links et al. 1988), BPD patients experienced in childhood more separation from caretakers than did control subjects. This early separation from parental figures in BPD patients is more likely to be due to marital separation than death of a parent. Although it is methodologically weak to ask adults about their memories of childhood, assuming the reality was as remembered, these studies reveal memories by BPD adults around themes that are different from those of memories of other patient groups. BPD patients report both parents as being less caring (Goldberg et al. 1985; Paris and Frank 1989), and especially fathers as being less interested and approving (Frank and Paris 1981). Relationships with parents are seen by BPD patients as conflicted and negative, and mothers are remembered as being overinvolved (Soloff and Millward 1983a).

There are data to suggest that the interaction between borderline patients and their parents is not only conflicted but hostile in nature, as would be expected from the psychodynamic formulations of BPO. For example, in one sample, although overinvolvement with the mother was characteristic of all pathological groups, borderline subjects were unique in reporting overinvolvement with a negative tone. Zweig-Frank and Paris (1991) have found that individuals with BPD, based on the Diagnostic Interview for Borderlines (DIB), report overprotective parental relationships. Along with others (Links 1992), we suspect that overinvolvement plus a hostile tone might be characteristic of the early environment of the borderline patient. This conceptualization, which is reminiscent of the concept of expressed emotion as has been designated in schizophrenic samples, is also characteristic of depressed patients, a group more like that of borderline individuals.

It is possible that recollections of specific childhood events, such as physical abuse and sexual abuse, are more reliable than those of general feelings and global impressions. In studies that assess the recollection of physical and sexual abuse of the BPD patient, the incidence seems high relative to that seen in other comparison groups. Numerous studies have linked sexual and physical child abuse to the development of BPD (Bryer et al. 1987; Herman et al. 1989; Links et al. 1988; Ogata et al. 1990; Stone 1990; Zanarini et al. 1989). In several samples, sexual abuse is reported for 25% of the sample, and physical abuse is reported for up to 50% of the sample. Most probably, prolonged and varied abuse is more detrimental than isolated events. In fact, Bryer et al. (1987), using a questionnaire and other self-report instruments, found that subjects who had experienced both physical and sexual abuse had higher mean borderline symptom scores than those with more limited abuse or those without abuse.

The prevalence of psychiatric disorders in the relatives of BPD patients is informative both from a genetic point of view and from the perspective of how these disturbed relatives might influence the family environment. In general, it appears that the incidence of schizophrenia is low and that the incidence of affective disorder is high (Soloff and Millward 1983a), especially if the borderline patient has a history of major depression (Pope et al. 1983). More specifically, however, the families of borderline patients have a higher incidence of borderline type behaviors (Loranger et al. 1982), alcoholism and alcohol abuse (Loranger and Tulis 1985), and antisocial personality disorder (Soloff and Millward 1983b) and other "dramatic cluster" (histrionic, borderline, antisocial) personality disorders (Pope et al. 1983). As might be expected, parental psychopathology and psychiatric disorders are linked to environmental events, and, in fact, in one sample these conditions increased the risk of childhood early loss or separation, sexual and physical abuse, and nonintact parental marriage (Links et al. 1990).

Summary

As data have accumulated on patients who meet DSM-III and DSM-III-R Axis II BPD criteria, it has become increasingly clear that this diagnosis or phenomenological description alone is inadequate. There are 93 ways to meet five, six, seven, or eight criteria out of a list of eight. Thus, patients who meet the categorical designation of BPD are quite heterogeneous. Most BPD patients also meet criteria for a number of comorbid conditions on both Axis I and Axis II. The overlap of the various Axis II disorders is so extensive as to call into question the separate existence of many of them.

Family history studies show a preponderance of borderline, substance abuse, and antisocial personality traits in relatives, which has led others such as Gunderson and Zanarini (1989) to suggest that the core problem for borderline individuals is impulse and action. Kernberg's underlying notion of BPO is quite congruent with these data. Given these limitations of the narrow, phenomenologically described BPD, we will consider the theoretical construction of BPO.

BORDERLINE PERSONALITY ORGANIZATION

Theoretical Background

A recent review (Gunderson and Zanarini 1989) suggests that there are three predominant psychodynamic etiologic theories concerning borderline personality pathology: Kernberg's theory emphasizing excessive aggression, a theoretical orientation emphasizing maternal withdrawal (Masterson and Rinsley 1975), and a position emphasizing introjective failure (Kohut 1971). Rather than simply review once more the same material and do justice to none, we will explicate the background to the formulation of BPO (Kernberg 1975) and its etiology.

In our view, BPO constitutes a broad spectrum of character pathology or personality disorders having in common a lack of integration of the concept of self and of the concept of significant others—that is, the syndrome of identity diffusion. This syndrome is characterized by chronic difficulties in assessing in an integrated way one's own motivations, behavior, and interpersonal interactions, and, by the same token, the motivation and integrated aspects of those others who are centrally significant in one's life. Identity diffusion underlies the chronic interpersonal difficulties of patients with BPO, their chaotic interactions in intimate relationships, and their failure in empathy and accurate assessment of their own and their significant others' intentions and actions. Identity diffusion differentiates patients with BPO, constituting the most severe spectrum of personality disorders, from neurotic personality organization—that is, patients with less severe character pathology or personality disorders who have an integrated sense of self and the capacity for integrated conception of significant others (i.e., normal identity formation).

A second major characteristic of BPO is the dominance of primitive defense mechanisms centering around the mechanism of splitting. These defense mechanisms have in common their dealing with unconscious intrapsychic conflict by mutual dissociation of contradictory aspects or motivations involved in such intrapsychic conflicts, and by a corresponding tendency toward oscillations between contradictory ego states that are respectively characterized by idealized "all good" and persecutory "all bad" experiences of self and others. These primitive defense mechanisms (i.e., splitting, projective identification, omnipotence, omnipotent control, primitive idealization, devaluation, and denial) are also characterized by behavioral components that tend to induce serious chaos and confusion in interpersonal relations. Clinically they are reflected in the apparent unpredictability, impulsivity, manipulativeness, blaming tendencies, arrogance, and helplessness typical of borderline patients, and, above all, in the lack of impulse control and of modulation of primitive affects, particularly anxiety, depression, and rage.

A third characteristic of BPO is the individual's maintenance of the capacity for reality testing—that is, the capacity for differentiating, when confronted with his or her behaviors, an intrapsychic origin from an external origin of stimuli; an awareness of differences between self and others; and the capacity for maintaining empathy with ordinary social criteria of reality. Reality testing differentiates BPO from psychotic disorders, including atypical psychotic conditions that may mask as personality disorders.

Structural Criteria

The Syndrome of Identity Diffusion

Clinically, identity diffusion is represented by a poorly integrated concept of the self and of significant others. It is reflected in the subjective experience of chronic emptiness, contradictory self-perceptions, contradictory behavior that cannot be integrated in an emotionally meaningful way, and shallow, flat, impoverished perceptions of others. Diagnostically, identity diffusion appears in the patient's inability to convey significant interactions with others to an interviewer, who thus cannot emotionally empathize with the patient's conception of himself or herself and others in such interactions.

Identity diffusion is also reflected in descriptions of significant persons in the patient's life that do not permit the interviewer "to put them together" in such a way as to gain any clear picture of them. The description of significant others is frequently so grossly contradictory that they sound more like caricatures than like real people.

An intimately related structural issue has to do with the quality of object relations: the stability and depth of the patient's relations with significant others as manifested by warmth, dedication, concern, and tactfulness. Other qualitative aspects are empathy, understanding, and the ability to maintain a relationship when it is invaded by conflict or frustration. The quality of object relations is largely dependent on identity integration, which includes not only the degree of integration but also the temporal continuity of the patient's concept of self and others. Normally, we experience ourselves consistently throughout time under varying circumstances and with different people, and we experience conflict when contradictions in our self concept emerge. The same applies to our experience of others. But in BPO, this temporal continuity is lost; such patients have little capacity for realistic evaluations of others. Borderline patients' long-term relations are characterized by an increasingly distorted perception of others. These individuals fail to achieve real empathy, and their relations with others are chaotic or shallow. In addition, intimate relations are usually contaminated by condensation of genital and pregenital conflicts.

Primitive Defense Mechanisms

Repression and such related high-level mechanisms as reaction formation, isolation, undoing, intellectualization, and rationalization protect the ego from intrapsychic conflicts by the rejection of a drive derivative or its ideational representation, or both, from the conscious ego. Splitting and other related mechanisms protect the ego from conflicts by means of dissociation or actively keeping apart contradictory experiences of the self and significant others. When such mechanisms predominate, contradictory ego states are alternatively activated. As long as these contradictory ego states can be kept separate from each other, anxiety related to these conflicts is prevented or controlled.

The mechanism of primitive dissociation or splitting and the associated mechanisms of primitive idealization, primitive types of projection (particularly projective identification), denial, omnipotence, and devaluation may be elicited in the clinical interaction of patients and diagnostician. These defenses protect the borderline patient from intrapsychic conflict but at the cost of weakening ego functioning, thereby reducing his or her adaptive effectiveness and flexibility in the interview and in life generally.

Splitting. Probably the clearest manifestation of splitting is the division of external objects in "all good" and "all bad," with the concomitant possibility of complete, abrupt shifts of an object from one extreme compartment to the other (i.e., sudden and complete reversals of all feelings and conceptualizations about a particular person). Extreme repetitive oscillation between contradictory self concepts is another manifestation of the mechanism of splitting.

Primitive idealization.   Primitive idealization complicates the tendency
to see external objects as either totally good or totally bad by increasing
artificially and pathologically their quality of "goodness" or "badness."
Primitive idealization creates unrealistic, all-good and powerful images;
this may be reflected in the interaction with the diagnostician by treating
him or her as an ideal, omnipotent, or godly figure on whom the patient
depends unrealistically. The interviewer or some other idealized person
may be seen as a potential ally against equally powerful (and equally
unrealistic) "all bad" objects.

Early forms of projection, especially projective identification.   In contrast to higher levels of projection characterized by the patient's attributing to the other an impulse he or she has repressed in himself or herself,
primitive forms of projection, particularly projective identification, are
characterized by 1) the tendency to continue to experience the impulse
that is simultaneously being projected onto the other person, 2) fear of
the other person under the influence of that projected impulse, and 3) the
need to control the other person under the influence of this mechanism.
Projective identification therefore implies intrapsychic as well as behavioral interpersonal aspects of the patient's interactions, and this may be
reflected dramatically in the diagnostic interview.

Denial.   Denial in borderline patients is typically exemplified by denial
of two emotionally independent areas of consciousness. (We might say
that denial here simply reinforces splitting.) Patients are aware that their
perceptions, thoughts, and feelings about themselves or other people at
one time or another are completely opposite to those they have had at
other times, but their memory has no emotional relevance and cannot
influence the way they feel now. Denial may be manifested in these
patients as a complete lack of concern, anxiety, or emotional reaction
about an immediate, serious, pressing need, conflict, or danger in their
lives, so that these patients calmly convey their cognitive awareness of the
situation while denying its emotional implications. Alternately, an entire
area of these patients' subjective awareness may be shut out from their
subjective experience, thus protecting them from a potential area of
conflict.

Omnipotence and devaluation. Both omnipotence and devaluation are derivatives of splitting operations affecting the self and object representations and are typically represented by the activation of ego states reflecting a highly inflated, grandiose self relating to depreciated, emotionally degrading representations of others. Narcissistic personalities, a special subgroup of BPO, present these defensive operations quite strikingly. Omnipotence and devaluation may become manifest in the patient's descriptions of significant others and his or her interactions with them and in his or her behavior during the diagnostic interview.

Reality Testing

Reality testing is defined by the capacity to differentiate self from nonself and intrapsychic from external origins of perceptions and stimuli, and the capacity to evaluate realistically one's own affect, behavior, and thought content in terms of ordinary social norms. Clinically, reality testing is recognized by 1) the absence of hallucinations and delusions; 2) the absence of grossly inappropriate or bizarre affect, thought content, or behavior; and 3) the capacity to empathize with and clarify other people's observations of what seem to them inappropriate or puzzling aspects of the patient's affects, behavior, or thought content within the context of ordinary social interactions.

Table 8–1 summarizes the differentiation of personality organization in terms of the three structural criteria of identity integration, defensive operations, and reality testing.

Nonspecific Manifestations of Ego Weakness

The "nonspecific" manifestations of ego weakness include the absence of 1) anxiety tolerance, 2) impulse control, and 3) developed channels of sublimation. These manifestations are to be differentiated from the "specific" aspects of ego weakness: the ego-weakening consequences of the predominance of primitive defensive mechanisms. *Anxiety tolerance* refers to the degree to which the patient can tolerate a load of tension greater than what he or she habitually experiences without developing increased symptoms or generally regressive behavior. *Impulse control* refers to the degree to which the patient can experience instinctual urges or strong emotions without having to act on them immediately against his or her better judg-

Table 9-2   Differentiation of personality organization

Structural criteria	Neurotic	Borderline	Psychotic
Identity integration	Self representations and object representations are sharply delimited. Integration identity: contradictory images of self and others are integrated into comprehensive conceptions.	Identity diffusion: contradictory aspects of self and others are poorly integrated and kept apart.	Self and object representations are poorly delimited or else there is delusional identity.
Defensive operations	Repression and high-level defenses: reaction formation, isolation, undoing, rationalization, intellectualization. Defenses protect patient from intrapsychic conflict. Interpretation improves functioning.	Mainly splitting and lower-level defenses: primitive idealization, projective identification, denial, omnipotence, devaluation.	Defenses protect patient from disintegration and self/object merging. Interpretation leads to regression.
Reality testing	Capacity to test reality is preserved: differentiation of self from nonself, intrapsychic from external origins of perceptions and stimuli. Capacity exists to evaluate self and others realistically and in depth.	Alterations occur in relationship with reality and in feelings of reality.	Capacity to test reality is lost.

ment and interest. *Sublimatory effectiveness* refers to the degree to which the patient can invest himself or herself in values beyond his or her immediate self-interest or beyond self-preservation—particularly to the degree to which he or she is able to develop creative resources in some area beyond his or her natural background, education, or training.

Chronic Interpersonal Difficulties

Chronic interpersonal difficulties are a direct consequence of identity diffusion—the incapacity to assess accurately others' behavior and the capacity to assess one's own behavior in interpersonal relations. As a general rule, the more intense the relations with others, the more contradictory and chaotic these relations become, leading to severe interpersonal conflicts at work and school, in intimate sexual relations, and in maintaining chronically inappropriate and ineffective relations with one's own family members.

Lack of Superego Integration

A lack of superego integration, another consequence of identity diffusion, descriptively relates to antisocial personality disorder diagnosis and features and to prognosis. The defensive lack of integration of self and object representations affects the integration of idealized and persecutory superego precursors as well. In other words, the internalized demands for ideal behavior and threats of punishment and of guilt feelings cannot be integrated into a harmonious, consistent, stable internalized system of morality. This lack of integration of superego varies across the spectrum of borderline patients, and its severity is related to the severity of prognosis for psychotherapeutic treatment. Superego integration can be evaluated by studying the degree to which the patient identifies with ethical values and has normal guilt as a major regulator. Regulation of self-esteem by excessively severe guilt feelings or depressive mood swings represents a pathological superego integration (typical of neurotic organization) in contrast to the modulated, specifically focused, self-critical functions of the normal individual in terms of ethical values. Superego integration is indicated by the degree to which the person is able to regulate his or her functioning according to ethical principles; to abstain from the exploitation, manipulations, or mistreatment of others; and to maintain honesty and moral integrity in the absence of external control.

Etiology

The internalization of object relations is a crucial organizing factor for both ego and superego development. Introjections, identifications, and ego identity formation constitute a progressive sequence in the process of internalization of object relations (Erikson 1950). The essential components of internalized object relations are self representations, object representations, and specific affect states or dispositions linking each self representation with a corresponding object representation. Two essential tasks that the early ego has to accomplish in rapid succession are 1) to differentiate the self representation from object representations and 2) to integrate self representations and object representations built up under the influence of libidinal drive derivatives and their related affects with their corresponding self representations and object representations that were constructed under the influence of aggressive drive derivatives and their related affects (Kernberg 1976).

The first task is accomplished in part under the influence of the development of the apparatuses of primary autonomy; perception and memory traces help to detect the origin of stimuli and gradually differentiate self representations and object representations. That first task fails to a major extent in the psychoses: a pathological fusion between self representations and object representations results in a failure in the differentiation of ego boundaries and, therefore, in the differentiation of self from nonself. In BPO, differentiation of self representations from object representations is sufficient to permit the establishment of firm ego boundaries and a concomitant differentiation of the self from others.

The second task, the integration of libidinally associated and aggressively associated self representations and object representations, fails to a great extent in borderline patients, mainly because of the pathological predominance of pregenital aggression. The resulting lack of synthesis of contradictory self representations and object representations interferes with the integration of the self concept and with the integration of object representations—that is, the establishment of total object relations and object constancy. The need to preserve the good self representations and the good object representations and good external objects in the presence of dangerous all-bad self representations and object representations leads to a defensive division of the ego. What was at first a simple defect in integration is used actively to keep good and bad self representations and object representations apart. This is, in essence, the mechanism of splitting. It is reinforced by subsidiary defensive operations, especially projective mechanisms, and thus results in an ego organization different from that in which repression and related mechanisms are used.

All-good and all-bad self representations and object representations seriously interfere with superego integration because they create fantastic ideals of power, greatness, and perfection, rather than the more realistic demands and goals of an ego ideal constructed under the influence of integrated, modulated, ideal self representations and object representations. Projection of bad self representations and object representations results, through reintrojection of distorted experiences of the frustrating and punishing aspects of the parents, in a pathological predominance of sadistic superego forerunners and a subsequent incapacity to integrate the idealized superego components with the sadistically threatening ones. All of this leads to a lack of superego integration and a concomitant tendency to reproject superego nuclei. Thus, dissociative or splitting processes in the ego are reinforced by the absence of the normal integrative contribution of the superego so that contradictory internalized demands, together with the insufficiency of the ego's repressive mechanisms, contribute to the establishment of contradictory, instinctually infiltrated, pathological character traits. This development is characteristic of BPO.

In contrast, when good and bad internalized object relations are so integrated that an integrated self concept and a related integrated representational world of object representations develop, a stable ego identity is achieved. At that point, a central ego core is protected from unacceptable drive derivatives by a stable repressive barrier, and the defensive character traits that develop have the characteristics of reaction formations or inhibitory traits. The development of that level of integration within the ego also creates the preconditions for the integration of the sadistically determined superego forerunners with the ego ideal and the subsequent capacity to internalize the realistic, demanding, and prohibitive aspects of the parents. This entire process fosters further superego integration and, eventually, depersonification and abstraction within the superego. The superego may then act as a higher level organizer of the ego, providing further pressures for a harmonious integration of any remaining contradictory trends within the ego. The modulation of such an integrated, more realistically determined superego permits a more flexible management of instinctual drive derivatives on the ego's part, with the appearance of sublimatory character traits.

The basic cause of these developments in borderline patients is their failure to integrate the libidinally and aggressively determined self and object representations. Such a lack of integration derives from the pathological predominance of aggressively determined self and object representations and a related failure to establish a sufficiently strong ego core around the (originally nondifferentiated) good self and object representations. The problem with borderline patients is that the intensity of aggressively determined self and object representations and of defensively idealized, "all good" self and object representations makes integration impossible. Because of the implicit threat to the good object relations, bringing together extreme loving and hateful images of the self and of significant others would trigger unbearable anxiety and guilt; therefore, there is an active defensive separation of such contradictory self and object representations. In other words, primitive dissociation or splitting becomes a major defensive operation.

Our view of the etiology of these psychostructural characteristics of BPO dovetail with Margaret Mahler's (Mahler et al. 1975) conception of early stages of psychosocial development predating the integration of the concepts of the self and of significant others (i.e., the stage of object constancy). In Mahler's conception, the normal stage of early symbiosis, characterized by lack of differentiation between self representations and object representations under conditions of extreme affect activation, may be pathologically maintained in psychotic conditions where self is not differentiated from others, self representation and representation of other are fused or nondifferentiated, and reality testing is therefore absent or lost. That symbiotic stage of development, probably active only during a few months in the first year of life, may become pathologically fixated and is characteristic of the psychic organization of psychotic disorders of childhood and adulthood, particularly schizophrenia, schizoaffective disorders, and major affective disorders.

In contrast, the stage of separation-individuation, normally dominant in the second half of the first year of life and up to the completion of the third year of life, is characterized by the differentiation between self and others under conditions of both extremely positive and extremely negative affect activation, so that reality testing is maintained. At the same time, however, self representations and object representations activated under conditions of idealized and persecutory experiences are dissociated or split off from each other so that an integration of the concept of self and an integration of the concept of significant others, and particularly the incorporation of their respective differential sexual characteristics, are not yet achieved. Pathology of this stage of separation-individuation results in the fixation of a pathological personality structure with these dissociated characteristics, precisely what we consider to be the case in BPO.

Margaret Mahler's stage of object constancy, normally initiated in the fourth year of life and under the dominance of advanced oedipal conflicts, characterizes neurotic personality organization. Because of the fixation at a structural level that precedes object constancy, patients with BPO enter the advanced oedipal phases with a strong persistence of preoedipal conflicts, particularly preoedipal aggression. This leads to a pathological condensation between preoedipal and oedipal conflicts under the dominance of preoedipal aggression, a characteristic clinically reflected in intense, aggressive affects and severe distortions in the sexual life of these patients. All these considerations summarize our theory of the psychological structure of patients with BPO and the psychodynamic origins of this pathology. Patients with BPD as defined in DSM-III-R constitute a central subgroup of the broad spectrum of severe personality disorders just described.

A frequent finding in patients with BPO is the history of extreme frustrations and intense aggression (secondary or primary) during the first few years of life. Excessive pregenital and particularly oral aggression tends to be projected and causes a paranoid distortion of the early parental images, especially of the mother. Through the projection of predominantly oral-sadistic but also anal-sadistic impulses, the mother is seen as potentially dangerous, and hatred of the mother extends to hatred of both parents, who are later experienced as a "united group" by the child. There is a "contamination" of the father image by aggression primarily projected onto the mother and a lack of differentiation between mother and father under the influence of a lack of realistic differentiation of different objects that is influenced by excessive splitting operations. These tend to produce, in both sexes, a combined and dangerous father-mother image, with the result that all sexual relationships are later conceived of as dangerous and aggressively infiltrated.

At the same time, in an effort to escape from oral rage and fears, premature development of genital strivings takes place; this effort often miscarries because of the intensity of pregenital aggression, which contaminates genital strivings as well, and numerous pathological developments take place that differ in both sexes.

Relationship Between Borderline Personality Organization and Borderline Personality Disorder

It is interesting to consider the empirically derived clusters of BPD symptoms with the conceptualization of BPO. This consideration is in part circular, as some of the criteria for BPD were derived from the writings of Kernberg. However, while initially derived from these writings, the criteria were also tested in a survey of practicing clinicians as to their estimated prevalence and accuracy.

BPD identity cluster and BPO identity diffusion.   The most obvious area of compatibility is between the identity cluster of DSM-III criteria and BPO identity diffusion. The BPD criterion of identity diffusion in DSM-III-R is stated in superficial terms in order (apparently) to arrive at some reliability. The BPO concept highlights a lack of coherent sense of self both cross-sectionally (i.e., patient feels like different person in different settings and with different people) and longitudinally (i.e., patient feels a lack of personal continuity across time, and estrangement from the past). The BPD criteria of feelings of emptiness and boredom and the intolerance of being alone are relatively poor criteria. In DSM-III-R, intolerance of being alone has been changed to frantic reaction to feared or real abandonment. This has more to do with the disrupted interpersonal attachment to others made by the BPD patient.

BPO primitive defenses and the BPD affect cluster.   The intense ambivalence of the borderline patient is managed by defensive splitting and concomitant idealization and devaluation of others. Thus, the patient is prone to stormy relationships in which rapid shifts of cognitive evaluation and mood are present. This theoretical description of BPO primitive defenses has some resemblance to the BPD affect cluster, most clearly with the criterion of unstable relations with idealization and devaluation. While in the cluster analysis the criterion of unstable relations correlates with anger, we have noted clinically that some patients have the former without overt anger. On a more theoretical level, the BPD affect cluster is a direct result of the identity diffusion.

The BPD impulse cluster.   The BPD actions of the impulse cluster (impulsivity and repetitive self-destructive behavior) are conceptualized in the BPO construct as the direct result of reduction in flexibility and ego strength. The self is split into contradictory aspects, and therefore the patient shows nonspecific aspects of ego weakness in the form of poor impulse control, decrease in anxiety tolerance, and decrease in sublimatory capacity. Impulsive actions, then, are the outward symptoms of the underlying structural ego weakness and primitive defensive operations.

BPO reality testing.   The BPO construct of reality testing is not represented in the BPD criteria. In some ways, this construct was separated in the schizotypal personality disorder criteria. In fact, this is a good illustration of the kind of splitting off of criteria (often related in individuals) into separate "disorders" on Axis II, one of the reasons for the massive Axis II "comorbidity" in clinical samples. There is a substantial group of BPD patients with comorbid schizotypal personality disorder (Fyer et al. 1988). These BPD/SPD patients probably include patients with borderline structure (variable reality testing) and those who have a psychotic structure.

BPO and Axis II comorbidity.   With the accrual of data on clinical populations using the phenomenological and behavior criteria of DSM-III-R Axis II, it has become apparent that the "overlap" of Axis II disorders is massive. In most clinical populations the average patient has from three to four personality disorders. It is very rare that a patient meets criteria for BPD alone. Using data from Widiger et al. (1991), we have examined the prominent overlap of BPD with other Axis II disorders. These data are in a sense a direct empirical investigation of the BPO hypothesis. That is, in the BPO system, neurotic personality organization is composed of the obsessive-compulsive, hysterical, and depressive/masochistic personality disorders, and the borderline level of organization includes BPD, narcissistic, antisocial, histrionic, schizoid, and paranoid personality disorders. Thus, we would expect a high comorbidity rate between Axis II BPD and narcissistic, antisocial, and histrionic personality disorders. Collapsing data across many studies, as was done in Widiger et al. (1990), it seems clear that the overlap is as predicted, not only in the patients but in their first-degree relatives.

COMPARISON AND COMBINED USE
OF THE BORDERLINE PERSONALITY DISORDER
AND BORDERLINE PERSONALITY ORGANIZATION SYSTEMS

The criteria of BPD are related to BPO as specific behaviors are related to the underlying organization of behavior. The two are articulated at different levels of abstraction and thus provide alternative advantages and disadvantages. At the present time we are in a neo-Kraepelinian revolution in which the emphasis is on phenomenological criteria that can be reliably assessed (Blashfield 1984). BPO is a structural analysis of the patient's personality organization. This conceptualization is in contrast to the Axis II BPD phenomenological description of the symptoms and behaviors of the borderline patient.

Following from the first point, the reliable assessment of Axis II BPD is quite possible and seems within reach with the use of semistructured interviews. At this level of assessment the main threat to reliable and valid assessment is the honest and accurate reporting of the patient. If need be, independent observation from family members may be obtained to either ascertain or substantiate the BPD diagnosis and description. The reliable assessment of BPO, on the other hand, is dependent upon the clinical sophistication of the assessor. Kernberg (1984) has articulated a structural interview that consists of a planned, clinical interview that uses probes from the interactional material to explore the three constructs related to BPO. In addition, our research team has constructed a self-report questionnaire that assesses BPO (Oldham et al. 1985).

Some BPD criteria are not personality traits but rather behaviors and symptoms that fluctuate over time. For example, the patient fluctuates in terms of impulsive behavior and self-destructive behavior. In contrast, the BPO structures are seen as relatively stable across time, and the outward behavior of the patient may change depending upon the circumstances at the moment.

The overlap of the Axis II disorders is so extensive in clinical samples as to mock the very meaning of the word "overlap," which implies some unity and distinctness in the entities that overlap. This overlap as determined empirically in clinical samples is consistent with that hypothesized by the BPO construct.

Finally, the eight isolated criteria of BPD are not helpful in conceptualization of the disorder and in treatment planning. The BPD criteria of Axis II were selected by a committee from the clinical writings of Kernberg and Gunderson. The short set of criteria does justice to neither of the authors. These particular criteria were probably selected with an eye to which characteristics could be most reliably assessed by the minimally trained clinician, a goal that may be useful for reporting to insurance companies but not for theoretical articulation or to guide research. An atheoretical melange of phenomenological and behavioral criteria is not helpful in providing a conceptual approach to intervention. This is not totally surprising, and, in fact, this situation was anticipated by the authors of DSM-III, who clearly state in the introduction that treatment planning necessitates much more than what is contained in each set of criteria. In fact, the current criteria focused at a behavioral level to ensure reliability are most useful for considering medication and possibly for behavioral treatments that can be used to focus on separate and multiple behavioral areas. More surprising is the fact that these behavioral criteria are not as useful for research, suggesting that a rampant atheoretical approach may ultimately be fruitless. As noted in our discussion in this chapter on the etiology of BPD and BPO, the research on family factors strongly suggests that the so-called overlap of multiple Axis II disorders (or some underlying construct such as BPO) must be taken into full account.

REFERENCES

American Psychiatric Association: Diagnostic and Statistical Manual of Mental Disorders, 3rd Edition. Washington, DC, American Psychiatric Association, 1980

American Psychiatric Association: Diagnostic and Statistical Manual of Mental Disorders, 3rd Edition, Revised. Washington, DC, American Psychiatric Association, 1987

Blashfield RK: The Classification of Psychopathology: Neo-Kraepelinian and Quantitative Approaches. New York, Plenum, 1984

Bryer JB, Nelson BA, Miller JB, et al: Childhood sexual and physical abuse as factors in adult psychiatric illness. Am J Psychiatry 144:1426–1430, 1987

Clarkin JF, Koenigsberg H, Yeomans F, et al: Psychodynamic psychotherapy of the borderline patient, in Borderline Personality Disorder: Clinical and Empirical Perspectives. Edited by Clarkin JF, Marziali E, Munroe-Blum H. New York, Guilford, 1992, pp 268–287

Cowdry RW: Psychopharmacology of borderline personality disorder: a review. J Clin Psychiatry 48(no 8, suppl):15–22, 1987

Erikson EH: Childhood and Society. New York, WW Norton, 1950

Frank H, Paris J: Recollections of family experience in borderline patients. Arch Gen Psychiatry 38:1031–1034, 1981

Fyer MR, Frances AJ, Sullivan T, et al: Comorbidity of borderline personality disorder. Arch Gen Psychiatry 45:348–352, 1988

Goldberg RL, Mann LS, Wise TN, et al: Parental qualities as perceived by borderline personality disorders. Hillside J Clin Psychiatry 7:134–140, 1985

Gunderson JG, Zanarini MC: Pathogenesis of borderline personality, in American Psychiatric Press Review of Psychiatry, Vol 8. Edited by Tasman A, Hales RE, Frances AJ. Washington, DC, American Psychiatric Press, 1989, pp 25–48

Herman JL, Perry JC, van der Kolk BA: Childhood trauma in borderline personality disorder. Am J Psychiatry 146:490–495, 1989

Hurt SW, Clarkin JF: Borderline personality disorder: prototypic typology and the development of treatment manuals. Psychiatric Annals 20:13–18, 1990

Hurt SW, Clarkin JF, Widiger T, et al: Evaluation of DSM-III decision rules for case detection using joint conditional probability structures. Journal of Personality Disorders 4:121–130, 1990

Kernberg OF: Borderline Conditions and Pathological Narcissism. New York, Jason Aronson, 1975

Kernberg OF: The structural diagnosis of borderline personality organization. Paper presented at the International Conference on Borderline Disorders. Topeka, KS, March 1976

Kernberg OF: Severe Personality Disorders. New Haven, CT, Yale University Press, 1984

Kohut H: The Analysis of the Self. New York, International Universities Press, 1971

Links PS: Family environment and family psychopathology in the etiology of borderline personality disorder, in Borderline Personality Disorder: Clinical and Empirical Perspectives. Edited by Clarkin JF, Marziali E, Munroe-Blum H. New York, Guilford, 1992, pp 45–66

Links PS, Steiner M, Offord DR, et al: Characteristics of borderline personality disorder: a Canadian study. Can J Psychiatry 33:336–340, 1988

Links PS, Boiago I, Huxley G, et al: Sexual abuse and biparental failure as etiologic models in borderline personality disorder, in Family Environment and Borderline Personality Disorder. Edited by Links PS. Washington DC, American Psychiatric Press, 1990, pp 105–120

Loranger AW, Tulis EH: Family history of alcoholism in borderline personality disorder. Arch Gen Psychiatry 42:153–157, 1985

Loranger AW, Oldham JM, Tulis EH: Familial transmission of DSM-III borderline personality disorder. Arch Gen Psychiatry 39:795–799, 1982

Mahler MS, Pine F, Bergman A: The Psychological Birth of the Human Infant. New York, Basic Books, 1975

Masterson JF, Rinsley DB: The borderline syndrome: the role of the mother in the genesis and psychic structure of the borderline personality. Int J Psychoanal 56:163–177, 1975

Ogata SN, Silk KR, Goodrich S: The childhood experience of the borderline patient, in Family Environment and Borderline Personality Disorder. Edited by Links PS. Washington, DC, American Psychiatric Press, 1990, pp 85–103

Oldham J, Clarkin J, Appelbaum A, et al: A self-report instrument for borderline personality organization, in The Borderline: Current Empirical Research. Edited by McGlashan TH. Washington, DC, American Psychiatric Press, 1985, pp 1–18

Paris J, Frank H: Perceptions of parental bonding in borderline patients. Am J Psychiatry 146:1498–1499, 1989

Pope HG Jr, Jonas JM, Hudson JI, et al: The validity of DSM-III borderline personality disorder: a phenomenologic, family history, treatment response and long-term follow-up study. Arch Gen Psychiatry 40:23–30, 1983

Soloff PH, Millward JW: Developmental histories of borderline patients. Compr Psychiatry 24:574–588, 1983a

Soloff PH, Millward JW: Psychiatric disorders in the families of borderline patients. Arch Gen Psychiatry 40:37–44, 1983b

Spitzer RL, Endicott J, Gibbon M: Crossing the border into borderline personality and borderline schizophrenia. Arch Gen Psychiatry 36:17–24, 1979

Stone MH: Borderline personality disorder (Chapter 17), in Psychiatry, Vol 2. Edited by Michels R, Cavenar JO Jr. New York, Basic Books, 1988

Stone MH: Abuse and abusiveness in borderline personality disorder, in Family Environment and Borderline Personality Disorder. Edited by Links PS. Washington, DC, American Psychiatric Press, 1990, pp 131–148

Waldinger RJ, Gunderson JG: Completed psychotherapies with borderline patients. Am J Psychother 38:190–202, 1984

Widiger TA, Frances AJ, Harris M, et al: Comorbidity among Axis II disorders, in Personality Disorders: New Perspectives on Diagnostic Validity. Edited by Oldham JM. Washington, DC, American Psychiatric Press, 1991, pp 163–194

Zanarini MC, Gunderson JG, Marino MF, et al: Childhood experiences of borderline patients. Compr Psychiatry 30:18–25, 1989

Zweig-Frank H, Paris J: Parents' emotional neglect and overprotection according to the recollections of patients with borderline personality disorder. Am J Psychiatry 148:648–651, 1991

An Ego Psychological View of the Borderline Patient

Michael Porder, M.D.

T HE TERM "BORDERLINE" WAS FIRST USED TO DESCRIBE patients by the psychoanalyst Adolph Stern (1938) more than 50 years ago. Since then, analytic theories about the etiology of the borderline syndrome have tended to parallel the idea that borderline pathology lies between neurosis and psychosis. Thus, the developmental basis of the syndrome has been assumed to arise in early childhood. In the present chapter I present a challenge to this view, which fails to take into account the complexity of developmental pathways to adult psychopathology.

Stern (1938) himself suggested that failures in early mothering were related to the pathological narcissism of the borderline individual, providing a "soil" from which other pathology would evolve. He also suggested that these patients experienced an anxiety that derived from early in development and that their idealization of the analyst and childlike self-image also pointed to disturbances in very early childhood.

Klein (1946) referred to schizoid mechanisms rather than borderline patients, but her ideas were influential in later formulations of borderline individuals using primitive defense mechanisms such as splitting and projective identification. These mechanisms seemed to have antedated neurotic defenses and were hypothesized to have developed in infancy.

Greenacre (1971) also speculated that ego development could be interfered with by anxiety and trauma in the first 2 years of life. Another ego psychologist concerned with early disturbances of this kind was Jacobson (1954). The work of Mahler and Furer (1968) suggested that there was a specific period of vulnerability in early childhood: the separation-individuation phase. Mahler (1971) later suggested that disturbances in this phase could apply to borderline phenomena. Masterson (1972) suggested a developmental approach to borderline adolescents based on Mahler's theories, and, in collaboration with Rinsley, he developed a specific theory in which the mother's resistance to individuation produced a pathological regressive tie between borderline individuals and their mothers (Masterson and Rinsley 1975).

Perhaps the best known psychoanalytic theorist on the role of early development in the borderline syndrome is Kernberg, whose views are summarized in Chapter 8. Kernberg (1984) drew parallels between borderline pathology and the developmental observations of Mahler and her co-workers (Mahler 1971; Mahler and Furer 1968). He modified the time frame for the development of borderline pathology so that he no longer adhered to the Kleinian schema (Klein 1946), which linked primitive defenses to the first year of life. He changed his developmental sequence to bring it into line with the "rapprochement" subphase of the separation-individuation process, which includes the end of the second year and the beginning of the third year of life. This shift allowed his ideas to coincide with the increasing capacity of the child to use language and imagery and to begin to develop an organized fantasy life. Overall, however, Kernberg adhered to a developmental sequence of psychopathology that places psychoses within the first year of life; "borderline personality organization" between 9 months and 3 years of age; and neurosis and neurotic character pathology after that time, when the oedipal phase would begin, higher level defenses would be activated, and mature superego pathology with the sense of internalized guilt would be in place.

Another group of authors could be arbitrarily called the "developmentalists." This is a heterogeneous group who have in common the premise that borderline pathology is the result of a defect mainly in the development of very early object relations. For most of these authors this concept refers to the mother-child relationship during the first 2 years of life. Of course, all of the authors described above could potentially be placed into this category, but they focus more on dynamic conflicts and less on the failures of the early mothering experiences. Many of the "developmentalists" base their ideas on the work of Mahler on separation and individuation, while others draw heavily on the work of Winnicott and Kohut. Winnicott and Kohut have developed their ideas in a way that is clearly applicable to borderline patients, so they can be included in this group. Mahler (1971), on the other hand, only mentioned the possible applicability of her work to borderline patients in one paper, although others have built their own hypotheses on her theoretical structure.

Winnicott (1953/1958, 1960/1965) has developed two concepts that have been of considerable importance to many psychoanalysts who have written about the treatment of borderline patients. These are 1) transitional objects and transitional phenomena, and 2) the holding environment. The concept of transitional objects/transitional phenomena describes the child's ability to creatively imagine a "me/not me," one form of which is the transitional object. This cognitive developmental leap may be used as a bridging phenomenon in the development of object relations. Many analysts conceptualize their own role as similar to that of a transitional object, because they see themselves as becoming a soothing and comforting extension of the patient. Most recently, Adler (1989) has hypothesized that the patient's ability to use the transference to the analyst as a fantasy repeats this early developmental step, which can be fostered or squelched by the analyst. The *holding environment,* on the other hand, describes a safe haven where the infant can be alone or alone in the presence of the other, a protected space such as a good mother would provide. Each of these concepts describes a setting in which a "mothering" analyst can allow the patient to make up for the failures of the patient's mother (see Kernberg, Chapter 13).

Bion (1959, 1967) also utilized a theory of object relations to describe the treatment of borderline patients. According to Bion, the analyst should function as a "container," a repository for the patient's projected impulses and painful affects. During treatment the analyst must accept these projected impulses and affects for a period of time before they can be reintrojected by the patient in a more modified form. This experience in the transference will undo the mother's failure to offer herself as a "container" for her infant's anxieties and impulses.

Kohut (1971) was another "developmentalist" whose theory emphasized that the analyst should function as a "selfobject" so that the patient could undo his or her psychological defects. Observing patients whom he described as "narcissistic characters," Kohut postulated that there was a developmental failure in these patients' capacity to form a "cohesive self." They demonstrated regressive narcissistic structures that he called the "grandiose self" and the "idealized parent imago." Although he insisted that his patients were not borderline, the grandiosity of these patients and the idealized image of the analyst in the transference fit beautifully into many of the clinical descriptions of borderline patients. For Kohut, the analyst must offer himself as a selfobject in order to undo the developmental defects that prevented the patient from forming a cohesive self. The developmental failure of these patients is due to the lack of appropriate empathic responses by their parents, but unlike most of the other authors, Kohut believed that many of these failures could take place as late as latency, after the major psychic structures had been relatively well integrated.

Adler and Buie (Adler 1985, 1989; Buie 1985; Buie and Adler 1982–1983) have drawn heavily on Winnicott and Kohut to support their hypothesis that the crucial problems of borderline patients relate to "aloneness," "abandonment," and the incapacity to maintain "evocative recall" of the object. They believe that these conflicts that are common to all borderline patients originate in failures of early mothering, so that these patients must use the analyst as a transitional object, or as a self-object, in order to develop the "self-soothing introjects" necessary for healthier emotional development.

Rinsley and Masterson (Masterson 1972; Masterson and Rinsley 1975; Rinsley 1977) have a different focus. They believe that their borderline patients demonstrate clearly that the mothers of these patients rewarded regressive behavior in their children and strongly disapproved of their childrens' attempts at separation and individuation. Rinsley and Masterson recommend a therapy geared to reverse this specific dynamic, a kind of corrective emotional experience in which the analyst acts to counteract the pathological effects of the mother.

All of these theorists seem to be in agreement that borderline pathology evolves at a very early developmental stage and is related to either maternal failure or excessive conflict during the first 2 years of life. Anxiety is extreme, and primitive defenses that protect the integrity of the early ego are activated. Object relationships are immature and/or narcissistic, and there is an incapacity to maintain a stable sense of self or identity. Moreover, there is a blurring between inside and outside such that reality testing is compromised, although neither this ego function nor any of the other maladaptations are as severe as those seen in psychotic patients.

Most of the conflict is thus rooted clearly in the preoedipal phase of development, with an absence of the following: oedipal, triangular conflict; the use of higher-level defenses; or more mature superego conflicts centering around internalized guilt.

These authors all believe that there is a definite distinction between the neuroses and borderline syndrome and that patients in both of these groups are clearly distinguishable from psychotic patients. Borderline patients may be said to have a defect in their development that distorts all of their later ego maturation. As a result of these beliefs, these analysts look to a special etiology for the borderline condition that is clearly different from that of the neuroses and that of the psychoses. In addition, all of these theorists recommend treatment approaches based on their developmental hypotheses.

The Kris Study Group of the New York Psychoanalytic Institute began a reassessment of these ideas in 1973, and Abend, Willick, and Porder (Abend et al. 1983, 1988) came to significantly different conclusions from most analysts. The study involved a review of the analytic literature on borderline patients and, more specifically, an intensive study of four borderline patients in psychoanalysis. The findings reported here also reflect our clinical experience in treating borderline patients in psychoanalysis. Although we did not apply DSM-III-R criteria (American Psychiatric Association 1987) to our patients, they would have met standard definitions of BPD. Although our patients varied somewhat from those studied by other authors in that they were analyzable, the analytic method gave us the opportunity to study their psychodynamics in great depth.

Because we believe that the term "borderline" describes a broad and varied group of patients, we are not convinced that all of these patients have specific, identifiable features in common. Therefore, we believe it is highly unlikely that the borderline category can be used to predict analytic results or to determine a specific treatment approach.

Furthermore, we believe that it is premature, in the light of current knowledge, to attribute the etiology of borderline conditions to failures in development that occur during a specific phase of life. Although speculation about early development is an honored psychoanalytic tradition, one of its major pitfalls is the idea that adult psychopathology reflects a direct, unmodified continuation of very early, preverbal developmental stages. Such theorizing contributes to fundamental errors in attributing the etiology of the psychoses to disturbances during the first 6 months of life, borderline conditions to the next 12 or so months, and the neuroses after the age of 3 years when so-called object constancy has been achieved. Such a simple schema is open to serious question. On the one hand, it discounts the role of biological factors that may be present in a certain number of borderline patients (see van Reekum et al., Chapter 1). On the other hand, it discounts the impact on fundamental ego capacities of serious trauma at later stages of development (see Chapters 6; Chapter 7).

While we agree with other analysts that preoedipal phases and conflicts may be extremely important in influencing degrees of psychopathology, we believe that at the present time there is not sufficient evidence to place the etiologic determinants for the borderline syndrome in any particular phase of development. All psychopathology, in our view, reflects major determinants from preoedipal and oedipal conflicts as well as superego pathology from several stages of development.

A corollary topic to phase specificity and etiology is the concept of ego defect. Many analysts believe that borderline patients have ego defects that have been caused by developmental failures in structure formation that are largely independent of intrapsychic conflict. As Stone suggests in Chapter 4, these ego deficits can be the result of constitutional factors. Whatever the organic factors in borderline patients might be, they will present a significantly different picture from that envisaged by those theorists who postulate psychogenic structural defects. It is likely that, at our current state of knowledge, all psychogenic ego impairments are inseparable from intrapsychic conflict. If this is so, then the concept of "defect," with its implication of irreversibility, is problematic. Furthermore, the hypothesis that regulatory functions from very early in infantile life are disturbed because of the failure of the caretaking person independent of psychic conflict, does not fit with the data as observed by many analysts. They observe similar disturbances but prefer to conceptualize them as the outcome of quite complicated interactions between unconscious wishes, defenses, and superego attitudes (Calef and Weinshel 1979). Early trauma is intertwined with conflicts from later developmental phases of childhood.

The concept of reality testing is important. The intactness of reality testing is one of the criteria that many theorists believe differentiates borderline patients from psychotic patients; it has been repeatedly stated

that borderline patients have intact reality testing or only transient failures in this ego function. We believe that such a simple formulation is
inaccurate for the same reasons that Freud's simple schema differentiating neurosis and psychosis could not be sustained by the clinical data.
Although prolonged psychotic episodes are not a prominent feature of
these patients, significantly long failures of reality testing may be present
in these patients, particularly around the person of the analyst. The function of reality testing is in itself an extremely complicated one that does
not lend itself to being described as "intact" or "defective" (Abend 1982).
It may well be that the disturbances in reality testing that do exist are the
result, in large measure, of the impact of conflict on various ego functions,
as well as of the influence of an extremely pathological environment that
distorts the "socialized reality" (Hartmann 1956) of these patients.

We also examined the object relations of our patients. All of our
patients had disturbed relationships with one or both parents that reflected conflicts from both preoedipal and oedipal eras, and they all had
experienced significant object loss. They had all made strong identification with the aggressor, particularly as involved taking on the sadistic
aspects of their parents' behavior. Their sexual lives and their relationships in general were permeated with aggression directed outward, toward the self, or both. Projections of aggression made them fear objects
and led to the need to control them. Oral, anal, and phallic phase issues
were all involved in these sadomasochistic features. We did observe severe
ambivalence, but we did not regularly encounter the dramatic and persistent division into "all good" and "all bad" self and object images that has
been emphasized in the literature (Kernberg 1984).

The extensive use of projection led to confusions between self and
other that disturbed these patients' reality testing in conflict areas. We did
not, however, observe the severe, gross psychotic distortions of selfobject
differentiation that one sees in schizophrenic regression. Projection of
aggression, envy, greed, homosexual impulses, heterosexual needs, impulses to control, enslave and exploit others, and superego condemnations and punishments were all present.

Our borderline patients demonstrated a profound degree of narcissism. They were more than usually concerned with gratifying their own
needs or subsuming their own needs to others in order to be the center of
the others' attention, rather than relating to other people in a more

mutual give-and-take manner. In their analyses, words and interpretations were clearly not sufficient; real gratification was demanded. They also used people for self-esteem regulation (Reich 1960), and they would react with extreme disappointment when people failed to supply them with libidinal and narcissistic gratifications. Usually, withdrawal or outbursts of rage would ensue. We did not find it helpful to view narcissistic problems as necessarily caused by failures of parental empathy, or to consider narcissism as having a separate line of development from object-related libidinal and aggressive drive maturation. Often we found that narcissistic traits were solutions to conflicts.

Most important for the understanding of these patients was the severity of their reactions to separation and loss, which has been emphasized by all analysts who write about more disturbed patients. Our case histories revealed a significant degree of actual object loss in childhood. However, it was clear to us that the day-to-day interactions between the child and his or her caretaker might well be more important than actual separation experiences. Fears of loss of the object and loss of the object's love were found to be present during each phase of psychosexual development. It was always important to analyze the specific, unique fantasies of the patients that provoked separation fears in order to understand the meaning of these fears and to trace their developmental roots. Separation reactions of our patients were more extreme than most, but not all, of our neurotic patients.

In contrast to much of the present literature on borderline patients, we observed intense superego conflicts. It is never easy to distinguish between more mature feelings of "internalized" guilt and those of fear of bodily damage, persecution, or punishment. It is true, however, that the fear of punishment or damage did play a larger role in borderline patients than in many neurotic patients. It is also true that the projection of greedy, controlling, and exploitative wishes allowed guilt feelings to be avoided until the projection had been modified. Nonetheless, it was clear that the borderline patients had developed strong superego condemnations.

Finally, we must consider the concept of primitive mechanisms of defense. Sigmund Freud and Anna Freud both thought that a hierarchical developmental view of defense mechanisms might be a helpful theoretical construct. Klein's list of primitive defenses and Kernberg's consolidation of those into splitting, projective-identification, denial, primitive idealization, and omnipotence and devaluation create a dichotomy between the primitive defenses of psychotic and borderline patients and those so-called higher-level defenses, such as repression, isolation, displacement, reaction formation, and others, that are utilized by neurotic patients. Our cases did not show this dichotomy. Our patients demonstrated many of the classical defense mechanisms in their analytical material, and they used more complex behaviors and psychological reactions for defensive purposes as well. These findings are consistent with a changing view of defenses, one in which defenses are seen less as stereotypical, fixed responses and more as ubiquitous phenomena in mental life that play a role in adaptation and normal development as well as psychopathology (Brenner 1982; Willick 1983). If one adheres to this newer hypothesis, then it is not necessary to postulate either a hierarchy of defenses or higher and lower levels within a defense mechanism (i.e., neurotic denial vs. primitive denial). In this later view, one should assess the patients' total ego functioning and not just their defense mechanisms when judging their degree of psychopathology. However, even utilizing the older conceptualization, we did observe that projection, denial, acting out, identification with the aggressor, the use of one drive derivative to defend against the other, and sadomasochistic libidinal regression were used extensively by our patients.

Finally, on the subject of defenses, Porder (1987) has offered an alternative hypothesis for what has been called "projective identification." What is observed clinically can best be understood as a compromise formation that includes as its major component an "identification with the aggressor" or a "turning passive into active." One can observe in the analytic setting a two-tiered transference-countertransference structure. On the surface is the familiar transference-countertransference picture of the analyst as the powerful parent and the patient as the helpless child. On another level, however, the patient enacts the role of the dominant parent, and the analyst experiences the feelings that the patient had felt as a child. It is the enactment of these conflicts within the analytic setting that produces feelings in the analyst. These feelings are not induced in the analyst as a result of the presence of primitive defenses from early in infantile life.

In summary, among psychoanalysts the whole question of the pathognomonic significance of the separation-individuation phase and the preoedipal era in the borderline individual is controversial. Kernberg remains the strongest proponent of the view that borderline personality is a discreet clinical entity with its own psychopathology of internalized object relations dating from a specific era of infantile development. However, this information does not take into account constitutional factors in borderline personality, the effects of physical and sexual abuse later in childhood, or the effects of a negative family environment during latency and adolescence. Our group believes that borderline patients are best described as being on a continuum between neurosis and psychosis and that they demonstrate admixtures of conflict from all developmental eras and have suffered chronic trauma in relation to their disturbed parent or parents.

REFERENCES

Abend SM: Some observations on reality testing as a clinical concept. Psychoanal Q 51:218–238, 1982

Abend SM, Porder MS, Willick MS: Borderline Patients: Psychoanalytic Perspectives. New York, International Universities Press, 1983

Abend SM, Porder MS, Willick MS: A response. Psychoanalytic Inquiry 8:438–455, 1988

Adler G: Borderline Psychopathology and Its Treatment. New York, Jason Aronson, 1985

Adler G: Transitional phenomena, projective identification, and the essential ambiguity of the psychoanalytic situation. Psychoanal Q 58:81–104, 1989

American Psychiatric Association: Diagnostic and Statistical Manual of Mental Disorders, 3rd Edition, Revised. Washington, DC, American Psychiatric Association, 1987

Bion WR: Attacks on linking. Int J Psychoanal 40:308–315, 1959

Bion WR: Second Thoughts: Selected Papers on Psychoanalysis. London, Heinemann, 1967

Brenner C: The Mind in Conflict. New York, International Universities Press, 1982

Buie DH: Book review of Borderline patients: psychoanalytic perspectives (by Abend SM, Porder MS, Willick MS). Int J Psychoanal 66:375–379, 1985

Buie DH, Adler G: Definitive treatment of the borderline personality. International Journal of Psychoanalytic Psychotherapy 9:51–87, 1982–1983

Calef V, Weinshel EM: The new psychoanalysis and psychoanalytic revisionism (book review essay on Borderline Conditions and Pathological Narcissism by Kernberg OF). Psychoanal Q 48:470–491, 1979

Greenacre P. Emotional Growth, Vol 1. New York, International Universities Press, 1971

Hartmann H: Notes on the reality principle. Psychoanal Study Child 11:31–53, 1956

Jacobson E: Contributions to the metapsychology of projective identifications. J Am Psychoanal Assoc 2:239–267, 1954

Kernberg OF: Severe Personality Disorders. New Haven, CT, Yale University Press, 1984

Klein M: Some notes on schizoid mechanisms. Int J Psychoanal 27:99–110, 1946

Kohut H: The Analysis of the Self. New York, International Universities Press, 1971

Mahler MS: A study of the separation-individuation process and its possible application to borderline phenomena in the psychoanalytic situation. Psychoanal Study Child 26:403–424, 1971

Mahler MS, Furer M: On Human Symbiosis and the Vicissitudes of Individuation. New York, International Universities Press, 1968

Masterson JF: Treatment of the Borderline Adolescent: A Developmental Approach. New York, Wiley, 1972

Masterson JF, Rinsley DB: The borderline syndrome: the role of the mother in the genesis and psychic structure of the borderline personality. Int J Psychoanal 56:163–177, 1975

Porder MS: Projective identification: an alternative hypothesis. Psychoanal Q 56:431–451, 1987

Reich A: Pathological forms of self-esteem regulation. Psychoanal Study Child 15:215–232, 1960

Rinsley DB: An object-relations view of borderline personality, in Borderline Personality Disorders: The Concept, the Syndrome, the Patient. Edited by Hartocollis P. New York, International Universities Press, 1977, pp 47–70

Stern A: Psychoanalytic investigation of and therapy in the borderline group of neuroses. Psychoanal Q 7:467–489, 1938

Willick MS: On the concept of primitive defenses. J Am Psychoanal Assoc (Suppl) 31:175–200, 1983

Winnicott DW: Transitional objects and transitional phenomena (1953), in Collected Papers: Through Pediatrics to Psychoanalysis. New York, Basic Books, 1958, pp 229–242

Winnicott DW: The theory of the parent-infant relationship (1960), in The Maturational Processes and the Facilitating Environment. New York, International Universities Press, 1965, pp 37–63

CHAPTER 10

The Borderline Personality: A Psychosocial Epidemic

Theodore Millon, Ph.D.

ONSTITUTIONAL DISPOSITIONS AND EARLY EXPERIENCE are essential ingredients in the formation of borderline personality disorder (BPD). However, they may not be sufficient in themselves to account for the increased incidence of the disorder in recent decades.

A number of phenomena suggest a role for social and cultural factors in BPD. Evidence for an increase in BPD prevalence is indirect but strong (Paris 1991) and is associated with increases in youth suicide, parasuicide, and substance abuse. A wide array of influences in Western societies since the Second World War have either set in place or further embedded those deficits in psychic cohesion that lie at the heart of the disorder. Specifically, the view is advanced that our contemporary "epidemic" of BPD can best be attributed to two broad sociocultural trends that have come to characterize much of Western life these past 40 years: 1) the emergence of social customs that exacerbate rather than remediate early, errant parent-child relationships, and 2) the diminished power of formerly reparative institutions to compensate for these ancient and ubiquitous relationship problems. Although early experience may set in place a vulnerability to future BPD development, the manifest character of the disorder may take clinical form because subsequent social forces either replicate these experiences or fail to remediate them. It is proposed that societal customs that served in the past to repair disturbances in early parent-child relations have declined in their efficacy and have been "replaced" over the past three to four decades with customs that exacerbate these difficulties.

Two central questions arise. First, what are the primary sources of influence that give rise to symptoms that distinguish BPD, namely, an inability to maintain psychic cohesion in realms of affect, intrapsychic structure, self-image, and interpersonal relationships? Second, which of these sources has had its impact heightened over the past three or four decades, accounting thereby for the rapid and marked increase in the incidence of the disorder?

It is the second question that calls for explication; it relates to which etiologic factors, each productive of the borderline individual's diffuse or segmented personality structure—constitutional disposition, problematic early nurturing, or contemporary social changes—have shown a substantial shift in recent decades. Is it some unidentified yet fundamental alteration in the intrinsic biological makeup of current-day youngsters; is it some significant and specifiable change in the character with which contemporary mothers nurture their infants and rear their toddlers; or is it traceable to fundamental and rapid changes in Western culture that have generated divisive and discordant life experiences (Kroll et al. 1982) while reducing the availability of psychically cohering and reparative social customs and institutions (Millon 1987; Segal 1988)?

Despite the fact that tangible evidence favoring one or another of these possibilities is not accessible in the conventional sense of empirical proof, the third "choice" is probatively more sustainable and inferentially more plausible. Toward these ends, two sociocultural trends generative of the segmented psychic structures that typify BPD will be elucidated. Although they are interwoven substantively and chronologically, these trends are separated for conceptual and pedagogic purposes.

INCREASINGLY DIVISIVE SOCIAL CUSTOMS

Readers of this chapter are immersed deeply in both our time and culture, thereby perhaps obscuring their ability to discern the many profound changes that have taken place in our society's institutions, changes often generative of unforeseen psychic and social consequences (Merton 1949; Parsons 1951). It is both intuitively and observationally self-evident that sweeping cultural changes can affect innumerable social practices, including those of an immediate and personal nature, such as patterns of child nurturing and rearing, marital affiliation, family cohesion, leisure style, entertainment content, and so on. To bolster our thesis that societal developments of the past half-century or so have created significant transformations in everyday life, we will turn next to a number of contemporary changes, narrowing our focus to those transitions conducive to the formation of psychic diffusion and division.

Social Discordance

It would not be too speculative to assert that the organization, coherence, and stability of a culture's institutions are in great measure reflected in the psychic structure and cohesion of its members (Durkheim 1953). In a manner analogous to the DNA double helix, in which each paired strand unwinds and selects environmental nutrients to duplicate its jettisoned partner, so too does each culture fashion its constituent members to fit an extant template. In societies whose customs and institutions are fixed and definitive, the psychic composition of its citizenry will likewise be structured; and when a society's values and practices are fluid and inconsistent, so too will its residents evolve deficits in psychic solidity and stability (Shils 1981).

This latter, more amorphous, state, so characteristic of modern Western life (Seabrook 1978; Thurow 1980), is clearly mirrored in the interpersonal vacillations and affective instabilities that typify BPD. Central to recent Western culture have been the increased pace of social change and the growing pervasiveness of ambiguous and discordant customs to which children are expected to subscribe (Hirsch 1976; Yankelovich 1981). Under the cumulative impact of rapid industrialization, immigration, urbanization, mobility, technology, and mass communication, there has been a steady erosion of traditional values and standards (Rosenberg 1980; Shils 1981). Instead of a simple and coherent body of practices and beliefs, children find themselves confronted with constantly shifting styles and increasingly questioned norms whose durability is uncertain and precarious (Fromm 1955; Reich 1970; Riesman 1971).

No longer do youngsters find the certainties and absolutes that guided earlier generations. The complexity and diversity of everyday experience play havoc with simple "archaic" beliefs and render them useless as instruments to deal with contemporary realities. Lacking a coherent view of life, maturing youngsters find themselves groping and bewildered, swinging from one set of principles and models to another, unable to find stability either in their relationships or in the flux of events (Cloward 1959; Heilbroner 1975). Few times in history have so many children faced the tasks of life without the aid of accepted and durable traditions. Not only does the strain of making choices among discordant standards and goals beset these children at every turn, but these competing beliefs and divergent demands prevent them from developing either internal stability or external consistency. And no less problematic in generating such disjoined psychic structures is the escalation in Western societies of emotionally capricious and interpersonally discordant role models.

Schismatic Families

Although transformations in family patterns and relationships have evolved fairly continuously over the past century, the speed and nature of transitions since the Second World War have been so radical as to break the smooth line of earlier trends (Zaretsky 1976). Hence, today the typical American child no longer has a clear sense of either the character or the purpose of his or her father's work activities, much less a detailed image of the concrete actions that comprise that work. Beyond the little there is of the father's daily routines to model oneself after, mothers of young children in modern Western societies have shifted their activities increasingly outside the home, seeking career fulfillments or needing dual incomes to sustain family aspirations (Moynihan 1986). Not only are everyday adult activities no longer available for direct observation and modeling, but traditional gender roles, once distinct and valued, have become blurred and questionable. Today, there is little that is rewarded and esteemed by Western society that takes place for children to see and emulate. What "real" and "important" people do cannot be learned from parents who return from a day's work too preoccupied or too exhausted to share their esoteric activities. Lost are the crystallizing and focusing effects of identifiable and stable role models that give structure and direction to maturing psychic processes. This loss contributes, then, to the maintenance of the undifferentiated and diffuse personality organization so characteristic of young borderline individuals.

With the growing dissolution of the traditional family structure in Western societies, there has been a marked increase in parental separation, divorce, and remarriage (Mizrachi 1964; Moynihan 1986). Children subject to persistent parental bickering and family restructuring not only are exposed to changing and destructive models for imitative learning but develop the internal schisms that typify borderline behaviors. The stability of life, so necessary for the acquisition of a consistent pattern of feeling and thinking, is shattered when erratic conditions or marked controversy prevails. There is an ever-present apprehension that a parent may be totally lost through divorce; dissension may lead to the undermining of one parent by the other, and a nasty and cruel competition for the loyalty and affections of children may ensue. Constantly dragged into the arena of parental schisms, the child not only loses a sense of security and stability but is also subjected to paradoxical behaviors and contradictory role models. Raised in such settings a child not only suffers the constant threat of family dissolution but, in addition, is often forced to serve as a mediator to moderate conflicts between the parents. Forced to switch sides and divide loyalties, the child cannot be "a coherent individual" but must internalize opposing attitudes and emotions to satisfy antagonistic parental desires and expectations (Millon 1987). The different roles the child must assume to placate the parents are markedly divergent; as long as the parents remain at odds, the child persists with behaviors, thoughts, and emotions that are intrinsically irreconcilable.

For many children divorce not only undermines the sense that one can count on things to endure, but it often dislodges formerly secure and crucial internalizations within one's psychic self, upsetting the fusions and integrations that evolved among once incorporated parental models and standards. With the children alienated from parental attachments, as well as often disillusioned and cynical, these internalized structures may now be totally jettisoned. Moreover, the confidence that one can depend in the future on a previously internalized belief or precept may now be seriously undermined (Wallerstein 1989). Devoid of stabilizing internalizations, such youngsters may come to prefer the attractions of momentary and passing encounters of high salience and affective power. Unable to gauge what to expect from their environment, how can they be sure that things that are true today will be there tomorrow? Have they not experienced capriciousness when things appeared stable? Unlike children who can predict their fate—good, bad, or indifferent—such youngsters are unable to fathom what the future will bring (Moynihan 1986;

Wallerstein 1989). At any moment, and for no apparent reason, they may receive the kindness and support they crave; equally possible, and for equally unfathomable reasons, they may be the recipient of hostility and rejection. Having no way of determining which course of action will bring security and stability, such youngsters vacillate, feeling hostility, guilt, compliance, assertion, and so on, shifting erratically and impulsively from one tentative action to another. Unable to predict whether their parents will be critical or affectionate, they must be ready for hostility when most might expect commendation, assume humiliation when most would anticipate reward. Eternally "on edge," emotions build up, raw to the touch, ready to react impulsively and unpredictably at the slightest provocation.

Other "advances" in contemporary Western society have stamped deep and distinct impressions as well, ones equally affectively loaded, erratic, and contradictory (Potter 1954). The rapidly moving, emotionally intense, and interpersonally capricious character of television role models, displayed in swiftly progressing half-hour vignettes that encompass a lifetime, add to the impact of disparate, highly charged, and largely inimical value standards and behavior models (Yankelovich 1981). What is incorporated is not only a multiplicity of selves but an assemblage of unintegrated and discordant roles, displayed indecisively and fitfully, especially among those youngsters bereft of secure moorings and internal gyroscopes. The striking images created by our modern-day flickering parental surrogate have replaced all other sources of cultural guidance for many; hence by age 18, the typical American child will have spent more time watching TV than in going to school or relating directly to his or her parents (Wilson 1980).

Although television may be nothing but simple pabulum for those with comfortably internalized models of gratifying human relationships, for those who possess a world of diffuse values and inconsistent standards, or one in which parental precepts and norms have been discarded, the impact of these "substitute" prototypes is especially powerful, and even idealized and romanticized. And what these TV characters and story plots present to vulnerable youngsters are the stuff of which successful "life stories" must be composed to capture the attention and hold the fascination of their audiences: violence, danger, agonizing dilemmas, and unpredictability, each expressed and resolved in an hour or less—precisely those features of social behavior and emotionality that come to character-

ize the impulsive actions and interpersonal capriciousness of the borderline individual.

To add to this disorienting and cacophonous melange are aggravations
consequent to drug and alcohol involvements. Although youth is a natural period for exploratory behaviors, of which many are both socially
adaptive and developmentally constructive, much of what is explored
entails high risks with severe adverse consequences in both the short and
long run. From the perspective of Western youngsters who see little in life
that has proven secure or desirable, the risks of these all-too-accessible
substances are experienced neither as intimidating nor perilous (Segal
1988). While they may be considered by many to be casual and recrea-
tional, their psychic effects are quite hazardous, especially among the
already vulnerable (Maris 1981). Thus, for borderline-prone individuals,
the impact of these substances will only further diminish the clarity and
focus of their feeble internalized structures, as well as dissolve whatever
purposefulness and aspirations they may have possessed to guide them
toward potentially reparative actions. Together, these mind-blurring effects add fresh weight to already established psychic diffusions.

DECREASING REPARATIVE AND COHERING CUSTOMS

The fabric of traditional and organized societies not only comprises standards designed to indoctrinate and inculcate the young but also provides
"insurance," that is, backups to compensate and repair system defects and
failures (Shils 1981). Extended families, church leaders, schoolteachers,
and neighbors provide nurturance and role models by which children
experiencing troubling parental relationships can find a means of substitute support and affection, thereby enabling these children to be receptive
to society's established body of norms and values. Youngsters subject to
any of the diffusing and divisive forces described previously must find one
or another of these culturally sanctioned sources of surrogate modeling
and sustenance to give structure and direction to their emerging capacities and impulses. Without such bolstering, maturing potentials are likely
to remain diffuse and scattered (Durkheim 1953; Millon 1987). Without
admired and stable roles to emulate, such youngsters are left to their own
devices to master the complexities of their varied and changing worlds, to

control the intense aggressive and sexual urges that well up within them, to channel their fantasies, and to pursue the goals to which they may aspire. Many become victims of their own growth, unable to discipline their impulses or find acceptable means for expressing their desires. Scattered and unguided, they are unable to fashion a clear sense of personal identity, a consistent direction for feelings and attitudes, or a coherent purpose to existence. They become "other-directed" persons who vacillate at every turn, overly responsive to fleeting stimuli, shifting from one erratic course to another (Riesman 1961). Ultimately, without the restitutive and remedial power of beneficent parental surrogates, they fail to establish internalized values to anchor themselves and to guide their future (Reich 1970).

This aimless floundering and disaffiliation may be traced in great measure to the loss in contemporary society of meliorative and reparative institutions (Wilson 1980). The customs of traditional culture ensured that deprived or abused children would have a second chance by finding compensatory sponsors who proclaimed values and conveyed purposes around which a rewarding or meaningful social life could be focused and oriented. It is these cultural losses to which we turn next.

Decline of Consolidating Institutions

The impact of much of what has been described previously might be substantially lessened if concurrent or subsequent personal encounters and social customs were compensatory or restitutive—that is, if they repaired the intrapsychically destabilizing and destructive effects of problematic early experiences. Unfortunately, the converse appears to be the case (Shils 1981). Whereas the cultural institutions of most societies have retained practices that furnish reparative stabilizing and cohering experiences, thereby remedying disturbed parent-child relationships, it is my thesis in this chapter that the changes of the past three to four decades not only have fostered an increase in intrapsychic diffusion and splintering but also have resulted in the discontinuation of psychically restorative institutions and customs, contributing thereby to both the incidence and exacerbation of features that typify borderline pathology. Without the corrective effects of undergirding and focusing social mentors and practices, the diffusing or divisive consequences of unfavorable earlier experi-

once take firm root and unyielding form, their structural weaknesses being displayed in clinical signs under the press of even modestly stressful events (Yankelovich 1981).

For example, one of the by-products of the rapid expansion of knowledge and education is that many of the traditional institutions of our society—such as religion, which formerly served as a refuge to many, offering "love" for virtuous behavior and caring and thoughtful role models—have lost much of their historic power as a source of nurturance and control in our contemporary world.

Similarly, and in a more general way, the frequency with which families in our society relocate has caused a wide range of psychically diffusing problems. We not only leave behind stability but with each move jettison a network of partially internalized role models and community institutions such as those furnished in church, school, and friendships (Wilson 1980). What is undone, therefore, is the psychic structure and cohesion that could have been solidified to give direction and meaning to what are otherwise disparate elements of existence. Not only do children who move to distant settings feel isolated and lonely in these unfamiliar surrounds, and not only are they deprived of the opportunities to develop a consistent foundation of social customs and a coherent sense of self, but what faith they may have had in the merits of holding to a stable set of values and behaviors can only have been discredited.

Disappearance of Nurturing Surrogates

The scattering of the extended family, as well as the rise of single-parent homes and shrinkage in sibling number, adds further to the isolation of families as they migrate in and out of transient communities (Moynihan 1986). Each of these factors undermines the once powerful reparative effects of kinship support and caring relationships. Contemporary forms of disaffection and alienation between parent and child may differ in their particulars from those of the past. But rejection and estrangement has been and is ubiquitous, as commonplace as rivalry among siblings. In former times when children were subjected to negligence or abuse, they often found familial or neighborly parental surrogates—grandmothers, older siblings, aunts or uncles, even the kind or childless couple down the street—who would, by virtue of their own needs or identifications, nurture or even rear them (Blumberg 1980). Frequently more suitable to parental roles, typically more affectionate and giving, as well as less disciplinary and punitive, these healing surrogates historically not only have served to repair the psychic damage of destructive parent-child relationships but have "filled in" the requisite modeling of social customs and personal values to which youngsters, so treated, would now be receptive to imitate and internalize.

In the past several decades in Western societies, estranged and denigrated children no longer find nurturing older siblings, aunts, or grandparents; nor are there the once accessible and nurturing neighbors (Shils 1981). With increased mobility, kinship separation, single-parenting, and reduced sibling numbers, Western society has few surrogate parents to pick up the pieces of what real parents may have fragmented and discarded, much less restore the developmental losses engendered thereby.

Reemergence of Social Anomie

For some, the question is not which of the changing social values they should pursue, but whether there are any social values that are worthy of pursuit.

Youngsters exposed to poverty and destitution, provided with inadequate schools, living in poor housing set within decaying communities, raised in chaotic and broken homes, deprived of parental models of "success and attainment," and immersed in a pervasive atmosphere of hopelessness, futility, and apathy, cannot help but question the validity of the "good society." Reared in these settings, one quickly learns that there are few worthy standards to which one can aspire successfully (Durkheim 1953; Rosenberg 1980; Seabrook 1978; Wilson 1980). Whatever efforts are made to raise oneself from these bleak surroundings run hard against the painful restrictions of poverty and the sense of a meaningless and empty existence and an indifferent, if not hostile, world. Moreover, and in contrast to earlier generations whose worlds rarely extended beyond the shared confines of ghetto poverty, the disparity between everyday realities and what is seen as so evidently available to others in enticing TV commercials and bounteous shopping malls is not only frustrating but painfully disillusioning and immobilizing (Blumberg 1980). Why make a pretense of accepting patently "false" values or seeking the unattainable goals of the larger society when reality undermines every hope, and social existence is so pervasively hypocritical and harsh?

Nihilistic resolutions such as these leave youngsters bereft of a core of inner standards and customs to stabilize and guide their future actions, exposing them to the capricious power of momentary impulse and passing temptation (Kenniston 1968; Seabrook 1978). Beyond being merely "anomic" in Durkheim's sense of lacking socially sanctioned means for achieving culturally encouraged goals, these youngsters have incorporated neither the approved customs and practices nor the institutional aspirations and values of our society (Durkheim 1953). In effect, they are both behaviorally normless and existentially purposeless, features seen in manifest clinical form among prototypal borderline individuals.

Until a generation or two ago, children had productive, even necessary, economic roles to fill within the family. More recently, when the hard work of cultivating the soil or caring for the home was no longer a requisite of daily life, youngsters were encouraged to advance their family's fortunes and status via higher education and professional vocations. Such functions and lofty ambitions not only were internalized but gave a focus and a direction to one's life as well, creating a clear priority to one's values and aspirations, and bringing disparate potentials into a coherent schema and life philosophy (Shils 1981).

Coherent aspirations are no longer commonplace today, even among the children of the middle classes (Mizrachi 1964; Wachtel 1983). In contrast to more disadvantaged youngsters, those of the upper middle class are no longer "needed" to contribute to the family's economic survival; on the other hand, neither can upwardly mobile educational and economic ambitions lead them to readily surpass the achievements of their already successful parents. In fact, such children are seen in many quarters as economic burdens, not as vehicles to a more secure future or to a more esteemed status for the family. Parents absorbed in their own lives and careers frequently view children as impediments to their autonomy and narcissistic indulgences.

The psychically cohering and energizing effects of "being needed" or of "fulfilling a worthy" family aspiration have increasingly been lost in modern Western societies. Without genuine obligations and real purposes to create intent and urgency in their psychosocial worlds, such

youngsters often remain diffused and undirected. At best, they are encouraged to "find their own thing," to follow their own desires and to
create their own aims. Unfortunately, freedoms such as these translate for
many as freedom to remain in flux, to be drawn to each passing fancy, to
act out each passing mood, to view every conviction or ethic to be of equal
merit, and, ultimately, to feel evermore adrift, lost, and empty.

Satisfying each momentary wish, consuming pleasures once shrouded
in mystery, today's youngsters have, nonetheless, been deeply deprived—
not of material wants but of opportunities to fulfill both the minor daily
chores now routinely managed by modern technology and the more
distant goals that kept the minds of yesterday's children centered around
a value hierarchy and oriented toward ultimate achievements (Kenniston
1968; Maris 1981).

While many of this generation have their bearings in good order, some
have submerged themselves in aimless materialism. Others remain adrift
in disenchantment and meaninglessness—a state of disaffected malaise.
Some have attached themselves to naive causes or cults that ostensibly
provide the passion and purpose they crave to give life meaning, but even
these "solutions" too often prove empty, if not fraudulent.

In earlier times, and in currently less advantaged societies, the disen-
chanted and disenfranchised, often dislocated from burdened homes or
cast out as unwelcome troublemakers, joined together in active protest
and rebellion. Problematic economic, social, and political conditions
were shared by many of the profoundly dissatisfied, who formed philosophical movements such as the German *Sturm und Drang* of the late 18th
century and the *Wandervogels* of the late 19th century. In 20th-century
Western societies, as well, we have witnessed similar though more benign
movements whose origins stemmed from an antipathy to parental ideals
and cultural norms, such as the American Beat and "Hippie" generations
of the 1950s and 1960s (Kenniston 1968; Mizrachi 1964).

Today, children of the West are "rebels without a cause." Whereas
earlier generations of disaffected youth, both here and elsewhere, were
bound together by their ressentiments, their opposition to economic or
political oppression, motivated by discernible and worthy common
causes that provided both group camaraderie and a path of action, today's
Western youngsters have no shared causes to bring them together (Wilson 1980). With middle-class youngsters materially well nourished and

clothed, unconstrained in an open society to follow their talents and aspirations freely, the purposelessness and emptiness are essentially an internal matter, a private rather than a collective affair, with no external agents against whom they can join with others to take to the streets (Kenniston 1968). It is these rebels without a cause, unable to forego the material comforts of home and ineffective in externalizing their inner discontents upon the larger scene, yet empty and directionless, who comprise a goodly share of today's borderline patients. Were it not for the general political, economic, and social well-being of Western life, many would band together, finding some inspiration or justification to act out in concert.

With advances in modern education we have seen a marked growth in Western psychological-mindedness, sufficient to encourage the parents of youngsters such as have been described to turn to our profession for guidance in solving the perplexing character of their children's emotional and social behaviors—for example, "I don't understand him; he has everything a young person could want." What in other times might have taken root as a social movement of disaffected young radicals has taken the form of an epidemic of materially nourished youth who possess the freedom to pursue abundance but who feel isolated, aimless and empty, and whom we "treat" for a deeply troubling psychological disorder (Potter 1954; Wilson 1980).

CONCLUSIONS

The sociocultural thesis presented here assumes that future borderline individuals are likely to possess troublesome constitutional proclivities and/or to have been subjected to early and repetitive experiences of a psychically diffusing or divisive nature. By contrast, youngsters endowed with an emotionally sturdy disposition and/or reared in a uniform, dependable, and stable manner are not likely candidates for BPD, whatever their encounters may have been with the social forces described herein.

The present thesis should be construed, then, as an addendum, one that seeks to affix the final ingredient of that trio of biopsychosocial influences that coalesce to form what we know as "borderline personality disorder."

REFERENCES

Blumberg P: Inequality in an Age of Decline. New York, Oxford University Press, 1980

Cloward RA: Illegitimate means, anomie, and deviant behavior. American Sociological Review 24:461–472, 1959

Durkheim E: Sociology and Philosophy. Glencoe, IL, Free Press, 1953

Fromm E: The Sane Society. New York, Holt, Rinehart & Winston, 1955

Kroll J, Carey K, Sines L, et al: Are there borderlines in Britain? A cross-validation of US findings. Arch Gen Psychiatry 39:60–63, 1982

Heilbroner RL: An Inquiry Into the Human Prospect. New York, WW Norton, 1975

Hirsch F: Social Limits to Growth. Cambridge, MA, Harvard University Press, 1976

Kenniston K: Young Radicals. New York, Harcourt, Brace & World, 1968

Maris R: Pathways to Suicide. Baltimore, MD, Johns Hopkins Press, 1981

Merton RK: Social Theory and Social Structure. Glencoe, IL, Free Press, 1949

Millon T: On the genesis and prevalence of the borderline personality disorder: a social learning thesis. Journal of Personality Disorders 1:354–372, 1987

Mizrachi EH: Success and Opportunity: A Study in Anomie. Glencoe, IL, Free Press, 1964

Moynihan DP: Family and Nation. New York, Harcourt Brace Jovanovich, 1986

Paris J: Parasuicide, personality disorders, and culture. Transcultural Psychiatry Research Review 28:25–39, 1991

Parsons T: The Social System. Glencoe, IL, Free Press, 1951

Potter D: People of Plenty: Economic Abundance and American Character. Chicago, IL, University of Chicago Press, 1954

Reich C: The Greening of America. New York, Random House, 1970

Riesman D: The Lonely Crowd. New Haven, CT, Yale University Press, 1971

Seabrook J: What Went Wrong: Why Hasn't Having More Made People Happier? New York, Pantheon, 1978

Segal BM: A borderline style of functioning: the role of family, society and heredity. Child Psychiatry Hum Dev l8:219–238, 1988

Shils E: Tradition. Chicago, IL, University of Chicago Press, 1981

Thurow L: The Zero Sum Society. New York, Basic Books, 1980

Wachtel PL: The Poverty of Affluence. New York, Free Press, 1983

Wallerstein JS: Second Chances: Men, Women, and Children a Decade After Divorce. New York, Ticknor and Fields, 1989

Wilson JO: After Affluence: Economics to Meet Human Needs. New York, Harper & Row, 1980

Yankelovich D: New Rules: Searching for Self Fulfillment in a World Turned Upside Down. New York, Random House, 1981

Zaretsky E: Capitalism, the Family, and Personal Life. New York, Harper & Row, 1976

Etiologic Theories of Borderline Personality Disorder: A Commentary

Jerome Kroll, M.D.

A COMMENTARY ON ETIOLOGIC THEORIES OF BORDERLINE personality disorder (BPD) requires a process of double bookkeeping: one to consider general problems about trying to discover and assign causality to any psychiatric condition, and a second one related to the specific problems regarding causality of a personality disorder, in this case, BPD. Underlying both tracks of the double process are several commonplace observations that, presumably, we all make, but which need to be spelled out, if for no other reason than that we do not take too much for granted.

The first general observation relates to the problem of pursuing and discussing the etiology of a condition while unable to agree whether the condition even exists as an entity, or, if it does "exist," how to define and delimit the condition in a satisfactory manner. How can we search for the cause of something when we do not know what this something is and, especially, when we do not know if it is a single something? Such a procedure of allowing the search for the causes of the condition to help establish and define the condition itself, however, has in fact been a very profitable method for the medical sciences and therefore is not as ludicrous as it may first appear. The process of searching for antecedent events and past and present correlations and of anticipating future developments helps to refine our constructs, to break up fortuitously merged groupings that turn out to be really quite unrelated, and to merge other groupings that we initially may have thought were fairly irrelevant to each other.

Nevertheless, there are hazards to the early search for etiologic factors that become particularly evident in consideration of the borderline conditions in the absence of an external gold standard or validation point. There is, of necessity, a certain circularity by which one decides which specific aspect of the rich borderline psychopathology will be considered as fundamental or prototypic of the disorder and which causal factors one is predisposed to search for and discover in evaluating the somewhat arbitrarily defined borderline individuals. If one defines BPD with a conceptual focus on affective symptoms, then one will likely find affective mechanisms underlying the disorder. If one defines BPD with a focus on dissociative symptoms and self-destructive behaviors, then one will likely find childhood sexual abuse experiences underlying the disorder. If one defines BPD in terms of impulse-ridden behaviors, then one will likely find a core theme of impulsivity connecting clinical symptoms and brain mechanisms.

Just as the borderline inpatient discovers and exposes the latent inconsistencies and ideological struggles between staff members on a psychiatric ward, and the borderline outpatient intuits and interacts with the vulnerabilities and blind spots of the therapist, so too does the institutional attempt to classify and explain the borderline disorder evoke more than the usual amount of interprofessional struggles over ideology, territory, and economics. The struggles are too obvious and well known to dwell upon, but briefly they involve the adversarial camps of biological psychiatrists, who see the major causes of mental illness as consisting of genetic and constitutional factors and the major treatment modalities as pharmacological interventions, and the psychological psychiatrists (and other health professionals), who see adverse life experiences as the major causes and corrective psychotherapeutic experiences as the major treatment modalities. Such a dichotomous situation, by no means unique to this generation or century, sets the stage for reductionistic theories of both a biological and an environmental etiology of the borderline disorder. At best, a true dialectic takes place, in which closer and closer approximations to a valid construct of "borderline" will emerge from a synthesis of the findings of each school. At worst, separate "Truths" are discovered and announced, and armed disciples (armed, that is, with words and reimbursement restrictions) will duke it out.

The second commonplace observation relates to the problems in psychiatry, as in all of medicine and indeed in life, of assigning specific causality to complex and ambiguous events and behaviors. If we grant that each human being is so individual, that each life experience is so rich and complex and the human species in general so plastic, and that our lives are lived out in very complex interpersonal networks within a still larger culture, and that we, the diagnosticians and assigners of causality, are ourselves sometimes narrowly involved in a therapeutic relationship with a patient and always broadly immersed within the larger culture such that we cannot obtain a proper perspective that several centuries of time passed by might afford us, then how, given all these problems of complexity and viewpoint and bias, can we expect to be able to come up with a simple "X causes Y" for any piece or pattern of human behavior?

Although in our calm reflective moments we can say that we know all these things and do not ever mean to reduce etiology to "X causes Y," nevertheless we also know that the whole thrust of science is to do precisely that, to elucidate the mechanisms by which X is both the necessary and sufficient antecedent of Y, such that if X, then Y. The questions of sufficiency and exclusivity as causal factors are, of course, far more problematic for the behavioral "sciences" than for physics or chemistry or even, perhaps, for other medical fields. To give an example relating to borderline individuals that might highlight this, we could not correctly say, "If an X, then a Y," when X = affective disorder and Y = borderline personality disorder, for we know that this is not so. If we reverse the order, however, could we say, "If a Y, then an X"?

This is fairly close to what is hypothesized by many biological psychiatrists. Even if the second statement were correct—namely, that all borderline patients have an affective disorder—we still recognize that, while having an affective disorder might be a necessary cause (or condition) to having a borderline disorder (i.e., one could not be borderline without having an affective disorder), having an affective disorder can certainly not be a sufficient cause for having a borderline disorder. For one may have an affective disorder and not have a borderline disorder—that is, not all persons with an affective disorder have a borderline disorder. Therefore, while it may be of pragmatic importance, in terms of treatment, to know if BPD were a subset of major affective disorder (MAD), we cannot speak of the affective disorder as the specific etiology of BPD. We still would have to search for those somethings that, in combination with an affective disorder, produce or cause BPD.

Paul Meehl (1977) has dissected this problem. In the present context of considering an etiology of borderline disorders, I would emphasize Meehl's notion of strong influence, in the sense of, "Without X, unlikely Y" and, further, "With X, most likely Y." The search for the etiology of BPD will have to involve a continuum of causative or contributory factors, ranging from those that strongly influence the likelihood that BPD will develop, to those that appear to be contributory but weakly influential in the development of BPD. The last clarification to make in this regard is that the X's must be nontrivial, that is, not belonging to the whole domain of conditions necessary to sustain life (e.g., breathing).

The final commonplace observation to make is that all etiologic theories must also acknowledge the cognitive-behavioral principle that behaviors that are reinforcing and reinforced become habitual and stabilized and thus become somewhat independent of the specific stimulus conditions under which they developed in essence. Behaviors such as cutting or bulimia can become generalized as successful tension-reduction mechanisms and no longer occur only in response to the specific stresses from which they originated. This particular segment of the causal chain is emphasized in Chapter 5 by Linehan and Koerner.

The range of etiologic hypotheses and the therapies derived from each of these theories reflect the entire gamut of theories about the determinants of human nature and behavior. Although it would not be accurate to say that to be human is to be borderline, one could say that to be human carries with it the very real possibility of being borderline, that is, of struggling with the same issues that borderline individuals struggle with, in ways not so very different at times from the ways of these individuals. An alternative phrasing is that there is a dimensional quality to the components of the borderline personality and that we all can be located somewhere on these dimensions. This means that borderline symptoms and styles, and their underlying causes, will differ only in degree from the behaviors, psychodynamics, and neurophysiology of those who are not borderline.

Essentially, the controversy among the etiologic theories of BPD represents the nature-nurture issue in yet one more modern garb. Is it the case that what we are, who we are, and how we act, are mainly determined by the types of life experiences that we have or by our genetic endowment and constitutional makeup? It will not do to dismiss the issue by stating that, obviously, it is neither one nor the other, but both. We all know this; only a fool would deny it. But the nature-nurture issue legitimately remains in the form of the question of what are the strong and what are the weak influences over particular pieces and enduring patterns of human behavior.

There are certain things that a theory of etiology should do if it is to have credibility. The theory should account for the major symptoms of the condition that it purports to explain by providing scientifically respectable evidence that links the symptoms to the underlying causes. The theory should accommodate the dimensional aspect of the disorder, namely, that the condition exists in varying degrees of severity, such that severity of the disorder is correlated with severity of the causal factors. The theory should explain or at least be compatible with the course of the disorder, including factors relating to the variability of the course. The presence and effects of moderating factors should be compatible with the action of major causal factors. Sex ratio, and other noteworthy demographic features if present, should be explained by the etiologic theory. Finally, response to therapies, including medication, should be explainable or at least compatible with the hypothesized etiologic factors.

Keeping in mind, then, the notions of specific etiology and of strong and weak influences, and the requirement that a credible hypothesis has to explain a substantial portion of the facts, we may proceed to evaluate the particular contributions set forth in the preceding chapters. The contributions of Paris and Zweig-Frank (Chapter 7), Perry and Herman (Chapter 6), Porder (Chapter 9), Millon (Chapter 10), and Linehan and Koerner (Chapter 5), set forth the evidence and arguments for various types of environmental or experiential theories of etiology of BPD, although most include constitutional factors as significant modulators of the individual's responses to environmental stressors. The contribution of van Reekum et al. (Chapter 1) presents the case for biological causal factors, with the work of Zanarini (Chapter 3) providing a middle ground from a particular perspective. All of the authors are aware that there is not a single etiologic agent, and they each make a case for their respective contenders in order to evaluate goodness of fit of hypotheses to evidence. Stone (Chapter 4) presents an integrative model in light of the contributions of the individual factors as strong and weak causal influences.

The contribution of van Reekum et al. (Chapter 1), presenting and evaluating the correlations between recent physiological and neuroscience findings and the clinical picture of BPD, is a particularly fair-minded analysis. What emerges is that the evidence is lacking for a narrowly conceived genetic transmission of BPD either sui generis or as an affective disorder. On the other hand, in terms of the recent findings of the Minnesota studies of twins reared apart (Bouchard et al. 1990) regarding the inheritance of temperament and personality traits or behavioral predisposition (constructs such as risk taking and inherent conservatism), and on the basis of other studies such as Kagan et al.'s (1988) work on shyness, it is only a matter of time before certain genetically influenced traits that underlie the development of BPD will emerge. The relative strengths of such basic traits in influencing the development of a borderline picture remain to be seen.

Perhaps the most interesting findings reviewed by van Reekum et al. (Chapter 1) are the various bits of evidence that some brain dysfunction occurs more commonly in BPD than in control cases. This makes some intuitive sense, considering that we are dealing with a population practically defined by impulsivity and oriented toward action. As van Reekum et al. point out, however, the evidence remains very nonspecific. Gold and Silk (Chapter 2) also soberly appraise the biological and pharmacotherapeutic evidence for a relationship between BPD and the affective disorders and finds it to be relatively weak.

Zanarini's contribution (Chapter 3) stands midway between biological and experiential explanations of BPD. To the extent that Zanarini and others have demonstrated a preponderance of impulsive-type behaviors (self-destructiveness, binging and vomiting, substance abuse, poorly controlled expression of strong emotions) in borderline patients and a degree of affinity to antisocial types, the findings are rather trivial, inasmuch as BPD is defined in the first place by impulsivity. The import of this hypothesis and of Zanarini's work, however, is to underscore the importance of looking for the biochemical and neurophysiological substrates of maladaptive personality traits such as impulsivity, a point also made by Soloff (1990). This needs to be done for the entire dimension of impulsivity and inhibition of behaviors; borderline individuals, by virtue of their more obvious difficulty with impulse control, serve as a good cohort for the study of such phenomena.

Picking up on this theme of biological substrates, Stone (Chapter 4) reviews brain mechanisms underlying a wide variety of human behaviors and speculates about their relationships to the component parts (impulsivity, overreactivity to seemingly minor stimuli, poor modulation of emotional expression) of the borderline picture. This will undoubtedly be a major area of research in the decade ahead. It must be emphasized at this early stage of inquiry, however, that not every discovery of a brain mechanism underlying intense emotionality or action proneness necessarily implies pathology.

Moving on to the environmental studies, the juxtaposition between Paris and Zweig-Frank (Chapter 7) and Perry and Herman's work (Chapter 6) is an interesting one. Both hypotheses obviously employ retrospective studies as evidence. Paris and Zweig-Frank are looking at relatively subtle factors, and Perry and Herman are focusing on more gross factors. Just in terms of this alone, the hazards of retrospective falsification are greater for Paris and Zweig-Frank's work, while the hazards of retrospective oversimplification are greater for Perry and Herman's work. I say the latter with some hesitation and hasten to add that I am not referring to the actual research done by Herman and others, but rather to the popularization and indiscriminate endorsement of the abuse hypothesis that draws a simple link between abuse and BPD. Nevertheless, it is clear that the evidence is fairly strong and impressive and provides the most robust "causal" or strong influence explanation of any single contender among the etiologic hypotheses at the present time. In fact, the evidence supporting abuse as the strongest environmental influence predisposing toward BPD is so strong that it is an embarrassment to acknowledge how long this evidence has been ignored while putative early developmental factors, on which there was no direct research evidence at all, were lightly bandied about (Masterson 1981). It represents an instructive lesson in the human tendency to prefer abstract thinking to concrete operations, an example of adherence to a Piagetian hierarchy with a vengeance.

The abuse hypothesis and its related research, however, is not without problems, the major one being, of course, that of specificity. Not all abused children become borderline, and not all borderline individuals, it appears, were abused. Nor are Perry and Herman and the other researchers claiming this. They, and we, recognize, first, that abuse is a generic term that needs to be exquisitely and painfully refined into its many different subtypes and dimensions. Second, and this has been pointed out by many, the abusive events do not take place in a vacuum. The contexts in which abuse occurs are themselves usually very abnormal and even, as Stone (1990) has written, grotesque. It is not just that a child or adolescent has been abused and, in many cases, continues to be abused, but rather that the entire atmosphere in which the child or adolescent is raised is poisoned by multiple boundary violations, reversal of mother-daughter caretaking roles, transfiguration of a safekeeper into a dangerous and feared figure, destructive uses of alcohol and drugs by various family members, disruption of a "normal" adolescence period as such, and, in general, repeated chaotic relationships and situations. In addition to these external events, the inner life of the child who has been abused is irrevocably changed. There are no longer any safe places; there is no getting away from one's own thoughts, one's dreams, one's stream of consciousness that plays and replays in the mind of the child the abuse and all its variations and imagined ramifications, the shame, guilt, confusion, and self-condemnation.

When one begins to consider the sequelae of child abuse on both total development and symptom formation, then the abuse hypothesis gains strength, for it links the childhood events with adult symptoms and personality. It is indirectly in recognition of this that the DSM-IV committee on Axis II is considering adding a ninth BPD criterion, namely, transient, stress-related psychotic-like experiences. This addition at least begins to approach the cognitive alterations and dissociative experiences of borderline patients that were ignored in DSM-III (American Psychiatric Association 1980), experiences that more and more appear to link BPD to a posttraumatic stress syndrome. If the evidence linking BPD to the affective disorders were half as solid as the data suggesting a relationship between BPD and posttraumatic stress disorder, the biological psychiatrists would have already declared the issue resolved.

Having extolled the relative strengths of the abuse hypothesis, however, a second problem with specificity, beside the observation that not all abused children go on to become borderline, must be discussed. This relates to a comparison of abuse experiences of borderline patients to those of patients with other psychiatric disorders. In essence, how does a control group stack up in this regard? Several studies have found that between 25% and 50% of general psychiatric female patients have been sexually or physically abused prior to their adulthood (Beck and van der

Kolk 1987; Briere and Zaidi 1989; Bryer et al. 1987; Carmen et al. 1984; Craine et al. 1988; Herman 1986; Jacobson 1989; Jacobson et al. 1987; Morrison 1989; Surrey et al. 1990; Winfield et al. 1990). The implications of such evidence for considering abuse to be a specific etiologic factor of BPD are clear; abuse alone, without further qualification, is insufficient, just as presence of an affective disorder alone is insufficient.

There is a need to study the details of abuse in order to correlate gender, types and intensities of abuse, frequencies, ages of onset, durations, and perpetrators of abuse with the actual clinical pictures that we see. This work has already been started by Perry and Herman, as reported here (see Chapter 6), and by Ogata and her colleagues (1990). While it is clear that not all abused children become borderline and that patients with other psychiatric disorders have also been abused, it may be that all (or almost all) children abused beyond certain thresholds of violence, coercion, intrusiveness, repetitiveness, and other heinous factors do in fact go on to become borderline—that is, to develop traits or styles of impulsiveness, self-injurious behaviors, mood lability, flashbacks, dissociative episodes, and boundary problems. Again, we may ask whether we are speaking of BPD or posttraumatic stress disorder.

The reverse side of the threshold of abuse consideration is the search for mitigating, ameliorating, or saving factors. In those children who have been abused and who do not go on to become symptomatic as adults, are we dealing with resilient children, perhaps on a genetic basis, who were also cushioned by a fortuitous, or sought after, relationship with another person (or even pet) who provided nurturance, attachment, and role modeling sufficient to compensate for the abuse and neglect? In the long sequence of factors leading to borderline development, the chain may well double back to the search for the biological foundations and mechanisms subserving impulse control and the influence of salient experiential factors themselves in establishing the stability, set point, and fine tuning of these basic evolutionary processes.

By comparison with the abuse data, the search for the more subtle, and, of necessity, harder to recover caretaker-child interactions, as exemplified by Paris and Zweig-Frank's study (see Chapter 7), is less dramatic but equally important. Nor are the two research areas (abuse and neglect, generally speaking) mutually exclusive. We need to try to obtain a well-rounded picture of experiential influences leading to the BPD configuration. Are there particular patterns of caretaker-child interactions that lead to the developmental deficits and aberrations that underlie borderline psychopathology? In terms of the methodological problems related to the "neglect" research, the major pitfall, in addition to that of specificity of influence, is the problem of retrospective falsification. We know that memories are subject to varying degrees of distortion. If the adolescent or early adult borderline patient is in conflict with the mother, is it not possible or even likely that, when asked what this mother was like in the early years, the answer will be very negatively formulated? Compounding this difficulty stands the basic observation that borderline patients tend to idealize and devaluate. We know from our immediate experience with these patients, such as their criticisms of therapists, that at least sometimes these criticisms are distortions. In these situations, we see devaluation at work firsthand. How much credibility, then, can we give to their memories of emotionally laden events of 15 or 20 years ago? It is not that some, or many, borderline patients may not have had awful childhoods with their parents; the question is how we are to know the distortions from the accurate memories.

The subject of the distortions of memory of childhood events serves as a natural introduction to psychoanalytic hypotheses of the etiology of the borderline syndrome. All of the earlier methodological problems that plague the other theories show up in greater degree with psychoanalytic theories. One does not have to be a Popperian positivist to recognize that there is an embarrassing lack of evidence in the territory between clinical observation and explanatory hypotheses. The several psychoanalytic theories associated with the names of Kernberg (1975), Masterson (1981), Rinsley (1989), and Adler (1985) all postulate some variation of a developmental disaster around the separation-individuation phase (age 18–30 months) of childhood. Essentially, the psychopathology of the mother does not allow healthy separation and individuation to occur, nor does it allow the development of a self-soothing introject, with the result that the libidinal and aggressive components of self and object (mental) representations are not integrated and negative emotions cannot be tolerated. This leads to a fragile sense of identity and the presence of primitive defenses (splitting and projective identification) into adult life. The problem, briefly, is that no evidence has ever been adduced to support such complex constructs or to bolster the underlying metapsychological assumptions. Do we know that borderline patients have in fact had trouble in their separation-individuation phase of development and that, furthermore, patients with other psychiatric problems have not, or have to a much lesser extent? Do we know that difficulties at ages 18–30 months are more important as causative factors in the development of the borderline disorder than are later (e.g., oedipal or latency-age) experiences? It is not that the evidence is equivocal; rather, it is that there is no evidence other than psychoanalytic reconstructions of adult patients' memories and reports. Kernberg's assumption that future borderline patients also had an excess of "aggression" as a biological given is too vague and undocumented at this point to salvage a hypothesis unsupported except by privileged data from within the analytic hour. Lest it seem that I am being unkind to this sort of psychoanalytic theorizing, the following points by Gedo (1986) (not made specifically in regard to the borderline hypotheses) will bear me out in this regard. He writes: "If one is committed to a set of theoretical assumptions, the potential use of observational data is restricted to an exercise comparable to trying on a number of ready-made suits for optimal fit" (p. 151), and again, ". . . the psychoanalytic controversies demonstrate that clinical innovators are quick to invent hypotheses about early childhood that are convenient for their purposes" (p. 160).

If we move on to Millon's thesis (see Chapter 10) of the social and cultural causes of the borderline condition, we once again bump into the problem of specific etiology, as well as the quandary of being caught up in, or limited by, our own cultural perspectives. Millon, of course, is sensitive to these issues and is not suggesting that either the emergence of social customs that exacerbate troubled parent-child relationships or the diminished power of previously stabilizing social institutions is the specific cause of BPD. Rather, Millon makes the point that these changed factors help to explain both the seeming increase in the borderline syndrome and perhaps the specific types of symptoms that constitute the borderline picture. While I am enormously sympathetic to Millon's appraisal of our contemporary loss of a sense of social values and personal integrity, nevertheless, I cannot help but be reminded that virtually every generation has viewed its younger generation as embodying some sort of deterioration of traditional values and as sadly reflecting a pervasive social discord. Who of us living in the second half of the 20th century cannot but feel that we have witnessed the most chaotic of times, the most determined and relentless slaughter of millions of people, the greatest sense that the individual is of absolutely no importance or effectiveness? But I have to wonder about the world view at the time of the fall of Rome and the barbarian invasions of Europe (from the viewpoint of those invaded, not from the barbarians'), or at the time of the Mongol invasions of Europe, or during the time of the Black Death epidemics of 1348 and after, when one-third to one-half the population of many regions died, or during the Thirty Years' War and other bloody events following the Reformation—and this is just considering the little subcontinent of Europe.

The problem is that, despite my sympathy with Millon's general appraisal, one suspects that the halcyon days of yesteryear tend to be romanticized. Nevertheless, and here must be Millon's point, while social conditions and failure of a coherent world view do not specifically cause the development of BPD, such disruptions of our social fabric do both underlie and reflect the existence of unstable families, lack of a strong moral sense, and glorification and psychological legitimization of selfishness that may predispose our youth to borderline styles and symptoms.

Because none of the authors specifically raised this next issue, I do so with some hesitation, but suggest that it belongs somewhere in a complete list of environmental factors that influence the development of BPD. I refer to the iatrogenic factor. We need to keep in mind that the borderline syndrome and its precursor, pseudoneurotic schizophrenia, seem to have increased in prevalence along with the growing influence and proliferation of long-term psychotherapy and therapeutic hospitalization and the shift of interest of psychiatric and psychological practitioners away from patients with schizophrenias and manic-depressive illness toward persons with characterological conditions and problems with quality-of-life issues. If we recall, the construct of pseudoneurotic schizophrenia (Hoch and Polatin 1949) was invented to describe the patient who became worse in psychotherapy, and the keen interest early on in borderline patients, and part of its very concept, was related to the notion of the difficult or special-problem patient (Burnham 1966; Main 1957). I would suggest that a certain segment of the borderline population has been encouraged in their acting out and their displaying of "borderline psychopathology" by the exciting and dependency-making interactions with their therapists. Again, as with Millon's general cultural factors, one cannot speak of specific etiology, but the iatrogenic influence needs to be considered.

To summarize, we have reviewed some very thoughtful work about the causal antecedents of BPD. All of these areas hold great promise for future research and refinement of the borderline construct. It may be that we will have to separate out two large classes (with some overlap) of borderline individuals: 1) those who have been abused and have a chronic form of posttraumatic stress disorder with characterological components, and 2) those who turn out, on follow-up, to have a relationship to an affective disorder and whose adolescent and early adult borderline symptoms subside by their fourth decade. We have to consider the role of subtle alterations in brain functioning underlying both groupings lest we make the errors of sociologists and forget that we are all evolutionarily produced biological creatures.

REFERENCES

Adler G: Borderline Psychopathology and Its Treatment. New York, Jason Aronson, 1985

American Psychiatric Association: Diagnostic and Statistical Manual of Mental Disorders, 3rd Edition. Washington, DC, American Psychiatric Association, 1980

Beck JC, van der Kolk B: Reports of childhood incest and current behavior of chronically hospitalized psychotic women. Am J Psychiatry 144:1474–1476, 1987

Bouchard TJ, Lykken DT, McGue M, et al: Sources of human psychological differences: the Minnesota study of twins reared apart. Science 250:223–228, 1990

Briere J, Zaidi LY: Sexual abuse histories and sequelae in female psychiatric emergency room patients. Am J Psychiatry 146:1602–1606, 1989

Bryer JB, Nelson BA, Miller JB, et al: Childhood sexual and physical abuse as factors in adult psychiatric illness. Am J Psychiatry 144:1426–1430, 1987

Burnham DL: The special-problem patient: victim or agent of splitting? Psychiatry 29:105–122, 1966

Carmen EH, Rieker PP, Mills T: Victims of violence and psychiatric illness. Am J Psychiatry 141:378–383, 1984

Craine LS, Henson CE, Colliver JA, et al: Prevalence of a history of sexual abuse among female psychiatric patients in a state hospital system. Hosp Community Psychiatry 39:300–304, 1988

Gedo JE: Conceptual Issues in Psychoanalysis. Hillsdale, NJ, Analytic Press, 1986

Herman JL: Histories of violence in an outpatient population: an exploratory study. Am J Orthopsychiatry 56:137–141, 1986

Hoch P, Polatin P: Pseudoneurotic forms of schizophrenia. Psychiatric Q 23:248–276, 1949

Jacobson A: Physical and sexual assault histories among psychiatric outpatients. Am J Psychiatry 146:755–758, 1989

Jacobson A, Koehler JE, Jones-Brown C: The failure of routine assessment to detect histories of assault experienced by psychiatric patients. Hosp Community Psychiatry 38:386–389, 1987

Kagan J, Reznick JS, Snidman N: Biological bases of childhood shyness. Science 240:167–171, 1988

Kernberg OF: Borderline Conditions and Pathological Narcissism. New York, Jason Aronson, 1975

Main TF: The ailment. Br J Med Psychol 30:129–145, 1957

Masterson J: Borderline and Narcissistic Disorders. New York, Brunner/Mazel, 1981

Meehl PE: Specific etiology and other forms of strong influence: some quantitative meanings. J Medical Philosophy 2:33–53, 1977

Morrison J: Childhood sexual histories of women with somatization disorder. Am J Psychiatry 146:239–241, 1989

Ogata SN, Silk KR, Goodrich S, et al: Childhood sexual and physical abuse in adult patients with borderline personality disorder. Am J Psychiatry 147:1008–1013, 1990

Rinsley DB: Developmental Pathogenesis and Treatment of Borderline and Narcissistic Personalities. Northvale, NJ, Jason Aronson, 1989

Soloff PH: What's new in personality disorders? An update on pharmacologic treatment. Journal of Personality Disorders 4:233–243, 1990

Surrey J, Swett C Jr, Michaels A, et al: Reported history of physical and sexual abuse and severity of symptomatology in women psychiatric outpatients. Am J Orthopsychiatry 60:412–417, 1990

Winfield I, George LK, Swartz M, et al: Sexual assault and psychiatric disorders among a community sample of women. Am J Psychiatry 147:335–341, 1990

SECTION II:
TREATMENT

INTRODUCTION

IN SPITE OF THE INCOMPLETENESS OF OUR KNOWLEDGE about the etiology of borderline personality disorder (BPD), we are still called upon to treat borderline patients. Somehow these patients have developed a reputation for being almost untreatable. This is far from the case, and every clinician who has worked with them consistently can report a few miraculous results, as well as a fair number of good outcomes. However, one cannot base therapy on testimonials. As with every psychiatric disorder, systematic empirical investigation of treatment methods is crucially important. But clinical trials for patients who tend to require extensive treatment are understandably rare. For this reason the reader will note that the treatment section of this book is shorter, more clinical, and contains fewer research citations than the etiology section.

However, we need to know if treatment for borderline patients is effective and whether it is cost-effective. BPD presents some special challenges for evaluation research. As with other personality disorders, its symptomatology is chronic and slow to change. Effective therapy therefore takes time, and randomized clinical trials could be prohibitively expensive. In particular, one cannot evaluate treatment without knowing the natural history of BPD.

The relation of outcome to treatment is the basis for McGlashan's discussion in Chapter 12. Useful clinical conclusions can be drawn by observing how patients recover over time from BPD. One of McGlashan's points is that by focusing on object relations rather than on global functioning, we may be emphasizing the weakest area of borderline functioning rather than capitalizing on strengths. Because borderline patients are often able to work in spite of their psychopathology, they can function in one relatively neutral sector. McGlashan's case vignettes bring to life the qualitative aspects of borderline functioning that can be lost in examining mean outcome scores.

McGlashan also draws some practical implications of outcome findings for treatment. He suggests that treatment be intermittent, continuous, and eclectic. The discouragement that therapists feel in treating BPD can be partly accounted for by their failure to understand the chronicity of the disorder. Intermittent treatment is more like general medicine: in the old adage, "To cure rarely, to help sometimes, to comfort always."

McGlashan's observations, based on his long-term follow-up study at Chestnut Lodge, are reasonably hopeful in showing that borderline patients will gradually improve and that patience and support over time will reap rewards. However, one of the problems in assessing long-term therapies of BPD is that natural history and therapeutic effects are confounded. When a patient improves after many years of therapy, is this BPD burning out, or the results of our hard work? The caveat has to be taken into account in considering the psychoanalytic therapy of BPD. "Natural" improvement is generally seen on 15-year follow-up, whereas after 5 years most borderline patients are unchanged (Paris 1988). Therefore, it may not be unreasonable to consider a patient who is dramatically improved after only 5 years of treatment as a therapeutic success.

Another problem in evaluating treatment options for BPD is the heterogeneity of clinical samples. What are the characteristics of the borderline patients who undergo psychoanalytic therapy, cognitive therapy, or psychopharmacological trials? Can we generalize successful results from one sample to another? If not, how can we identify what kind of borderline patient we are dealing with in order to rationally individualize treatment? There are no easy answers to any of these questions, and we must therefore interpret even rigorously evaluated treatment results with caution.

Long-term analytically oriented psychotherapy is one of the most frequently recommended treatments for BPD in psychiatric settings. In Chapter 13, Kernberg presents the rationale. Long-term therapy has not been systematically evaluated for BPD (or for any other disorder) because of the enormous expense that would be required to do so. Kernberg describes an approach that has been presented in a manual and is now being empirically investigated, although the results are not yet in. He also demonstrates that his method is similar to those described by a number of other authors, such as Adler, Volkan, and Searles.

In the absence of clinical trials, we fall back on clinical wisdom, and it is the analytically oriented therapists who have provided most of that wisdom, often inspirationally so, for burgeoning therapists. Kernberg, like McGlashan, is far from starry-eyed about what can be done for borderline patients. He is well aware of how often we fail and how discouraging those failures can be after years of effort (e.g., Kernberg 1984). However, he provides clinicians with a very clear conceptual framework for working with borderline patients and, in doing so, replaces chaos with order.

However, there is not an absolute consensus about the psychoanalytic treatment of BPD. Kernberg tends to be conceptual and confrontative, emphasizing active interpretation. Other writers have suggested a softer and more supportive approach, providing the holding environment that these patients need to recover (e.g., Adler 1985). Whatever one's theoretical system, working long-term with borderline patients requires some framework so that the therapist can tolerate the dysphoria until such time as the patient gets better.

Which borderline patients benefit from long-term treatment? This question, which again raises the issue of how to subgroup borderline patients, has been well reviewed by Waldinger (1987). The clinical literature suggests that only a minority of borderline patients are candidates for intensive psychotherapy. This approach requires ego strength to benefit from long-term treatment, and we need more accurate assessment before beginning a therapy that will be taxing for both patient and therapist. However, because long-term outcome studies suggest that the treatment of BPD is rather unpredictable (Paris 1988), we cannot expect that such assessment will be more than a way of excluding those cases that are least likely to benefit. One possibility, which has not been empirically tested but would be congruent with the work of McGlashan, is that borderline patients who are able to work consistently in their outside life may have a greater capacity to work in psychotherapy. Because psychotherapy is work, such patients should be expected to form a stronger working alliance.

For both clinical and practical reasons, long-term psychoanalytically oriented psychotherapy may not be a practical alternative for more than a minority of borderline patients. Fortunately there are important alternatives. Some of these involve an entirely different theoretical rationale, such as Linehan's application of cognitive-behavioral therapy. In Chapter 14, Shearin and Linehan apply the Linehan model of BPD (described in Chapter 5) to treatment. It is a new approach, geared to dealing directly with the most disturbing borderline behaviors, such as suicidality and self-mutilation.

It is possible that Linehan's approach could be combined with other forms of treatment. In fact, with the exception of the absence of reconstructive interpretations, the technical approach has many overlaps with the recommendations of psychodynamic therapists such as Gunderson (1984), Kroll (1988), and Kernberg (1984). A great deal of emphasis is put on getting under control behaviors that threaten the treatment alliance, and confrontation is used in the context of a positive relationship with the patient.

Linehan calls her treatment *dialectical behavior therapy* (DBT). What she means by "dialectical" is the exquisite balance between acceptance and autonomy in the treatment, dynamic issues that have been considered crucial in the development of the borderline personality (Melges and Swartz 1989). Another point of overlap with other authors is the importance of validating the experiences of borderline patients, including their frequent traumatic histories. The preliminary findings of the effectiveness of DBT by Shearin and Linehan are quite encouraging, although, as they point out, only short-term outcome has so far been assessed. Another question is to what extent the patients who are able to contract to enter DBT are typical of BPD patients as a whole.

The question whether sample bias prevents generalization about effectiveness demonstrated in clinical trials can be asked about all the forms of psychotherapy that have been recommended for BPD. One is always left with the question of whether reported success is a function of which patients agreed to start in a specific treatment modality, and which patients stayed in treatment long enough to have their outcome assessed. In addition, clinical trials may not be designed to compare the relative efficacy of different treatments. We do not yet have any comparative studies, and until we do, the choice of treatment is more art than science.

In choosing among psychotherapies, we should remember that different borderline patients have different needs. As Waldinger (1987) points out, the controversy about intensive versus supportive therapy for BPD may simply reflect subgroups of patients, some of whom can benefit from intensive therapy and some of whom cannot. Furthermore is there any reason to believe that all borderline individuals need continuous therapy? As Gunderson et al. (1989) have shown, most BPD patients do not tolerate such therapy for long, and the majority of them drop out (probably to return at a later date when a crisis arrives). Dropping out is the rule even when the patient undergoes long-term psychotherapy, as shown in a study by Waldinger and Gunderson (1984). This goes along with outcome research demonstrating the long-term chronicity of BPD. As McGlashan emphasizes, we need not feel uncomfortable with intermittent therapy; on the contrary, it could be considered the norm for this population.

The dynamics of BPD may interfere with the capacity to tolerate the dependency and intensity of a continuing therapeutic relationship. Silver (1985) and Perry (1989) have suggested capitalizing on this phenomenon, moving from a continuous therapy to an intermittent one. However, in their models one begins with intensive therapy that then becomes intermittent when the patient's need for separation and autonomy warrants a change.

There are also borderline patients who never enter therapy at all but turn up from time to time in a crisis. Many of these cases are managed by multiple crisis intervention, and the outcome studies indicate that most of these patients will recover in time if they do not commit suicide. In this context the sometimes frustrating work done with borderline patients in hospital emergency rooms and outpatient clinics is better grounded than is immediately apparent. There are patients who self-select out of psychotherapy, and we have no reason to consider that their decision is the wrong one. In a model that parallels the medical management of chronic illness, the therapist tolerates pathology, remains available, and works toward rapid remobilization. Some borderline patients gravitate toward continuous supportive treatment. (This modality can be defined as therapy in which the operative element is the relationship with a therapist rather than specific interventions such as interpretation or behavioral shaping.) It is possible that supportive therapy is the most widely used option for the management of BPD, particularly in settings such as community clinics or social agencies. Patients can also shift from continuous to intermittent therapy. There seems to be a population of borderline patients who are most comfortable with this approach, although as reported by Wallerstein (1986), there are a few who will become "lifers."

Finally, there are borderline patients who may or may not be manageable in psychotherapy but whose symptoms are so severe that these must be targeted pharmacologically. Some will be treated primarily with medication, but many borderline patients who are in therapy will need medication from time to time in the course of treatment to manage their impulsivity and dysphoria. There has therefore been a great deal of interest in applying the proven success of psychopharmacological research to the borderline patient.

Soloff's review in Chapter 15 of the role of medication in BPD is both comprehensive and cautionary. Psychopharmacological agents have a limited, but by no means dramatic, effect on the phenomena of BPD. Tricylic antidepressants are not particularly effective. The best documented (if marginal) improvement is with neuroleptics. Concerning the use of fluoxetine in BPD, there are encouraging open trials but no double-blind studies; thus the jury is still out. It may be that we will have to understand a great deal more about the constitutional factors in BPD before we develop effective treatment with drugs. Alternatively, if we were to discover a medication that produces dramatic effects in BPD, it might lead us to a better understanding of etiology (as has happened so many times before in psychiatry).

As Silver and Rosenbluth point out in Chapter 16, many borderline patients will have at least one hospitalization in the course of their illness. In most cases this will be precipitated by a suicide attempt or threat. There are several areas of controversy around inpatient treatment. Polar views have been presented by Kernberg (1984), who argues for long-term hospitalization of the more difficult cases in order to make outpatient psychotherapy possible, and Dawson (1988), who thinks we should never hospitalize borderline patients. Silver and Rosenbluth, taking an intermediate view, suggest that short-term hospitalization is the norm and present a practical program for limiting regression and making adequate discharge plans. They also discuss some of the common complications of inpatient treatment and how to work around them.

Although borderline patients are usually hospitalized for their suicidality, they tend to be chronically suicidal over extended periods. Because one cannot constantly readmit patients every time they threaten suicide, therapists working with BPD patients have to develop an approach for dealing with chronic suicidality. As is evident by the high suicide rate documented in outcome studies of BPD, it is by no means clear that we know how to prevent suicide. A number of suggestions have been made in the clinical literature for how to balance safety with effectiveness in handling the suicidal borderline patient. This thorny area of management is reviewed in Chapter 17 by Paris.

In Chapter 18, Gunderson and Sabo place the emphasis on eclecticism in treatment. Essentially clinicians need to be aware that each borderline patient's condition is a unique clinical problem and that the options have to be individualized. Thus, there are borderline patients who are best controlled with medication; those who benefit from intermittent crisis intervention; those who need hospitalization, or at least partial hospitalization; and those who do surprisingly well in psychotherapy. It should be added, as Frances et al. (1984) have pointed out, that there are probably borderline patients who are best not treated at all.

Although we cannot say whether borderline patients improve because of or in spite of our treatments, treating borderline patients can nevertheless be rewarding. Every clinician who has carried out a series of long-term uncovering psychotherapies with borderline patients can report complete recoveries. Although this anecdotal evidence needs support from clinical trials, it is reasonable to assume that borderline patients do respond to treatment, albeit unpredictably. This might be one final occasion to consider the heterogeneity of BPD. If we knew which patients to offer which treatment on the basis of clinical assessment, we could save ourselves grief and be cost-effective in management. Until that time, we have to depend on clinical judgment.

The emphasis of this book has been on empirical evidence, but it must be clear by now that systematic evaluation of treatment for borderline patients is just beginning. The best studies are in psychopharmacology, which is essentially an adjunctive treatment, and even then we draw inferences from mostly short-term outcomes. For the overall clinical management of BPD, which whether continuous or intermittent is likely to stretch over years, we lack meaningful data. We need research at least on the model of the Boston study of the psychotherapy of schizophrenia (Stanton et al. 1984), in which treatments are compared for long-term outcome. That model of research would require both patient researchers and generous granting agencies.

In the interim, the variety of treatments available for BPD requires clinicians to be broadly knowledgeable. "Borderline personality disorder" exists on the borderline of biological, psychological, and social phenomena, and one needs to be comfortably eclectic to effectively manage patients with this disorder. Above all, the bad reputation of the borderline patient in treatment is due to unrealistic expectations on the part of the therapist. When one has a good sense of what one can and cannot do with BPD patients, there is no need to burn out.

REFERENCES

Adler G: Borderline Psychopathology and Its Treatment. New York, Jason Aronson, 1985

Dawson DF: Treatment of the borderline patient, relationship management. Can J Psychiatry 33:370–374, 1988

Frances A, Clarkin J, Perry S: Differential Therapeutics in Psychiatry: The Art and Science of Treatment Selection. New York, Brunner/Mazel, 1984

Gunderson JG: Borderline Personality Disorder. Washington, DC, American Psychiatric Press, 1984

Gunderson JG, Frank AF, Ronningstam EF, et al: Early discontinuance of borderline patients from psychotherapy. J Nerv Ment Dis 177:38–42, 1989

Kernberg O: Severe Personality Disorders. New Haven, CT, Yale University Press, 1984

Kroll J: The Challenge of the Borderline Patient. New York, WW Norton, 1988

Melges FT, Swartz MS: Oscillations of attachment in borderline personality disorder. Am J Psychiatry 146:1115–1120, 1989

Paris J: Follow-up studies of borderline personality disorder: a critical review. Journal of Personality Disorders 2:189–197, 1988

Perry S: Treatment time and the borderline patient. Journal of Personality Disorders 3:230–239, 1989

Silver D: Psychodynamics and psychotherapeutic management of the self-destructive character-disordered patient. Psychiatr Clin North Am 8:357–375, 1985

Stanton AH, Gunderson JG, Knapp PH, et al: Effects of psychotherapy in schizophrenia. Schizophr Bull 10:520–598, 1984

Waldinger RJ: Intensive psychodynamic therapy with borderline patients: an overview. Am J Psychiatry 144:267–274, 1987

Waldinger RJ, Gunderson JG: Completed psychotherapies with borderline patients. Am J Psychotherapy 38:190–202, 1984

Wallerstein R: Forty-two Lives in Treatment. New York, Guilford, 1986

Implications of Outcome Research for the Treatment of Borderline Personality Disorder

Thomas H. McGlashan, M.D.

T REATMENT OF MENTAL ILLNESSES PROCEEDS IN A VACUUM of understanding about the very nature of these disorders. This is not by choice or design; we simply do not know how or why things go awry in the majority of the identified mental diseases. In fact, we frequently even have difficulty identifying these disorders with much mutuality beyond random agreement. Nowhere in our discipline has this been more apparent than with borderline personality disorder (BPD). Its labyrinthine nosologic history has seen the disorder meander through several definitions to its current uneasy placement as a personality disorder. There does, however, seem to be a trajectory of progress midst this Babylonian landscape. As we gather observations over the years and record them into an expanding bibliography of perspective, the disorder becomes more distinct. As our focus sharpens, it also becomes more polymorphic and complex. We discern a plausible etiology for case A and a reasonable pathophysiology for case B, but recognize that neither model fits cases C, D, E, or F. And so on.

In the past decade our bibliography and perspective have been enriched by a number of longitudinal studies that tracked the long-term course and outcome of patients identified as having BPD based on contemporary diagnostic criteria (McGlashan 1986a; Paris et al. 1987; Plakun et al. 1985; Stone 1990a). Although this chapter focuses on the findings emerging from only one of these studies (McGlashan 1984a, 1984b), thus far the findings have been relatively consistent across investigations (see

Paris 1988). This set of longitudinal data is new and therefore in need of replication and further scrutiny, but its consistency suggests that it can and should be used to inform treatment strategies now. The good news is that we can see what we are trying to treat with greater clarity. The bad news is that our expanded and more realistic perspective demands we abandon comfortable theoretical dogmas and relinquish the notion that the hard-won understanding and successful treatment of one BPD patient can be applied to the next BPD patient.

LONG-TERM COURSE AND OUTCOME PROFILES FROM THE CHESTNUT LODGE FOLLOW-UP STUDY

What do we know about the natural history of residentially treated BPD patients? In the Chestnut Lodge follow-up study, 81 patients were identified at index admission as having BPD by DSM-III (American Psychiatric Association 1980) and Gunderson and Kolb (1978) criteria. The courses of their treatment and long-term (average of 15 years) outcomes have been detailed in numerous publications (Bardenstein and McGlashan 1988; Heinssen and McGlashan 1988; McGlashan 1985, 1986a, 1986b, 1987, 1992; McGlashan and Heinssen 1988, 1989). The outcome in BPD patients was superior to that of patients with schizophrenia, schizoaffective psychosis, bipolar affective disorder, and schizotypal personality disorder, and comparable to that of patients with unipolar affective disorder.

Focusing on the BPD cohort, the following clinical profile emerged (McGlashan 1986a). The majority of our BPD patients were single and female. Onset of disorder was usually in late adolescence, with illness escalating through the 20s. Onset was seldom precipitated by specific stress but appeared more in the nature of a pattern change in response to altered developmental demands. Prior to first psychiatric contact, BPD patients were more likely to be at least moderately impaired in all adaptive spheres (i.e., social, sexual, and instrumental). First treatment contact occurred in the third decade. Like most patients referred to Chestnut Lodge, the BPD cohort were chronically ill and had experienced many prior treatment exposures without remarkable success. For the BPD patients, however, this was more likely to be in the form of outpatient psychosocial treatment as opposed to inpatient and somatic treatments, which were more usual for the patients with psychosis. Also, in keeping with their classification as having Axis II personality disorders, our BPD patients were less ill at their index (Chestnut Lodge) admission in the nature and degree of productive symptomatology.

Although treated residentially without time limitations, the BPD patients at Chestnut Lodge did not tend to become institutionalized. Their inpatient time was the shortest of the diagnostic groups, and they were among the least likely to require transfer to other institutions. They were also far less passive and compliant (traits characteristic of the "institutionalized patient"), as evidenced by a high rate of signing out of the hospital against medical advice (Heinssen and McGlashan 1988).

Overall Outcome

At follow-up, the BPD patients were doing well in their basic living situations. Most lived autonomously, some with intimate partners and some with children. They were similar to patients with unipolar affective disorder in this arena and strikingly divergent from patients with schizophrenia.

The hospitalizations required by some of the BPD patients after Chestnut Lodge were frequently brief and crisis oriented. Although medication was not used extensively after discharge, psychosocial outpatient treatments (usually individual or group psychotherapy) were very common, with nearly half of the patients requesting or requiring further therapeutic support.

Instrumentally, BPD patients proved quite productive in terms of both the amount and the quality of work, and they generally had accumulated good work records. In fact, many appeared to work diligently despite an otherwise difficult existence. Also, BPD patients scored a mean of 2.9 on Hollingshead and Redlich's (1957) scale of occupational level at follow-up, indicating that jobs were being held equivalent to administrative managers, small business owners, minor professionals, etc. Although this may simply reflect good baseline socioeconomic status, the BPD patients were able to use such resources productively.

One of the cornerstones of BPD psychopathology rests in the area of relationships, which tend to be stormy, conflict ridden, and labile in intensity. Therefore, the outcome of these patients' relationships in the social sphere was of particular interest. At follow-up, the Chestnut Lodge BPD patients proved to be moderately active socially. Here, however, the distribution of scores was bimodal. One group functioned well and managed to create and maintain meaningful relationships with stability over time. This group further clustered roughly into three subgroups: 1) good social but no intimate relations, 2) partial intimate but no generative relations, and 3) intact intimate and generative relations. The other cluster in the bimodal distribution of patients, however, essentially dealt with this problematic area by studious avoidance of relationships. They appeared to be people who had concluded that their emotional equilibrium required abstinence in object relations. Overall, these patients' characteristic labile relationships appeared to resolve with time in one or the other direction, that is, either steadily social or regularly distant.

Symptomatically, most BPD patients demonstrated distinct evidence of persisting psychopathology. They often managed to compartmentalize and effectively prevent their symptoms from intruding on their instrumental capacities, but they were less successful in sequestering conflicts from the social sphere. The nature of their continuing psychopathology was consistent with the signs and symptoms leading to the initial diagnosis. Depressive signs and symptoms were very common, as was substance abuse.

Outcome as a Function of Age at Follow-up

In contrast to the patients with schizophrenia and affective disorder, the outcome scores for the BPD patients varied significantly with time postdischarge. Their global outcome profile traced an inverted U, with the apogee occurring in the second postdischarge decade when the average subject was in his or her 40s (McGlashan 1986a). We also found, upon closer scrutiny, that male and female BPD patients differed in several aspects of their clinical profiles. This finding plus the variability in functioning over time prompted an investigation into the long-term natural history of BPD by gender (Bardenstein and McGlashan 1988).

Our principal findings were as follows. At baseline (Chestnut Lodge admission), more female BPD patients were married than were the males, and they related better heterosexually than did the males. Their manifest illness presented with more depressive symptoms and self-destructive behaviors. The male BPD patients, on the other hand, were more antisocial and uncooperative (i.e., more AMA discharges). Over lengthening follow-up intervals, the female BPD patients retained an ever-married status more frequently, but the male BPD patients proved to be consistently more active socially. Both male and female BPD patients advanced occupationally, symptomatically, and globally with time. The female BPD cohort that was followed up 20 or more years after discharge fell off in their symptomatic and global functioning, but this sample was small ($n = 9$) and likely biased by cohort effects.

When outcome was good, no gender differences emerged. When outcome was bad, however, the female patients were more self-damaging at baseline and follow-up, and the male patients were more antisocial at baseline and prone to alcohol abuse at follow-up.

Prediction of Outcome

While a certain consistency emerged in the temporal vicissitudes of our BPD patients, especially within gender, it was also clear that these patients still comprised a heterogeneous sample with variable presentations, functional abilities, and long-term outcomes. Certain key baseline dimensions were identified, however, that predicted long-term course and reduced this variance in longitudinal profile (McGlashan 1985).

Three variables emerged most frequently and consistently as predictors of global outcome: IQ, affective instability, and length of previous hospitalizations. Higher IQ was associated with better global outcome. The mean IQs for the group with poor global outcome and for the group with good global outcome were 112 and 120, respectively. Affective instability, which indicates marked shifts from normal mood to depression, irritability, or anxiety over brief periods of time (typically hours, rarely more than a few days), was present in 53% of the poor-outcome subjects compared with only 16% of the good-outcome patients. Length of previous hospitalizations was the third strong predictor of global outcome. Prior to index admission, the poor-outcome group averaged 10 months in other institutions, whereas the good-outcome group averaged exactly one-half that amount of time.

Several more variables emerged as predictive when multidimensional outcome was considered: hospitalization, work functioning, social functioning, intimate relations, symptomatology, and global functioning. Among the characteristics associated with better outcome were male gender, less family history of substance abuse, better premorbid heterosexual functioning, absence of magical thinking, presence of felt affect (e.g., dysphoria, elation), and control of aggression in relationships.

We also found that BPD characterized by narcissistic and antisocial traits did not differ in longitudinal profile from BPD without these traits (McGlashan and Heinssen 1989). This finding was somewhat at variance with Stone's (1990a) long-term follow-up of BPD patients from the New York State Psychiatric Institute. He found below-average outcomes for BPD patients with concomitant antisocial personalities or with a history of having been in jail. BPD patients with schizotypal personality disorder comorbidity, or who were victims of parental brutality or rape, also did poorly. Better-than-average outcomes in his sample were associated with high artistic talent, "exceptional" attractiveness (in females), higher IQ, and alcohol abuse under control through involvement in Alcoholics Anonymous.

None of the above characteristics have been used to define BPD, yet all of them serve the clinically useful purpose of estimating prognosis and generating actuarial approximations of the treatment resources and strategies that will be needed case by case.

TREATMENT IMPLICATIONS

Overall, BPD can be a serious and disabling, even lethal, mental disorder. This was especially true for the Chestnut Lodge cohort. Here were patients who had failed with a large variety of prior therapeutic strategies. Yet their long-term trajectory was surprisingly favorable considering the depth of their psychopathology at admission. Time was kind to them if they stayed alive (only two committed suicide). Many got better who remained in therapy; many got better who did not. Some managed to cultivate native talents; others became more savvy about choosing people they could depend on. Action gave way to hesitation and became informed more often by experience. No longer hovering in neutral, development shifted back into gear. Adolescence was often still in force, but it faded eventually as life extended into the fourth and fifth decades. For many of these patients, their parents' fondest hopes came true: they finally grew up.

Highly condensed life stories of five patients from the Chestnut Lodge follow-up study BPD cohort are presented below. These profiles of the natural history of the illness have been selected as being prototypically illustrative of what happened to these patients over time, especially the time periods before and after Chestnut Lodge. Because we are interested in the life story in its larger, longitudinal perspective, we will not focus on the details of their treatment at Chestnut Lodge or elsewhere. Suffice it to say that most BPD patients from this era at Chestnut Lodge received exploratory interpersonal psychotherapy and active, largely inpatient, milieu therapy. Treatment was long-term, with lengths of stay measuring in months and years. Continuity of care with the primary psychotherapist beyond inpatient and day patient phases was encouraged. Very few patients received medication or psychosocial interventions that were supportive, behavioral, or rehabilitative in nature. The therapy of BPD patients at Chestnut Lodge today, however, incorporates all of the above and has been described in more detail elsewhere (Fenton and McGlashan 1990).

The implications of these illness natural history profiles are difficult to condense and generalize because each patient to be described, like each patient in the entire cohort, achieved his or her adaptation in highly individual ways. Nevertheless, we feel that the following treatment attitudes and/or strategies emerge from these profiles: 1) an attitude of optimism and patience, and 2) a commitment to providing protection, to encouraging work, to discouraging intimacy, and to applying an eclectic range of interventions pragmatically. Each will be elaborated with an illustrative follow-up story.

Maintaining Treatment Attitude of Optimism and Patience

Officially, "borderline" is a diagnostic label. Unofficially, in clinical parlance, it is synonymous with "anathema." The new longitudinal data, however, offer a welcome counterpoint to this pejorative colloquial caste. These patients may be among the most trying and difficult in our professional practices, but there is reason for optimism about their likely course and outcome over many years.

Case Example: Jeffrey

Jeffrey was a single 21-year-old when admitted to Chestnut Lodge in the mid-1960s. Difficulties became apparent when he was in college, marked by falling grades, anxiety, and difficulty concentrating. Jeffrey was socially isolated, and he alienated peers with his rudeness and arrogant intellectualizing. After being evicted from a dormitory suite, he lived alone. He never dated, nor did he participate in school activities. Jeffrey began outpatient psychotherapy, but after the first of three suicide attempts at age 19, he had to be hospitalized. Eight hospitalizations followed, mostly for manipulative suicidal gestures, in between which he became more and more anxious and nonfunctional. At index admission, Jeffrey was described as unrealistically demanding, rejecting, and unable to tolerate criticism or change. He was often depressed and suicidal and complained of loneliness. Socially, he was initially cold, superficial, and suspicious. Jeffrey was also prone to anxiety attacks and was intensely disturbed by therapy, during which he would regress to abject dependency upon the therapist, whom he would begin calling at all hours of the day and night.

After several months of inpatient treatment, Jeffrey was discharged from Chestnut Lodge while AWOL. Thereafter, he traveled for 6 months, allegedly to find jobs, but found none. He returned to the Rockville area to visit staff and patients at Chestnut Lodge. After tutoring math at a local university for two years, he returned home and entered college full time. For a long time after his discharge, he engaged in heavy marijuana smoking and was arrested in a drug raid after three semesters of college. He was convicted but not jailed. Jeffrey left school and worked odd jobs while living at home. He eventually resumed his education and received a bachelor of science degree in physics and math. Jeffrey subsequently worked for several electronics firms, started an unsuccessful consulting firm, and finally accepted a high-paying job with a computer company.

At follow-up, Jeffrey was 29 years old, single, and living alone. He dated occasionally, but not seriously. He saw people regularly, but his relationships were superficial. Jeffrey visited his parents monthly. No problems with drug or alcohol abuse were present. Jeffrey complained of a slight depression most of the time but was never rehospitalized. He had received no psychiatric treatment since his discharge from Chestnut Lodge.

Jeffrey's chronically self-destructive, haughty, and hostile presentation, as well as his unauthorized exit from Chestnut Lodge, would not engender much trust in his prospects for the future. Yet without further treatment he settled down after some initial meandering geographically and chemically. He negotiated school and employment with increasing stability and responsibility. Although living alone, he was socially engaged and on good relationships with his family. Overall, he was back on a track not at all unusual for an ambitious bachelor in his late 20s. Furthermore, queries to Jeffrey about what led to this turnaround in his life's path elicited no specific catalysts or influences; his explanations dovetailed into a single theme: "got older." And indeed he had.

Knowing Jeffrey's story and those of others like him we can, as psychoeducators, teach and encourage our patients with BPD that their lot is likely to improve with time, that life does not consist of an endless extension of the present. Their disorder, like their developmental level, is not stagnant but dynamic, fluid, and capable of being interred beneath successive levels of accrued maturity. During times of travail and despair, such reminders can be motivating, if not lifesaving.

Making Commitment to Protecting the Patient

If time is on the side of the BPD patient, then one of the primary aims of any treatment effort in the here and now is to prevent irreversible, untoward consequences of the psychopathology. Unfortunately, BPD is a disorder characterized frequently by the borderline individual's faulty judgment and poor impulse control as well as by his or her driven, self-destructive behavior. Although most of the time this activity has some interpersonal manipulative aim, the game can be desperate and, if lost, can result in permanent damage. Death by suicide, loss of reputation by sexual and/or substance excesses, or loss of freedom because of antisocial behavior are all too common in this disorder and are the more tragic considering such behavior may be a transitory aberration in the patient's life trajectory.

The treatment implications are clear. BPD patients should be protected from the negative consequences of their behaviors whenever possible. This usually amounts to intermittent but active intervention at times of crisis, using hospitalization if necessary to offer safety. When the seriousness of a patient's "dangerous" behavior or threat is in doubt, treaters should err on the side of being manipulated. A therapist's injured narcissism is far more reversible than a patient's injured flesh. For some BPD

patients, a therapeutic relationship, or even the promise of one, is sufficient protection. For others, crisis intervention and short-term hospitalization are necessary. For still others, these treatment approaches prove to
be inadequate, and long-term forms of asylum are required. Here too,
treaters worry about being manipulated by BPD patients who are perceived as wanting only to "regress" and to be coddled. Again, it is better
for the therapist to be duped than for the patient to be dead. Furthermore,
the natural history of BPD patients who have been given this form of
extended care is quite encouraging. The data indicate rather strongly that
institutionalization is not a danger as it can be with psychotic patients. In
the Chestnut Lodge follow-up study, the vast majority of even the most
dependent BPD patients eventually left the hospital on their own initiative
and did not have to chronically depend on the "good graces" of society.

Case Example: Fred

Fred was a single 21-year-old when admitted to Chestnut Lodge. Onset of
his illness began at age 12 with symptoms of social isolation and increasing friction with peers. A psychiatrist recommended he attend boarding
school, which led to some years of better functioning. Then Fred's favor-
ite teacher committed suicide, an event that initiated a series of petty
thefts requiring punishment. At age 16, after the birth of a sister, Fred
began to have violent temper tantrums or to lie on his bed and stare at the
ceiling most of the day. He barely graduated high school. He ran away
from home, had a homosexual encounter, and was picked up by the
police for vagrancy. Fred began psychotherapy and entered another
boarding school to prepare for college.

After admission to college, he fell behind in his studies, depledged his
fraternity, and quit school. He entered another university but was rejected
by the fraternity he wanted to join. When his parents refused to accept a
collect telephone call from him, he hot-wired a car, stole money from the
fraternity, shot and wounded a drugstore clerk, and was arrested. After
serving 13 months in jail, Fred received a psychiatric evaluation that
eventually led to his transfer to Chestnut Lodge.

On admission, he reported feelings of loneliness and despair. He often
abused alcohol and could become oppositionally silent and manipulative.
Fred was discharged from Chestnut Lodge against medical advice after
years of treatment divided equally between inpatient and day patient
phases.

After discharge, Fred married and divorced twice, having had two children by his first wife. At follow-up 23 years postdischarge, he reported working full time in real estate after having worked in several previous jobs. He lived alone in his own home. He was not in treatment, nor was he taking medication. Fred was, however, socially active, dated regularly, and participated in political groups and clubs. His friendships were moderately close and satisfactory. He did not keep in touch with his children.

Fred described episodic depressions that he had treated with alcohol until he developed adult-onset diabetes. He replaced alcohol with self-help psychology books and was a devotee of a television evangelist. He considered seeing a therapist for "problem solving" but found self-motivation tapes and books just as helpful. When asked in which areas he felt he had improved, he stated that he had much better control of his temper and was able to tolerate frustration without losing control. Fred described thinking through situations and considering alternatives instead of taking impulsive action.

Fred came to Chestnut Lodge in lieu of spending further time in the state penitentiary. In retrospect, it appears to have been a good move. Although Fred's sojourn at Chestnut Lodge was no picnic, either for him or for the hospital, it probably served to protect him from the negative consequences of his antisocial impulsivity. Perhaps it was in jail or in the hospital when Fred began to develop temper control, frustration tolerance, and the ability to learn from his behavior—that is, developmental capacities that are a specific antidote to psychopathic behavior. As such, both jail and Chestnut Lodge protected him from further aggressive behaviors that could have permanently maimed him and/or others. It is also possible that Chestnut Lodge protected him from the negative consequences of jail, although this is hard to assert because the developmental maturation demonstrated by Fred also occurs frequently in criminals who spend all of their time in jail and never receive any psychiatric treatment. Perhaps Fred's transfer to a hospital from the penitentiary at least ensured that he would not emerge a more learned and ruthless criminal.

Encouraging Work

In psychotic disorders, especially schizophrenia, work disability is almost universal. In striking contrast, we found the capacity to work largely unimpaired in our BPD patients. In fact, this capacity came to play a central role in their recovery and maturation. The structure and responsibility of work served as a steady track leading them out of the woods of meandering lability, unstable relationships, and chaotic impulsivity. Work productivity often provided them with their richest source of self-esteem, sometimes the only source. Equally important, the structure of work provided daily human contact to assuage loneliness, but through relationships that were safely regulated by role.

Case Example: Janice

Janice was a married 35-year-old when admitted to Chestnut Lodge. When she was 10 her father died, after which she periodically starved herself, became anxious, and had difficulty concentrating. Although active socially, she was described as unpredictably snobbish with her friends. Shortly after graduating from college she met her future husband. They married, but Janice was embarrassed by, and avoided, sexual intercourse as much as possible. She often felt irritable, depressed, inadequate, and inferior. She criticized her husband constantly. She was hospitalized for marked lability of mood at age 28. During her stay, she discovered she was pregnant. After discharge, her relationship with her husband deteriorated. She began experiencing homosexual feelings along with periods of depression and hostility. She developed frequent, violent temper outbursts, often directed toward her mother or toward her young son, whom she whipped and fantasized about destroying. After the delivery of her second child, a daughter, Janice behaved suicidally, developed somatic complaints, and neglected her appearance. At age 35 she was admitted to Chestnut Lodge, where she was described as labile in mood, critical, overweight, and somatically preoccupied. Staff found her manipulative and splitting.

After years of inpatient and day patient treatment, Janice was discharged from Chestnut Lodge with medical advice. She had separated from her husband and her mother had died. Upon leaving the hospital, she passed a Civil Service examination and worked full time thereafter, supporting herself completely. She became a placement specialist for the unemployed and received awards for her work, an accomplishment of which she was very proud. Over the years, Janice had two prolonged sexual affairs, one with a married man and the other with a man 10 years her junior. She did not feel close to her daughter and avoided her son, who she suspected was gay. At follow-up she lived alone in an apartment, socialized rarely, and had to struggle just to attend church on Sunday mornings. She had one or two casual friends whom she visited monthly and on holidays. Janice was never rehospitalized, but she had engaged continuously in intensive psychotherapy with four successive therapists. She also took medication for depression and somatic complaints. She experienced suicidal ideation and had made several innocuous, "passive" attempts. She had mild difficulty with drinking and overeating. She experienced phobias about crossing bridges, riding elevators, and other outside activities to the extent that she was often unable to attend psychotherapy. She seldom, however, missed work. She felt resigned to being the victim of a bad life.

It is clear that Janice continued to struggle. She used treatment continuously, yet remained symptomatic and interpersonally estranged from those with whom others would have been close. In the midst of this, however, work was a steady, positive endeavor, something to which she remained loyal and the only thing about which she spoke without a bitter edge to her voice. The same could be said about Jeffrey and Fred above. For them as well, life became organized initially around work and remained a core source of orientation and predictability.

It is hard to know how to manipulate work therapeutically for BPD patients, because in most cases they seek work on their own initiatives. Perhaps it is sufficient to encourage such developments and to ensure that part-time instrumental industry is a component of any treatment plan, even during periods of crisis and regression. A treatment milieu that explicitly values work is also necessary. For example, patients should be exhorted actively to initiate or hang onto jobs. Or, when privileges are rescinded for manipulative and/or impulsive behaviors, the privilege to work should be exempt, or should be the very last privilege to go. Some BPD patients may possess the desire to work but not the talent. A careful diagnostic assessment of vocational capacities can help rehabilitative counselors steer patients toward jobs that match their level or toward training opportunities that enhance their level.

Discouraging Intimacy

As noted, for many of our BPD patients intimate relationships remained a major source of stress, symptom development, and painful failure. The borderline vulnerability to forming unstable relationships often contin-ued and stubbornly resisted the buffer of time. The female BPD patients, in particular, were drawn to intense one-to-one closeness (or driven to it by loneliness) again and again. By follow-up, 100% of the female BPD patients had been married at least once, compared with about 50% of the male BPD patients (Bardenstein and McGlashan 1988). At follow-up, however, most of the female patients, such as Janice, were divorced from their spouses or estranged from their lovers. Many, like Janice, were also distant from their children. The same, of course, was true of Fred, but many of the other male BPD patients avoided this maelstrom by develop-ing relationships that were numerous but superficial. They avoided inti-macy, sometimes from the start, sometimes after one or two disastrous romances. As noted elsewhere (Bardenstein and McGlashan 1988), male patients from this era (1950–1980) were blessed by the easy availability of careers to cathect and about which to orient their lives. They were not boxed into finding meaning primarily through exclusive long-term rela-tionships. They had a choice and chose nonintimacy. Today, however, this can serve as a model for both sexes.

Case Example: Luanne

Luanne was a single 20-year-old when admitted to Chestnut Lodge. Her first symptoms began when she went away to college. She became increas-ingly withdrawn and preoccupied and was unable to finish the year. She was employed twice briefly but quit each job because she was convinced she could not succeed. She began psychotherapy and soon vacillated between hating her therapist one day and refusing to leave his office the next. She was hospitalized psychiatrically twice for a total of 8 months. Few details were given of her treatment or her mental state except a note about her being very hot tempered.

On admission to Chestnut Lodge, Luanne was hostile, assaultive at times, and "impulsive." She devalued her therapist, constantly telling him he was insignificant. She did not appear to be motivated for therapy but nevertheless settled into a long-term stay as an inpatient and day patient. Luanne was discharged with medical advice in the late 1950s.

While still a day patient at Chestnut Lodge, Luanne met and married her husband, a former patient from another psychiatric hospital. She became pregnant twice and had a son each time. She described these pregnancies as the greatest times in her life. She was physically well and felt that having children gave her a reason to live. Her marriage, however, was quite unstable, as her husband was frequently psychotic and hospitalized. After 5 years, Luanne left her husband and moved to another city to be near her parents. At this time she was depressed, anxious, panicky, and occasionally suicidal. She screamed at and hit her children. She drank three to four beers per night and went on heavier "drinking binges" periodically. She entered psychotherapy, felt that her doctor was a "lousy therapist," and became more disturbed instead of less. Her therapist eventually refused to treat her anymore, sending her for consultation elsewhere.

For several years, Luanne was not in treatment and worked as a secretary while she raised her sons alone. She was involved with several different men over the years and reported suffering feelings of great loss when the relationships ended. She began to have difficulty with her children and entered therapy again, seeing a female therapist once a week for 3 years. At first she felt they had good rapport, but with time her depression increased and she began feeling more and more out of control. She finally decided to quit therapy because it seemed to stir up more feelings than she thought she could manage. For the 3 years prior to the follow-up interview, Luanne was not in treatment and reported feeling "much more together and much less anxious."

At follow-up Luanne was 48 years old, divorced, and living alone in an apartment. She worked full time as a secretary. She was not thrilled with the job but managed to support herself. She was quite active socially, although most of her relationships were rather superficial. She belonged to several theater and singing groups, serving as a "den mother" for members rather than performing. She opened up her home as a "commune" of sorts where young adults who were involved in the groups would stay for short intervals, sometimes up to a month or more. She had two "faithful" women friends whom she could "trust" if she "wanted to," but never risked getting very close with them. She no longer dated, stating that she had "ruled out sex," but did have several men friends. She felt she had good relationships with her sons now that they lived in different localities. She felt much more relaxed since they had left home and were functioning well on their own. Symptomatically, Luanne experienced only slight degrees of anxiety and depression. She drank alcohol occasionally but no longer abusively.

Luanne was one of the female BPD patients who learned the hard way to restrict intimacy in her life. With virtually everyone—friends, lovers,

children, and therapists—she found closeness a liability, ultimately burdened with more conflict and dysphoria than reward. Her latter-day
adaptation was a compromise: a commune of acquaintances, and friendships that were robust in number but truncated in depth. Also she was
quite aware of the trade-off, that she had relinquished trust and romance
for feeling "much more together and much less anxious." Many of our
BPD patients, especially the males, negotiated a similar deal with themselves. They frequently met, at least partially, their strong needs for
attachment through active involvement in groups where contact was
ubiquitous but a certain interpersonal distance was also guaranteed by the
context.

The most common group, of course, was the work scene, with relationships carefully regulated by rules and hierarchy. Almost as common
were religious, political, or therapeutic self-help groups like Narcotics
Anonymous or Alcoholics Anonymous.

Thus, many BPD patients learned to settle for superficiality. Whether
this can be taught as an active, adaptive strategy in treatment, however,
remains a question. Actively counseling BPD patients to avoid intimacy,
in fact, seems counterintuitive to the psychotherapeutic process as traditionally conceived. Perhaps what is useful is for treaters to recognize that
closeness and intimacy may stir up domains of psychopathology in many
BPD patients that are relatively impervious to the traditional strategies of
understanding. Gunderson et al. (1989) noted, for example, that between 25% and 66% of borderline patients unilaterally dropped out of
individual psychotherapy within the first 6 months. When and if such
resistance appears regnant, it may be wise for therapists to avoid pursuing an exploration of the patient's defenses against intimacy in the context of a close and intense therapeutic relationship, especially if such an
endeavor has been tried unsuccessfully one or more times in the past.
More may be gained at less risk of failure and injury by exploring alternate ways of being with others and/or encouraging the patient's participation in groups and a wide social network. At the very least, such
patients should be helped to clarify what is for them the most comfortable interpersonal distance, that is, what depths of relatedness they can
and cannot tolerate. This may mean going with the flow of the BPD
patient's crisis-oriented life-style and accepting that treatment may be
sought only on an "as needed" basis. It is important to remain steady,

letting the patients control the distance and remembering that they can be resourceful too.

Applying an Eclectic Range of Interventions

The discussion to this point has been based on some of the characteristics we found to be relatively common among our BPD patients over the long term: their tendency to get better, to adapt well to work, and to handle continuing interpersonal deficits with compromise. We also found a vast heterogeneity. From individual to individual, differences were more striking than similarities, and this must be taken into account when drawing up any guidelines for treatment. Stone (1990b) suggests that we must deal with such complexity with eclecticism and pragmatism. Our collection of BPD life stories strongly endorses this attitude and overall strategy. The extraordinary variance within and among BPD patients demands that treatment be multimodal, opportunistic, and driven by continuous assessment of outcome (i.e., of the ratio of benefits to risks). For some patients this will mean recommending no treatment (Frances and Clarkin 1981); for others it will mean suggesting long-term inpatient or residential care (Fenton and McGlashan 1990). For some it will mean using medication (Cowdry and Gardner 1988), for others intensive psychotherapy (Kernberg 1984), for still others cognitive-behavioral therapy (Linehan et al. 1991), and so forth. What, for example, would be the treatment of choice for the following patient?

Case Example: Debbie

Debbie was a single 17-year-old when admitted to Chestnut Lodge in the mid-1950s. She was noted to have had almost a lifelong history of being "intensely suspicious, distrustful, dictatorial, and at times furiously angry. She was very anxious, lonely, and isolated . . . moody, distressed, and depressed." She was continuously demanding of people and very dependent.

At age 9, following the death of her adoptive mother, Debbie began having night terrors during which she "sensed a presence in her room." At 10 she started what became more-or-less continuous outpatient treatment. At age 15, she lost interest in school, began to have rages, and was delinquent (i.e., went out to bars with a rough crowd of boys). She began work with a new therapist and talked of suicide and wrist slashing. She complained of loneliness and isolation and began to pursue sex, first with her adoptive brother, and then with any man that entered the home. Debbie believed she saw and heard Martians who could communicate with her deceased adoptive mother. With all this, her therapist became convinced that hospitalization was required.

Debbie was hospitalized for 8 months at age 16, during which time she received electroconvulsive therapy (ECT) and "massive doses of Thorazine," none of which produced any positive results. She was then transferred to Chestnut Lodge. At admission Debbie was noted to be intensely hostile and threatening, at times throwing things. She was in and out of Chestnut Lodge many times and was finally discharged with medical advice 8 years after admission.

While still in the Washington, D.C. area, Debbie married and worked as an art therapist and held several other part-time positions. She reported her initial functioning as good, but her marriage deteriorated and she separated and moved West. She divorced about $3\frac{1}{2}$ years later. After her move, she taught school for a while, then began working in a beauty salon. She held that job for about 1 year before a rehospitalization forced her to quit. Debbie had been hospitalized twice briefly prior to this for depression. She also entered psychotherapy, which she attended with varying frequencies of four times a week to once a month over a 4-year period. It appears that phenothiazines again were attempted during this time, but a worsening of symptoms prompted their discontinuation.

At some point, approximately 10 years after discharge from Chestnut Lodge, Debbie learned of her ex-husband's suicide and said that this prompted her third hospitalization. At admission she weighed only 95 pounds and had been drinking a fifth of wine a day. During her hospitalization she was given 20 treatments of electroconvulsive therapy and was discharged as improved 5 months later. She reentered outpatient therapy, returned to work at the beauty salon, and reported doing fairly well for about 1 year. Over the next 5 years, however, she was admitted over 30 times to the same institution. These admissions were usually brief, often lasting only a day or two. Overdoses most often prompted the staff to admit her, only to see her sign out AMA a day or so later. On one occasion she stepped in front of a car in an unsuccessful suicide attempt. It is not clear when Debbie was started on Elavil, but she reports that she received high doses of this medication for quite a while until a seizure led to a reduction in dosage and ultimately to discontinuation. Elavil was later tried once more but again stopped because of fluid buildup. Debbie also spent 4 years on Dilantin, 300 mg qd, presumably for the control of seizures. At the time of follow-up she was taking Valium prn.

At follow-up, Debbie was 51 years old, divorced, and living alone in a house. She was in psychoanalytic psychotherapeutic treatment at a frequency of once every 2 weeks and was taking Valium prn. She had been hospitalized twice in the past year for drug overdoses. She was not working and was living on a modest trust fund. When she had last worked, which was about 1 year prior to follow-up, she held a public relations position for about 3 months. Socially, Debbie was relatively uninvolved. She described her social activity as consisting of nightly visits to a local restaurant where she had gotten to know some people superficially. She dated infrequently. She said wistfully that her friends from previous places rarely visited but then added that she would rather be by herself.

Symptomatically, Debbie was experiencing periodic psychotic symptoms that included hallucinations, derealization, and depersonalization. She said she felt like "Alice in Wonderland—bigger, smaller, walls closing in on me." She heard voices in her house and saw visions of people (all deceased) standing at her bedside. She said they would tell her things to do such as rewrite her will. These episodes were transient. She also complained of depression. Debbie had a severe problem with alcohol and was likely intoxicated on several occasions when contacted for follow-up. She also had overdosed on medication many times and described these as attempts to commit suicide. On one occasion she attempted to strangle herself with a belt.

During the follow-up telephone interviews, Debbie seemed intoxicated and her speech was slurred. Affect was somewhat flat, consistently depressed, and had an edge of bitterness and despair. She expressed little sadness or humor. Debbie was oriented to all spheres, and content was appropriate and intellect intact. However, she was vague and concrete at times. Debbie presented herself as a victim who had no sense of enjoyment or fullness in her life and was struggling to function at a minimal level.

Debbie, without question, represents one of the poorest outcomes in our follow-up sample of BPD patients. By displaying unremitting disability, she was unusual but not unique. By the age of 51 she had seen and been seen by literally dozens of mental health workers, and she had been

prescribed the gamut of treatments ranging from outpatient psychotherapy and pharmacotherapy to inpatient care and ECT, from long-
term residential treatment with intensive, exploratory psychotherapy to
outpatient aftercare. None of it seemed to help her escape her vicious
spiraling between entitled, hostile dependency on the one hand, and
bitter withdrawal on the other, played out largely with "helping" professionals.

It is hard to know what to recommend for Debbie given this grim
legacy of therapeutic failure. Perhaps she is a prime candidate for Frances
and Clarkin's (1981) prescription of "no treatment," because treatment so
predictably provoked negative reactions. Certainly this option stands as
the one not yet attempted in her case. Even so, of what would this "no
treatment" consist, especially at times when she entered an emergency
room having taken an overdose? Ultimately we must confront the fact
that we do not know, because virtually all of the available treatment
strategies were tried, in adequate doses, by adequate practitioners.

Debbie's case advocates for an eclectic treatment approach by highlighting the limitations of our therapeutic expertise. She defeated all com-
ers. Her story should keep us humble, skeptical about what we "know,"
and continuously searching for different solutions.

THE RATIONALE FOR INTERMITTENT, CONTINUOUS, AND ECLECTIC THERAPY

The patient with BPD presents us with a difficult yet challenging task. As
Aronson (1989) concluded in his recent review of the use of psychotherapy in treating BPD, "despite the voluminous treatment literature of the
last 50 years, it still appears that borderline patients remain on the border
of treatability" (p. 525). Given this, it is heartening to know that the newly
gathered natural history data suggest that time can offer further normal
development to serve as an ally in our mutative efforts with these patients.
At the same time, we must be cognizant of the limits to which we can
generalize our data about natural history to the larger universe of BPD
patients. The information gathered from the Chestnut Lodge follow-up
study derives from a sample with unique characteristics that must be kept
in mind. On the one hand, they were disadvantaged in being severely ill

and experiencing repeated "treatment failures." On the other hand, they were advantaged in being well off financially, generally quite intelligent, and often endowed with marketable talents. Our natural history profiles do not come from an untreated epidemiological sample of people with BPD. They come from a sample of well-treated hospitalized patients. Our observations and inferences, therefore, may not apply to some populations—for example, to healthier BPD patients who can be treated as outpatients and who never require hospitalization, or to disadvantaged BPD patients whose dismal economic circumstances constantly undermine any and all potential treatment effects.

In devising therapies it is crucial to begin with the limits of what we know. We do not know the etiologies of BPD, but guess they are multifactorial. We also do not know the pathophysiologies of BPD, but guess they are pleomorphic. We do not even have a prototypic description of the malady because no characteristic proves pathognomonic or specific. We do not know if BPD is a manifestation of affective disorder or an atypical form of psychosis (McGlashan 1983). Jeffrey, for example, could have been suffering from a behaviorally expressed recurrent depression and Debbie, from schizoaffective disorder with histrionic traits.

Therefore, because we do not know what makes a "borderline," how can we endorse any unitary model that purports to unmake a "borderline"? Stone (1987, 1988) has written cogently about this dilemma. He suggests that while BPD appears to be an entity, it is also very heterogeneous in both etiology and pathogenesis. Therefore, because the borderline patient's problems are eclectic in their source, treatment must be eclectic in its application. Stone (1987) suggests, for example, that only one in three hospitalized BPD patients can use psychoanalytic psychotherapy. In another communication Stone (1988) explores an etiologic hypothesis of psychobiological hyperirritability for some BPD patients and suggests that certain treatment strategies follow. For example, the first phase of any treatment for such patients would be a reduction of irritability, initially with medications such as carbamazepine or lithium, and subsequently with a variety of psychosocial approaches (such as cognitive-behavioral therapy, Alcoholics Anonymous, or rehabilitative problem solving, etc.) to increase the patient's mastery over "psychodynamically obvious" but uncontrollable impulses. Once impulsivity has been mastered, various forms of psychotherapy may be useful, beginning with those that are supportive in tone, that are flexible in length, and that try to educate the patient about what can and cannot be reasonably expected of others. The emphasis is on developing a comfortable working relationship and learning to solve problems jointly. If progress can be made in these domains, more in-depth analytic work may be attempted, assuming that the patient is sufficiently interested and resilient.

The borderline patient's chaotic impulsivity and tendency to split elicits complementary strategies from therapists, that is, treatments that are dogmatically overcontrolling and split between the extremes of neglect and intensive involvement. For many years the treating professions (especially within psychoanalysis) were divided between those who felt that continuous treatment offered the only hope and those who felt that continuous treatment offered only danger. Of late, the split seems to be disappearing beneath an emerging integrative strategy known as *intermittent continuous treatment*. Silver (1983, 1985) may have been the first to write about this form of treatment explicitly as "long-term intermittent" therapy. It consists of short-term intermittent psychotherapeutic treatment offered on a long-term basis. Perry (1989) has recently termed this "intermittent continuous" therapy. It is consistent with the medical model of a chronic disease with acute exacerbations. The primary aim of treatment is to support the patient in crises to decrease self-injury. Such availability is offered on a long-term or continuing basis, hopefully to prevent further exacerbations, minimize irreversible setbacks, and foster the natural growth that comes with time. Continuous active treatments such as intensive psychotherapy are reserved only for those who successfully negotiate or survive this matrix and who initiate the effort fully cognizant of the risks inherent with exploratory work.

In the borderline war of split acronyms it may be said that the broadest and most flexible approach to the fire of BPD is ICE, or a treatment that is Intermittent, Continuous, and Eclectic. With this model, the precise prescription will vary from patient to patient, sometimes dramatically, because BPD patients are different, sometimes astoundingly. At the same time it capitalizes on an apparent long-term maturational or healing tendency that seems to be common across many BPD patients despite their differences. Although we may not have a clear grasp of what we are dealing with, there is reason to hope that time offers a reward for our continued interpersonal availability and investment.

References

American Psychiatric Association: Diagnostic and Statistical Manual of Mental Disorders, 3rd Edition. Washington, DC, American Psychiatric Association, 1980

Aronson TA: A critical review of psychotherapeutic treatments of the borderline personality: historical trends and future directions. J Nerv Ment Dis 177:511–528, 1989

Bardenstein KK, McGlashan TH: The natural history of a residentially treated borderline sample: gender differences. Journal of Personality Disorders 2:69–83, 1988

Cowdry RW, Gardner DL: Pharmacotherapy of borderline personality disorder: alprazolam, carbamazepine, trifluoperazine, and tranylcypromine. Arch Gen Psychiatry 45:111–119, 1988

Fenton WS, McGlashan TH: Long-term residential care: treatment of choice for refractory character disorder? Psychiatric Annals 20:44–49, 1990

Frances A, Clarkin JF: No treatment as the prescription of choice. Arch Gen Psychiatry 38:542–545, 1981

Gunderson JG, Kolb JE: Discriminating features of borderline patients. Am J Psychiatry 135:792–796, 1978

Gunderson JG, Frank AF, Ronningstam EF, et al: Early discontinuance of borderline patients from psychotherapy. J Nerv Ment Dis 177:38–42, 1989

Heinssen RK, McGlashan TH: Predicting hospital discharge status for patients with schizophrenia, schizoaffective disorder, borderline personality disorder, and unipolar affective disorder. Arch Gen Psychiatry 45:353–360, 1988

Hollingshead AB, Redlich FC: Social Class and Mental Illness. New York, Wiley, 1957

Kernberg OF: Severe Personality Disorders: Psychotherapeutic Strategies. New Haven, CT, Yale University Press, 1984

Linehan MM, Armstrong HE, Suarez A, et al: Cognitive-behavioral treatment of chronically parasuicidal borderline patients. Arch Gen Psychiatry 48:1060–1064, 1991

McGlashan TH: The borderline syndrome, II: is it a variant of schizophrenia or affective disorder? Arch Gen Psychiatry 40:1319–1323, 1983

McGlashan TH: The Chestnut Lodge follow-up study, I: follow-up methodology and study sample. Arch Gen Psychiatry 41:573–585, 1984a

McGlashan TH: The Chestnut Lodge follow-up study, II: long-term outcome of schizophrenia and the affective disorders. Arch Gen Psychiatry 41:586–601, 1984b

McGlashan TH: The prediction of outcome in borderline personality disorder: part V of the Chestnut Lodge follow-up study, in The Borderline: Current Empirical Research. Edited by McGlashan TH. Washington, DC, American Psychiatric Press, 1985, pp 61–98

McGlashan TH: The Chestnut Lodge follow-up study, III: long-term outcome of borderline personalities. Arch Gen Psychiatry 43:20–30, 1986a

McGlashan TH: Schizotypal personality disorder: Chestnut Lodge follow-up study, VI: long-term follow-up perspectives. Arch Gen Psychiatry 43:329–334, 1986b

McGlashan TH: Borderline personality disorder and unipolar affective disorder: long-term effects of comorbidity. J Nerv Ment Dis 175:467–473, 1987

McGlashan TH: The longitudinal profile of borderline personality disorder: contributions from the Chestnut Lodge follow-up study, in Handbook of Borderline Disorders. Edited by Silver D, Rosenbluth M. New York, International Universities Press, 1992, pp 53–86

McGlashan TH, Heinssen RK: Hospital discharge status and long-term outcome for patients with schizophrenia, schizoaffective disorder, borderline personality disorder, and unipolar affective disorder. Arch Gen Psychiatry 45:363–368, 1988

McGlashan TH, Heinssen RK: Narcissistic, antisocial, and non-comorbid subgroups of borderline disorder: are they distinct entities by long-term clinical profile? Psychiatr Clin North Am 12:653–670, 1989

Paris J: Follow-up studies of borderline personality disorder: a critical review. Journal of Personality Disorders 2:189–197, 1988

Paris J, Brown R, Nowlis D: Long-term follow-up of borderline patients in a general hospital. Compr Psychiatry 28:530–535, 1987

Perry S: Treatment time and the borderline patient: an underappreciated strategy. Journal of Personality Disorders 3:230–239, 1989

Plakun EM, Burkhardt PE, Muller JP: Fourteen-year follow-up of borderline and schizotypal personality disorders. Compr Psychiatry 26:448–455, 1985

Silver D: Psychotherapy of the characterologically difficult patient. Can J Psychiatry 28:513–521, 1983

Silver D: Psychodynamics and psychotherapeutic management of the self-destructive character-disordered patient. Psychiatr Clin North Am 8:357–377, 1985

Stone MH: Psychotherapy of borderline patients in light of long-term follow-up. Bull Menninger Clin 51:231–247, 1987

Stone MH: Toward a psychobiological theory of borderline personality disorder: is irritability the red thread that runs through borderline conditions? Dissociation 1:2–15, 1988

Stone MH: The Fate of Borderline Patients: Successful Outcome and Psychiatric
    Practice. New York, Guilford, 1990a
Stone MH: Treatment of borderline patients: a pragmatic approach. Psychiatr
    Clin North Am 13:265–285, 1990b

CHAPTER 13

The Psychotherapeutic Treatment of Borderline Patients

Otto F. Kernberg, M.D.

WITH THE IMPACT OF NEW CLINICAL EXPERIENCES AND empirical research in the last 20 years, the psychodynamic psychotherapy for patients with borderline personality disorder (BPD) has evolved in a more exploratory, expressive direction. The supportive psychotherapy approaches that were formerly recommended as the treatment of choice have been losing their appeal. Differences persist, however, regarding the extent to which the psychotherapy should be purely analytic, exploratory, or expressive, or should combine expressive and supportive features, at least in the initial stages of treatment.

Waldinger (1987) has provided a comprehensive review that is at once a synthesis and a summary of the differences and common features among the views of the leading contributors in this field, including Buie and Adler (1982–1983), Chessick (1977), Giovacchini (1979), Gunderson (1984), Kernberg (1982), and Masterson (1976). All of these individuals adopt an essentially interpretive or expressive approach, although they vary 1) in the degree to which they consider supportive techniques helpful or even central in the early stages of treatment; 2) in the degree to which providing a holding environment early in the treatment is crucial; and (3) in the degree to which the therapist needs to structure the boundaries and the framework of the treatment.

Waldinger and Gunderson (1987), in their conclusions regarding the study of five borderline patients treated with long-term psychoanalytic psychotherapy, propose the following general strategies:

1. The treatment must include a stable framework that defines the boundaries of its setting.
2. The therapist must be more active than he or she would be with
   neurotic patients because of the borderline patient's problems in reality
   testing, projective mechanisms, and distortions.
3. The negative transference has to be tolerated.
4. The patient must be helped via interpretation to establish bridges
   between his or her actions and feelings.
5. Self-destructive behavior needs to be discouraged by clarification and
   confrontation.
6. Acting out has to be blocked by setting limits on actions that endanger
   the patient, others, or the treatment.
7. In the early phases of treatment, clarifying and interpreting the transference in the here and now should be viewed as preferable to making
   genetic interpretations.
8. Countertransference analysis must be treated as a crucial aspect of the
   interpretive work.

Adler (1989), in comparing the models of Kernberg (1984), Masterson
(1981) and Rinsley (1982), Adler (1985) and Buie and Adler (1982–1983),
Gunderson (1984), and Searles (1986), also stresses the importance of
analyzing the countertransference, the processes and problems in building the therapeutic alliance, the problems posed by getting the patient to
comply with treatment schedule and boundaries, and the complications
presented by self-destructive actions and inadequate social and family
support. He concludes that, in contrast to Kernberg's "relatively clear
distinctions between supportive and expressive psychotherapy, most of
the literature defines a mixture of supportive and expressive/exploratory
techniques" (p. 62).

In what follows, and in order to highlight some potentially alternative
strategies within the common frame of psychodynamic psychotherapy for
borderline patients, I am selecting a few representatives from this field.
Because of the basic similarity of my own approach to that of Gunderson
and Waldinger and of Masterson and Rinsley, I shall utilize my own
approach as representing that general strategy, while underlining the fact
that there are significant differences between what I do and what others
do in the early stages of the treatment. These differences reside in my

emphasis on early interpretations of the negative transference, whereas the others stress the importance of the therapist's holding function and of building up the therapeutic alliance at that time.

Because Volkan (1987) has integrated my ideas with ideas stemming from Winnicott (1953, 1956, 1960), I shall outline Volkan's approach. The significant difference between Adler and Buie's approach to my treatment strategies has led me to choose Adler's (1985) formulations for a more detailed analysis. And, finally, because of Harold Searles' (1986) significant utilization of concepts from interpersonal psychoanalysis, I have selected him as another major representative of contemporary psychodynamic psychotherapy with borderline patients. In the final section of this chapter, I summarize some contributions to the psychodynamic psychotherapy of borderline patients derived from my recent work.

AN APPROACH TO THE TREATMENT OF THE BORDERLINE PATIENT: THE WESTCHESTER DIVISION–NEW YORK HOSPITAL BORDERLINE PSYCHOTHERAPY RESEARCH PROJECT

We have constructed a theory of psychodynamic treatment of borderline patients that derives from the theory of psychoanalytic technique but modifies this technique by creating a general strategy aimed at resolving the specific disturbances of borderline patients (Kernberg 1984; Kernberg et al. 1989). Our basic objectives are the diagnosis and psychotherapeutic resolution of the syndrome of identity diffusion, and, in the process, resolution of primitive defensive operations characteristic of these patients and their primitive internalized part-object relationships into "total" object relationships characteristic of more advanced, neurotic, and normal functioning. Primitive internalized object relations are constituted by part-self representations relating to part-object representations in the context of a primitive all-good or all-bad affect state. They are part-object relations precisely because the representations of self and object have been split into an idealized and a persecutory component—in contrast to the normal integration of good or loving, and bad or hateful representations of self and significant others. These primitive, or part-object, relations emerge in the treatment situation in the form of primitive transferences characterized by the activation of such self and object representations and their corresponding affect as a transference "unit" enacted defensively against an opposite primitive transference unit under completely opposite affect valence or dominance.

In essence, the *psychotherapeutic strategy* in the psychodynamic treatment of borderline patients consists of a three-step procedure:

1. *Diagnosis of an emerging primitive part-object relationship in the transference and the interpretative analysis of the dominant unconscious fantasy structure that corresponds to this particular transference activation.* For example, the therapist may point out to the patient that their momentary relationship resembles that of a sadistic prison guard and a paralyzed, frightened victim.

2. *Identification of the self and object representation of this particular primitive transference and the typically oscillating or alternating attribution of self and object representation by the patient to himself or herself and to the therapist.* For example, the therapist may point out, in expanding the previous intervention, that it is as if the patient experienced himself or herself as a frightened, paralyzed victim, while attributing to the therapist the behavior of a sadistic prison guard. Later on in the same session the therapist may point out to the patient that now the situation has become reversed, in that the patient behaves like a sadistic prison guard, while the therapist has been placed in the role of the patient as a frightened victim.

3. *Linking of this particular object relationship activated in the transference and an entirely opposite one activated at other times but constituting the split-off idealized counterpart to this particular, persecutory object relationship.* For example, if at other times the patient has experienced the therapist as a perfect, all-giving mother, while experiencing himself or herself as a satisfied, happy, loved baby who is the exclusive objective of mother's attention, the therapist might point out that the persecutory prison guard is really a bad, frustrating, teasing, and rejecting mother and the victim an enraged baby who wants to take revenge but is afraid of being destroyed because of the projection of his or her own rage onto mother. The therapist might add that this terrible mother-infant relationship is kept completely separate from the idealized rela-

tionship out of the fear of contaminating the idealized one with the persecutory one, and of the destruction of all hope that, in spite of the rageful, revengeful attacks on the bad mother, the relationship with the ideal mother might be recovered.

The successful integration of mutually dissociated or split-off, all-good and all-bad primitive object relations in the transference includes the integration not only of the corresponding self and object representations but also of primitive affects, leading to affect modulation, to an increase in the capacity for affect control, to a heightened capacity for empathy with both self and others, and to a corresponding deepening and maturing of all object relations.

This psychotherapeutic strategy also includes a particular modification of three basic tools derived from standard psychoanalytic technique. First, there is a modification in the tool of *interpretation*—that is, the process of establishing hypotheses about unconscious determinants of the patient's behavior.— In contrast to standard psychoanalysis, interpretation here involves mostly the preliminary phases of interpretative interventions: 1) a systematic *clarification* of the patient's subjective experience; 2) the tactful *confrontation* of the meanings of those aspects of his or her subjective experience, verbal communication, nonverbal behavior, and total interaction with the therapist that express further aspects of the transference; and 3) a restriction of the unconscious aspects of interpretation to the *unconscious meanings in the here and now only*. In contrast to standard psychoanalysis, where interpretation centers on unconscious meanings both in the here and now and the "there and then" of the unconscious past, in the psychodynamic psychotherapy of borderline patients psychodynamic interpretations of the unconscious past are reserved for relatively advanced stages of the treatment, when the integration of primitive transferences has transformed primitive transferences into advance transferences (more characteristic of neurotic functioning, and more directly reflective of actual experiences from the past).

Second, the *transference analysis is modified,* in each session, so that it can be guided by the therapist's ongoing attention to the long-range treatment goals with any particular patient and the dominant, current conflicts in the patient's life outside the sessions. To ensure that the treatment does not excessively gratify the patient's transference, thus undermining the patient's initial motivation and treatment objectives, the therapist has to keep in touch with the long-range treatment goals. Also, in order to prevent splitting off of external reality from the treatment situation, and severe acting out expressed by such dissociation between external reality and the treatment hours, transference interpretation has to be linked closely to the present realities in the patient's life. In short, then, in contrast to psychoanalysis, in which a systematic focus on the transference is a major treatment strategy, in the psychodynamic psychotherapy of borderline patients transference analysis is modified by attention to initial treatment goals and present external reality.

Third, *technical neutrality may have to be limited.* Insofar as interpretations require a position of *technical neutrality*—that is, the therapist's equidistance from the forces in mutual conflict in the patient's mind—this neutrality is an important aspect of the psychodynamic psychotherapy of borderline patients, as well as of standard psychoanalysis. However, given the severe acting out of borderline patients inside and outside the treatment hours, technical neutrality may have to be limited by indispensable structuring (i.e., limit setting) of the treatment situation, which (at least temporarily) reduces technical neutrality and requires its reinstatement by means of interpretations of the reasons that the therapist moved away from a position of technical neutrality.

Our strategy also requires a set of *tactical considerations* regarding the interventions in each treatment hour, which give a particular coloring to this psychotherapy that differentiates it both from standard psychoanalysis and from supportive psychotherapy.

In contrast to supportive psychotherapy, in our treatment approach the therapist refrains, as much as possible, from technical interventions such as affective and cognitive support, guidance and advice giving, direct environmental intervention, and any other technical maneuver that would reduce technical neutrality—with the exception of necessary structuring or limit setting in or outside the treatment hours. As mentioned before, whenever such limit setting becomes necessary, it also requires a systematic effort to analyze the reasons for setting these limits, the interpretation of the underlying transference conflicts, and the gradual resolution of the need to set such limits by means of interpretative resolution of these underlying conflicts. In contrast to supportive psychotherapy, transferences are not utilized for enhancing the therapeutic alliance, patient

compliance, or symptom resolution, but both positive and negative transferences are interpreted (with the exception of milder aspects of the
positive transference, which may be left untouched, in order to foster the
therapeutic alliance, particularly in early stages of the treatment). Our
treatment approach includes a systematic effort to interpret the patient's
primitive idealizations of the therapist because of their counterpart to
dissociated primitive negative transferences.

In each session, it is important to assess the patient's capacity to
differentiate fantasy from reality and to carry out interpretation of unconscious meanings only after the confirmation of commonly shared views of
reality on the part of the patient and therapist. This may require consistent and tactful confrontation of the patient with immediate reality before
interpreting the unconscious meaning. The patient's attribution of fantastic meanings to the therapist's interpretive interventions also needs to be
clarified and interpreted. It is important to assess secondary gain of severe
symptoms and behaviors, to interpret such secondary gain, and, if necessary, to reduce or eliminate it by limit setting, with the corresponding
need to reassess and interpret any slippage of technical neutrality. The
analysis of unconscious sexual conflicts must include the analysis of contamination of sexuality with aggression in order to help the patient to free
his or her sexual behavior from the control by aggressive impulses.

The interpretation of unconscious meanings must often start out
being formulated in a metaphorical, "as if," or atemporal way before
linking the interpretation with a particular aspect of the patient's past. For
example, to say "It is now as if an enraged child were defiantly provoking
his father to show that he is not afraid of him" may be a better way of
initiating an interpretation that links present and past than a direct implication that the patient is concretely repeating an experience of the past.
Premature and forceful interpretation of the unconscious past may reinforce the confusion between present and past and induce transference
psychosis, not to mention risking the danger of artificially indoctrinating
the patient. In contrast, the formulation of interpretations in a metaphorical, atemporal, or "as if" mode facilitates the emergence of new, previously unsuspected material.

Another crucial aspect of tactical interventions is the need to interpret
primitive defenses systematically as they emerge in each hour. The interpretation of primitive defenses tends to strengthen reality testing and

overall ego functioning. In contrast to previous conceptions of primitive defenses, these defenses do not "strengthen" the frail ego of the borderline patient but are the very cause of chronic ego weakness. Interpretation of primitive defenses is a major tool for increasing ego strength and reality testing and facilitates the interpretation of primitive transferences. In this connection, primitive transferences and more advanced or realistic transferences that characterize later stages of the treatment may alternate, so that patients sometimes present primitive and advanced transferences within the same session. The general principle is to interpret, as much as possible, primitive transferences before the advanced ones.

Given the severe tendencies toward acting out on the part of borderline patients, dangerous complications in their treatment may derive from their characterologically based, "nondepressive" suicide attempts, drug abuse, self-mutilating and other self-destructive behaviors, and aggressive behaviors that may be life-threatening to themselves and others. An important aspect of each session, and not just a part of the overall structuring of the treatment, is the assessment of whether there are emergency situations that require immediate interventions. On the basis of our general treatment strategy and the specific experiences in the treatment of severely ill borderline patients, we have constructed the following set of priorities of intervention that reflect the need to assess, diagnose, and treat these and other complications.

A threat of imminent suicidal or homicidal behavior has the highest priority in each session. If there seem to be immediate threats to the continuity of the treatment, these constitute the second highest priority to be taken by the therapist. If the patient appears to be communicating in deceptive or dishonest ways, this becomes the third highest priority: psychodynamic psychotherapy demands honest communication between patient and therapist and, by the same token, the interpretation of the transference meanings that underlie the patient's dishonesty or deceptiveness. Acting out in the sessions as well as outside the sessions constitutes the next highest priority, already signaled in our earlier statement that transference analysis must include the consideration of dominant conflicts outside the hours of therapy.

With these priorities considered, the therapist may then concentrate fully on the analysis of the transference along the lines already outlined. There are times when the dominant affects in the hours are linked with developments outside the hours—that is, "affective dominance" may not always center in the transference. If that is so, affective dominance determines the focus of the therapist's attention, with an awareness that affect-laden conflicts outside the treatment situation also may have transference implications that may become clearer and more dominant later on.

Finally, trivialization of the patient's communication requires attention: the therapist's sense that "nothing is going on" in the hours implies either trivialization, deceptiveness, a dominance of narcissistic resistances, or perhaps a period of respite and working through—or simply the therapist's temporary disorientation. The therapist has to decide which of these causes of real or apparent trivialization he or she should take up.

This psychodynamic psychotherapy for borderline personality organization (BPO) (see Chapter 8) requires that the therapist see the patient in face-to-face interviews and maintain his or her natural behavior but refrain from communicating anything about his or her private life to the patient as part of the general psychodynamic principle of not gratifying transference needs but analyzing them. To be technically neutral and to maintain a natural, objective stance while remaining "in role" does not mean "studied indifference"; to the contrary, the therapist must examine his or her own emotional reactions to the patient on an ongoing basis in order to detect undue involvement or undue distancing on his or her part and to be able to diagnose any countertransference implications. The analysis of what Racker (1968) described as concordant and complementary identifications in the countertransference is an important aspect of the psychodynamic psychotherapy of borderline patients. We assume that, particularly under conditions of complementary countertransference—that is, when the therapist's countertransference reflects his or her unconscious identification with a repressed, dissociated, or projected self representation or object representation of the patient—the diagnosis of this identification in the countertransference is an extremely helpful tool for diagnosing the dominant primitive object relation activated in the transference. The therapist's utilization of the countertransference consists in his or her silent analysis of the corresponding meanings, whether it stems from the patient or from himself or herself, and the utilization of this understanding in his or her interpretative interventions. Rather than communicating the countertransference directly to the patient, the therapist utilizes it in the formulation of his or her transference interpretations.

Patients with BPO, like all patients with severe characterological pathology, tend to communicate significantly in nonverbal ways, in addition to the content of their verbal communications. The therapist must be alert to the content of the patient's communications, to his or her nonverbal communication, and to the total atmosphere expressed in the moment-to-moment relationship between patient and therapist. We also assume that an underlying, nonverbalized, constant aspect of the relationship between patient and therapist is an important potential "channel" for transference communication, together with the moment-to-moment shifting verbal and nonverbal communications. The therapist has to be alert to all these sources of information: they constitute the raw material for his or her constructions of interpretative interventions. This therapeutic alertness toward the total communication of the patient is particularly helpful when the sessions have prolonged silences, a resistance that may be interpretatively resolved by the analysis, at such points, of predominately nonverbal and general relational "channels" of communication.

Our approach also considers the analysis of severe regressions in the transference, particularly strong paranoid regressions, microparanoid psychotic episodes, and transference psychosis in general. Because under such conditions reality testing may be temporarily lost in the therapeutic communication, a tactical intervention mentioned before—that is, to clarify reality fully before interpreting the unconscious elements in the transference—now becomes operational. Therefore, when the patient is deeply regressed, most of the psychotherapeutic interventions may be focused on analyzing the distortions of immediate reality in the patient-therapist interaction and their potential meanings. Transforming a breakdown of common reality boundaries into the hypothesized activation of an unconscious object relationship involving patient and therapist at that point is one more application of the first step of our psychotherapeutic strategy (see above) involving the strategic analysis of primitive transferences.

Advanced stages of the psychodynamic psychotherapy of borderline patients resemble the psychodynamic psychotherapy, and even the psychoanalytic treatment, of neurotic patients. At such advanced stages of the treatment, more subtle and specific characterological pathology and corresponding transference resistances may be explored and resolved, particularly the more subtle aspect of narcissistic pathology. Severe negative therapeutic reactions, especially in patients with significant narcissistic pathology, may complicate the treatment and require focusing once more on the more primitive transference developments (e.g., unconscious envy of the therapist) implied in these reactions. In short, the analysis of primitive transferences, while gradually receding throughout the duration of the treatment, still remains as a therapeutic task to the very end of the treatment.

THE APPROACH OF GERALD ADLER

Adler (1985) divides treatment of borderline psychopathology into three successive phases. In *phase I,* the therapist tries to establish and maintain a dyadic relationship in which he or she can be steadily used over time by the patient as a holding selfobject. The aim is to allow the patient to acquire a solid evocative memory of the therapist as sustaining holder, which serves as a substrate out of which the patient can then form adequate holding introjects.

The inevitable development of rage, however, interferes with this process. This rage has three sources: first, holding is never enough to meet the patient's felt need to assuage aloneness, and the patient is inclined to vengefully destroy the offending therapist. Hence, the patient fears that he has lost or killed the therapist and that he is threatened by the therapist's responding to his rage by turning from "good" to "bad." Second, the frustrating holding selfobject is distorted by projection of "hostile introjects" so that the patient "carries out what he experiences as an exchange of destructiveness in a mutually hostile relationship" (Adler 1985, p. 50). Third, the patient's envy of the object that is so endowed with the potential for holding sustenance produces hateful destructive impulses toward the therapist. Finally, the patient may also feel a primitive guilt because he feels undeserving of the therapist's help owing to his own evilness.

Treatment in phase I aims to reduce these impediments by means of clarification, confrontation, and interpretation. The therapist, as a holding selfobject, provides "transitional objects" (a term Adler uses to refer to the therapist's providing the patients, for example, with vacation addresses and postcards), telephone calls, and extra appointments to reaffirm that the therapist continues to exist. The patient thus learns that the therapist is an enduring and reliable holding selfobject, or that the therapist is indestructible as a "good object" (here Adler refers to Winnicott [1958]).

In *phase II*, the major task is to help the patient, by means of what Kohut (1971) has called "optimal disillusionment," to gradually become aware of the unrealistic aspects of the holding introjects established in phase I. While the patient is still heavily dependent on a continuing relationship with holding selfobjects, he needs to be weaned for a viable setup for adult life "in which selfobjects cannot realistically be consistently available and must over the years be lost in considerable number" (Adler 1985, p. 59).

In *phase III*, to help the patient become optimally autonomous in regard to secure holding and a sense of worth, the therapist's focus is on helping him develop a realistic superego that is not inappropriately harsh. Also, the patient's ego must develop a capacity for pleasurable confidence in the self and for directing love toward the self that is similar to the affectionate nature of object love rather than narcissistic love.

THE APPROACH OF VAMIK VOLKAN

Volkan (1987) agrees, essentially, with Kernberg's (1975, 1984) formulations regarding the predominance of primitive defensive operations— particularly what Volkan calls "defensive splitting," in contrast to "developmental splitting"—as a central feature of the most severely ill borderline patients. Volkan points out that splitting is not limited to the borderline patient and that it finds expression in adult life, particularly under socially facilitating circumstances involving ethnicity, nationality, and so forth. By the same token, borderline patients also present repressive mechanisms together with splitting, although they utilize splitting more than repression. Regarding the question of etiology, Volkan also agrees with Kernberg about the condensation of oedipal and preoedipal conflicts in the borderline patient.

Volkan focuses particularly on the psychosis-prone borderline patient and discusses nine such patients in some detail. These nine patients were treated over several years, seven of them successfully, and all nine showed marked improvement in stabilizing their object relationships and their vocations, and in learning to tolerate being alone. The seven patients who were successfully treated showed, in addition, significant resolution of their object conflicts, advanced along the preoedipal-oedipal continuum, and they gradually shifted into a more advanced defensive organization.

Volkan specifically tolerates and welcomes a transference regression in his patients, acknowledging his debt to Boyer (1983), Giovacchini (1979, 1986), and Searles (1979, 1986). Volkan assumes that such regression brings about a dedifferentiation of self and object representations, similar to what occurs in a transference psychosis. This dedifferentiation is then followed by a progressive development in which self and object representations are differentiated, and the patient experiences "developmental splitting" in the transference instead of the previous defensive splitting.

Volkan outlines six steps in treatment:

1. *Establishing with the patient a reality base for the treatment.* Volkan provides explicit information about the nature of the treatment and of the task for the two participants, and sets necessary limits in a tactful, "nondrastic" way.

2. *Appearance of the first split transference.* Here Volkan is alert to early manifestations of splitting in the transference. He brings his observation to the patient's attention without genetic interpretations or an active effort to resolve this splitting process. He also concentrates on preserving the therapeutic relationship and maintaining a "holding function" by focusing on the patient's psychic operations in the here and now. The therapist helps the patient see how sharply split percepts of others are a characteristic phenomenon in the patient's experience, without attempting to interpret and resolve them at this stage. He also agrees with Rosenfeld (1987) in avoiding interpretation of manifest oedipal material at this stage, which might serve a defensive function as an "upward resistance." Volkan also pays attention to the patient's experience of the therapist's analyzing functions in order to clarify significant distortions in the perception of the therapist.

3. *Appearance of a focalized psychotic transference leading to reactivated and transference-related transitional phenomena.* It is at this point that Volkan stresses the importance of tolerating and facilitating psychotic regression in the transference. He uses the concept of psychotic "therapeutic stories," an affectively lived drama, a here-and-now version of a real or fantasized event in the past that includes considerable action

inside and outside the sessions. Now transference psychosis and delusional relatedness may emerge, processes that may last for a few weeks or months. Optimally, the patient now develops new transitional objects or phenomena, which have the potential to become a new bridge to reality. Volkan here uses concepts of Winnicott (1953, 1956, 1960) and Greenacre (1970).

4. *Appearance of a second split transference.* This transference now becomes the focus of the work and includes the possibility of mending the patient's opposing object-relations units. At this point, the interpretation of the meaning of splitting of all-good from all-bad images includes genetic material as it appears in the transference, in the patient's daily activities, and in dreams. The emphasis now is also on identification with the analyst's integrative functions.

5. *Development of the transference neurosis.* The patient may develop profound depression as part of the integration of mutually split-off object representations in the transference, and the vicissitudes of the Oedipus complex begin to dominate the material. Volkan has found that with the development and resolution of these issues, patients show an increased capacity for repression, and that some of the elements of split-transference manifestations that are not mended are repressed.

6. *Appearance of the third split transference and termination.* This final step is a stage of repetition and working through of previously explored issues. This step approximates that of classical analysis and working through of the termination phase of treatment. Volkan quotes Modell's (1976) writing on the termination stages with patients with narcissistic character disorder; Volkan agrees that, in a similar way, borderline patients may present atypical terminations characterized by the return of primitive splitting.

THE APPROACH OF HAROLD SEARLES

Perhaps the most central concept in Searles' (1986) formulations is the idea that the borderline patient, by means of projective identification, projects his pathogenic introjects onto the therapist, who, experiencing the consequences of these projective mechanisms in the countertransference, tends in turn to activate, as part of his countertransference regression, his own primitive dissociated introjects. The condensation of projected transference elements (the patient's introjects) and the therapist's reactivated transference dispositions (the therapist's primitive layer of pathogenic introjects) permits the therapist to identify with experiences that the patient cannot tolerate in himself and to share with the patient his understanding of the nature of these primitive introjects. In interpreting the transference, the therapist shares with the patient aspects of his countertransference that reflect his understanding and acceptance of this joint world of projected and reactivated introjects.

On the negative side, Searles goes on, the danger exists that the therapist may not be able to tolerate the reactivation of his own past introjects within his countertransference. This may lead to premature interpretations of the transference and a consequent perpetuation of projection and reprojection by interpretation, leading to stalemates in the treatment. Another negative possibility is that the therapist may become fixated in his own countertransference regression and fail to extricate himself interpretatively from that situation.

Searles warns against the danger of "brainwashing" the patient with premature interpretations but also refers to the patient's temptation to project his own brainwashing tendencies onto the therapist. He stresses the need for the therapist to accept the countertransference consequences of the patient transferences as an indispensable precondition for the patient's eventual acceptance of the therapist's interpretations. Searles offers abundant clinical evidence throughout to illustrate his proposal that every bit of psychopathology in the patient has a counterpart somewhere in the therapist's functioning and that there are always nuclei of real intuitions in the transference developments.

Another, and related, important concept is that of the therapeutic symbiosis as an indispensable precondition for psychotherapeutic work to proceed. Searles' concept of symbiosis is a relatively broad one, including both actual merger phenomena (such as are characteristic of transference regression in schizophrenic patients) and those confusions or interchanges of aspects of personality that are products of projective identification operating mostly in the patient but also in the therapist.

The therapeutic symbiosis, in Searles's view, includes the patient's multiple identifications with self and objects, projected and introjected, and is characterized by profound ambivalence because of the mutually contradictory nature of these identifications. This ambivalent symbiosis serves both as a defense against threatening primitive aggression associated with the relationship to pathogenic introjects, and as a potential for emotional growth as tolerance and working through of these mutually split-off internalized object relations are achieved in the transference experience and analysis. Searles illustrates the many and complex forms these transference-countertransference developments may take: for example, the patient's defensive detachment with the therapist's approaching vacation may reflect, in part, his identification with the analyst's defensive detachment because the latter cannot fully acknowledge his own dependency on his patient. The patient's narcissistic withdrawal therefore interacts with the analyst's defenses against his own dependency needs toward the patient as a transference object. Or perhaps, oedipal-triangular relationships may be played out, for example, by the patient's jealousy of a thriving plant in the therapist's office. At times the therapist who feels "irrelevant" to his patient may represent the patient's own projected "irrelevant" self. The therapist, in short, may become the patient's self, his multiple introjects, live and dead, human and nonhuman. Searles reminds us of his earlier work regarding the differentiation of the animate and inanimate world on the basis of the normal introjection of mother during the symbiotic period of development; he points to the deepest levels of loss of orientation toward external reality when the most primitive maternal introjects are split off and projected.

Searles questions some standard assumptions of psychoanalytic psychotherapy, such as the autonomous development of the "real" relationship to the therapist in the early years of treatment. He points out that this "real" relationship more often than not may be a split-off, symbolically meaningful transference relationship that differs from other, dissociated transference relationships: the "real" relationship can emerge only in advanced stages of the treatment as the consequence of working through split-off, primitive object relations in the transference.

In an attempt to provide some general characteristics of Searles' technique, I would stress 1) the emphasis on the communication of countertransference; 2) the very careful and gradual development of transference interpretations against the background of the tolerance and silent analysis, within the therapist's mind, of the symbiotic relationship; 3) the general tendency to tolerate lengthy silences; 4) the use of a long-range time frame for giving the patient the "space" to experience himself or herself as different from the therapist in the relationship, to gradually hear more realistically what is being said, to listen to it, and to associate to it; and 5) the therapist's parallel process of growth in his or her capacity to hear, listen, and understand.

Searles' emphasis, that one can interpret only within the symbiosis—to do otherwise is to risk sterile intellectualizations—is the counterpart to his stress on the therapist's need to tolerate split-off, internalized, projected object relations from the patient in his or her countertransference before interpretation can proceed.

Searles explores the very limits of the psychotherapeutic relationship in proposing that the patient can abandon his or her illness only if the therapist has come to cherish it too so that the patient's improvement becomes an experience of loss for both patient and therapist. This idea touches on some of the most complex and subtle aspects of the developments in long-term treatment of severely regressed patients. Searles also suggests that, just as the therapist must become the patient's mothering shield against the outside world so that the patient can submerge himself or herself protectively within the therapist, the therapist must be able to submerge himself in the patient, the patient thus assuming the function of the maternal shield for the therapist as a precondition for the patient's abandonment of his or her own autistic stance. In other words, within the therapeutic symbiosis, the patient, by identification with the therapist, must accept his or her roles as both protected infant and protective mother who helps the patient to differentiate and individuate.

RECENT DEVELOPMENTS IN THE APPROACH OF KERNBERG: THE TRANSFERENCE IMPLICATIONS OF SEVERE SUPEREGO PATHOLOGY

Some degree of superego pathology is frequent in the personality structure of patients with BPO. The severe distortions in ego development, the predominance of splitting mechanisms, and the lack of integration of internalized object relations influence the setting up of various layers of the superego. The normal integration and mutual toning down of idealized preoedipal superego precursors and of aggressive, persecutory preoedipal superego precursors fail to some extent, with a consequent weakening of the internalization of the later, more realistic superego internalizations of the oedipal period. The effects of these distortions in superego developments include some degree of failure to develop stable, integrated value systems, the ordinarily solid fundament of built-in autonomous morality.

These superego failures cause a weakness of normal superego regulation by means of differentiated self-criticism, a tendency toward regulation of self-esteem by violent mood swings, and a dissociation between states of intense exaggerated guilt feelings and despair, on the one hand, and rageful, inconsiderate, self-serving flaunting of ordinary considerations for other peoples' rights and for objective considerations of fairness and justice, on the other. In addition, borderline patients may present some degree of passive or parasitic and aggressive antisocial behavior, which is of particular importance regarding the prognosis for their psychotherapeutic treatment. In fact, as I have stressed throughout my contributions to this field, the quality of object relations and extent to which antisocial features are present are the two overriding prognostic factors in the treatment of BPO.

Superego pathology becomes an important issue in the treatment strategy, particularly in dealing with transferences that evolve as a consequence of its expression. As mentioned before, in our research project on the psychodynamic psychotherapy of borderline patients, we have established a list of priorities of subject matters that require urgent attention.

The highest priority is dealing with imminent threats to the life of the patient, of other individuals, or of the therapist, so that violent and potentially destructive behavior needs to be focused upon and dealt with first.

A second priority is represented by indications that, probably, the treatment is about to be disrupted, and it is essential that the therapist focus on the transference implications of such potentially imminent breakdown of the therapeutic relationship. In my view, two major factors involved in the high rate of early dropout in the psychotherapy of borderline patients are 1) lack of attention to setting up the initial treatment contract and 2) lack of attention to the transference implications of threats of disruptions of the treatment.

The third highest priority, finally, is the evidence of deceptiveness in the patients' communication—that is, the conscious suppression or alter-ation of essential information to the therapist—so that the therapist must necessarily be in error in his or her assessment of the patient's present emotional state and reality. This deceptiveness may take the form of suppression of information, of feeding the therapist false data (i.e., out-right lying), and/or using manipulative behavior intended to disorient the therapist or to exploit him or her in some way. All of these behaviors are carried out in clear consciousness by the patient and are not a conse-quence of unconscious denial or confusion.

It is striking how difficult it is for therapists to acknowledge to them-selves and to their patients that their patients are lying to them or treating them in a dishonest, deceptive way. Typically, patients who develop such behaviors also project such tendencies onto the therapist. Indeed, the more dishonest the patient, the more dishonest he believes his therapist to be, and the less he can trust what his therapist says to him. In some cases, verbal communication is vitiated to such an extent that it becomes a mockery of ordinary psychotherapeutic communication.

I have coined the term *psychopathic transference* to refer to periods in the treatment when such conditions of deceptiveness prevail in the trans-ference. In my view, it is essential to explore such transferences in great detail and to resolve them interpretatively before proceeding with other material (except the two higher priorities—imminent threats to life, po-tential disruptions in treatment—mentioned earlier). The psychopathic transferences tend to infiltrate and corrupt the entire psychotherapeutic process and are a major reason for psychotherapeutic stalemates and failure. To treat a patient psychotherapeutically requires total commu-nication between patient and therapist, and it is for this technical rea-son—and not for any "moralistic" one—that the therapist has to work on opening the field of communication by resolving psychopathic trans-ferences.

The therapist should share with the patient his or her concern at the patient's lying or consciously distorting information. This confrontation may bring about an immediate, angry attack on the part of the patient, who may in turn accuse the therapist of aggression or dishonesty. By means of projective identification and omnipotent control, the patient may unconsciously try to provoke the therapist to behavior that the patient may then interpret as dishonest.

These cases illustrate patients' intrapsychic conflicts between a desire for honesty and a corruption of this desire, conflicts that usually reflect an unconscious identification with a parental image perceived as profoundly inconsistent or dishonest. In cases with narcissistic personality disorder, the enactment of a sadistically infiltrated, pathologically grandiose self that operates against the healthy, dependent part of the patient's self constitutes a frequent dynamic underlying psychopathic transferences.

In other cases, a stubborn and silent protracted tendency to lying may defy the therapist's efforts to explore the very reasons for this deceptiveness. Still other patients may insist, over an extended period of time, that there are issues that they will not discuss with the therapist, which is honest and may permit the therapist to analyze the reasons for that fearfulness and distrust.

In somewhat different yet related cases, there seems to be open communication, except that the patient treats all other people with total ruthlessness and lack of consideration, expects the psychotherapist to treat him or her in the same way, and acts as if there were no such thing as an honest mutual commitment between two people. Here, rather than deceptiveness, the patient's assumption is that any closeness or commitment is deceptive and that the therapist, by pretending to be interested— beyond any financial, scientific, or prestige benefits he or she may gain from the patient—is really dishonest. This may be an unconscious dynamic as well as a consciously experienced fear.

What I have been describing are patients suffering from a deep corruption of the capacity for closeness, dependency, emotional commitment, and love. Typically, following the exploration of the origins of these psychopathic transferences and their effects on the therapeutic relationship, the transferences tend to shift, after a time, into a different disposition. The patient gradually begins to understand that complete openness may be necessary for psychotherapeutic work to proceed but that this exposes him or her to the danger of rejection, criticism and attack, as he or she sees it, on the part of the therapist. The patient who, after maintaining crucial information secret for an extended period of time, finally "confesses" what he did not dare to discuss before, typically experiences fears of attack, depreciation, or abandonment on the part of the therapist. The patient who treats all other people as "objects" typically fears that the abandonment of that protective distance from the therapist will endanger his or her security. In short, psychopathic transferences gradually are transformed into paranoid ones.

There are many patients with BPO whose predominately negative transferences contain strong paranoid elements from the beginning of the treatment. Although, on the surface, severely paranoid borderline patients may appear to be more difficult treatment challenges than more smoothly functioning patients with psychopathic transferences, it is much easier to explore the corresponding projective identifications of primitive internalized persecutory objects in the paranoid transferences. What is of particular importance here is that when such paranoid transferences are the outcome of previously worked-through psychopathic transferences, the paranoid elements may be particularly powerful and be expressed as serious distortions in the therapeutic relationship, even to the extent of the development of transference psychosis.

When this occurs, the technique I have described in earlier work (Kernberg 1984) to deal with paranoid regression in the transference may be particularly helpful. If the patient seriously distorts the reality of the therapist's behavior, the therapist may communicate to the patient that, in the therapist's view, the reality of their interaction is completely different and that, in some very specific ways, the therapist is convinced of something diametrically opposite to the patient's conviction. Simultaneously, the therapist continues, he accepts the patient's conviction regarding that issue, so that they have reached a state in which both are convinced of what turn out to be "incompatible realities." This reproduces the situation that occurs when a "mad" person and a "normal" person try to communicate with each other without an outside witness or arbitrator to clarify the reality of the situation. The only alternative, of course, is that the therapist might be lying to the patient, and if the patient is convinced of that, this assumption would need to be explored further. The analysis of what the assumed dishonesty of the therapist means to the patient may lead directly to very primitive psychopathic transferences and their antecedent object relationships in the patient's early life. In other cases, the therapist now must examine the patient's paranoid regression in terms of the activation of a "psychotic nucleus" in the transference, sorting out the extent to which unresolved psychopathic transferences (e.g., the patient's assumption that the therapist is lying) need to be reexplored later on.

In my experience, when the therapist communicates his tolerance of incompatible realities and fully examines the patient-therapist relationship under such conditions, it may gradually lead to the resolution of the psychotic nucleus and of the paranoid transference itself. Paranoid transferences typically reveal the presence of severe primitive aggression in the form of "purified" aggressive internalized part-object relations that are split off from the patient's idealized self and object representations.

The decrease of projective mechanisms and of paranoid transferences by interpretation brings about a gradual recognition by the patients of the intrapsychic sources of their own aggression, and the development, for the first time in the treatment, of authentic experiences of guilt, remorse, concern for the therapist, and anxiety over the possibility of repairing their relationship. Patients become aware that their attacks were directed not at the bad, sadistic, tyrannical, or dishonest therapist, but at the good therapist who was trying to help them. This development marks the beginning of depressive transferences, characteristic of advanced stages of the psychodynamic psychotherapy of borderline patients, indicating that a significant degree of integration is taking place. At this point in the treatment, patients begin to be able to reflect on the implications of their own behavior and to integrate the previously split-off images of the idealized and the persecutory therapist, in the context of also developing an integrated view of their parental images in terms of the idealized and persecutory aspects of their representations.

The most important problem at this advanced stage of the treatment may be the therapist's unawareness of the beginning of change in the patient. The early manifestations of such a depressive potential may show in the patient's more considerate behavior toward others and in his or her sublimatory functioning outside the treatment situation. The therapist may miss the development of such a new potential, especially in patients who had evinced severely paranoid transferences over an extended period of time. One additional reason why such an improvement may go undetected is that the patient may develop negative therapeutic reactions from an unconscious sense of guilt. This is a higher-level negative therapeutic reaction than that which obtains in the case of narcissistic personalities, in whom negative therapeutic reactions usually reflect unconscious envy of the therapist.

The most dramatic indicators of depressive transferences in the advanced stages of the treatment of borderline patients will be the growing evidence of the patients' capacity to empathize with the therapist's feeling states (sometimes they develop an uncanny capacity to interpret the therapist's behavior), their concern for "maintaining alive" what is being learned in the psychotherapy, their capacity for independent work on the issues developed within the treatment outside the treatment hours, and their expression of dependency on and love for the therapist rather than a superficial "as if" show of cooperation in the search for additional gratifications.

The outline presented here is necessarily schematic and oversimplified. Given the periods of chaotic condensation of transferences from many sources and levels of development in the treatment of borderline patients, depressive, paranoid, and psychopathic features may coexist or intermingle. The importance of the outlined sequence, however, lies in orienting the therapist to the order of priority in which he or she should explore such chaotic transferences. I have found it extremely helpful to first take up and resolve psychopathic transferences before focusing on the paranoid aspects of the material, and then to resolve persistent paranoid elements before examining the depressive developments in the transference.

REFERENCES

Adler G: Borderline Psychopathology and Its Treatment. New York, Jason Aronson, 1985

Adler G: Psychodynamic therapies in borderline personality disorder, in American Psychiatric Press Review of Psychiatry, Vol 8. Edited by Tasman A, Hales RE, Frances AJ. Washington, DC, American Psychiatric Press, 1989, pp 49–64

Boyer LB: The Regressed Patient. New York, Jason Aronson, 1983

Buie D, Adler G: The definitive treatment of the borderline patient. International Journal of Psychoanalytic Psychotherapy 9:51–87, 1982–1983

Chessick RD: Intensive Psychotherapy of the Borderline Patient. New York, Jason Aronson, 1977

Giovacchini PL: Treatment of Primitive Mental States. New York, Jason Aronson, 1979

Giovacchini PL: Developmental Disorders: The Transitional Space in Mental Breakdown and Creative Integration. New York, Jason Aronson, 1986

Greenacre P: The transitional object and the fetish with special reference to the role of illusion. Int J Psychoanal 51:447–456, 1970

Gunderson JG: Borderline Personality Disorder. Washington, DC, American Psychiatric Press, 1984

Kernberg OF: Borderline Conditions and Pathological Narcissism. New York, Jason Aronson, 1975

Kernberg OF: The psychotherapeutic treatment of borderline personalities, in Psychiatry 1982: The American Psychiatric Association Annual Review, Vol 1. Edited by Grinspoon L. Washington, DC, American Psychiatric Press, 1982, pp 470–487

Kernberg OF: Severe Personality Disorders: Psychotherapeutic Strategies. New Haven, CT, Yale University Press, 1984

Kernberg OF, Selzer MA, Koenigsberg HW, et al: Psychodynamic Psychotherapy of Borderline Patients. New York, Basic Books, 1989

Kohut H: The Analysis of the Self. New York, International Universities Press, 1971

Masterson JF: Psychotherapy of the Borderline Adult. New York, Brunner/Mazel, 1976

Masterson JF: The Narcissistic and Borderline Disorders. New York, Brunner/Mazel, 1981

Modell AH: "The holding environment" and the therapeutic action of psychoanalysis. J Am Psychoanal Assoc 24:285–307, 1976

Racker H: Transference and Countertransference. New York, International Universities Press, 1968

Rinsley D: Borderline and Other Self Disorders. New York, Jason Aronson, 1982

Rosenfeld H: Impasse and Interpretation. London, Tavistock, 1987

Searles HF: Countertransference and Related Subjects. New York, International Universities Press, 1979

Searles HF: My Work With Borderline Patients. New York, Jason Aronson, 1986

Volkan V: Six Steps in the Treatment of Borderline Personality Organization. Northvale, NJ, Jason Aronson, 1987

Waldinger RJ: Intensive psychodynamic therapy with borderline patients: an overview. Am J Psychiatry 144:267–274, 1987

Waldinger RJ, Gunderson JG: Effective Psychotherapy with Borderline Patients. New York, Macmillan, 1987

Winnicott DW: Transitional objects and transitional phenomena: a study of the first not-me possession. Int J Psychoanal 34:89–97, 1953

Winnicott DW: On transference. Int J Psychoanal 37:386–388, 1956

Winnicott DW: Collected Papers: Through Pediatrics to Psycho-analysis. New York, Basic Books, 1958

Winnicott DW: The theory of the parent-infant relationship (1960), in The Maturational Processes and the Facilitating Environment. New York, International Universities Press, 1965, pp 37–55

Dialectical Behavior Therapy for Borderline Personality Disorder: Treatment Goals, Strategies, and Empirical Support

Edward N. Shearin, Ph.D.
Marsha M. Linehan, Ph.D.

THE THEORY OF *DIALECTICAL BEHAVIOR THERAPY* (DBT) FOR patients with borderline personality disorder (BPD) has been described by Linehan and Koerner in Chapter 5. In the current chapter we focus on the application of this therapy, including the general framework of treatment, its goals, the strategies used to achieve these goals, and the effectiveness of the treatment (Shearin and Linehan 1989).

TREATMENT FRAMEWORK

Dialectical behavior therapy has a structural side that is similar in form to, but different in exact detail from, other therapies. These elements include its format, settings, patient and therapist characteristics, use of supervi-

Because DBT was developed with parasuicidal borderline women and has to date undergone empirical tests just with that group, we have used only the pronoun "she" in the following sections when referring to individuals with borderline personality disorder. This usage does not imply that the disorder is limited to women or that the statements made might not also apply to men with the disorder.

Preparation of this chapter was supported in part by National Institute of Mental Health Grant MH34486 to Marsha Linehan.

sion, and emphasis on orientation given to new patients. The elements of this framework are described below.

Format

Dialectical behavior therapy uses the format of both an individual and a group treatment session each week. During the first year of treatment, the group is used to teach behavioral coping skills. Thereafter, it becomes a combined support and interpersonal process group that augments the individual treatment. The individual session is usually 1 or 1.5 hours in length, and in some crisis situations it may also temporarily become necessary to meet twice a week. The group meets for 2 or 2.5 hours depending upon its needs. The group has generally been led by two co-therapists, who have at times also been individual therapists for some of the patients. During the first year of treatment, patients are required to be in both individual therapy and behavioral skills training. Under usual circumstances the skills training is conducted in the group setting. Maintaining group therapy after the first year is a matter of individual preference and need. In no case, however, can a patient be in group therapy without concomitant individual therapy.

Settings

Dialectical behavior therapy imposes no unusual setting requirements beyond what might be customary in a conventional behavior therapy practice. For adult patients, individual sessions have generally been in the offices used for regular clinical practice by the therapists. In some instances, the requirements of a specific treatment temporarily led to different settings. For example, patients who problematically avoided locations necessary for employment or social contacts (behaviors that interfered with quality of life) were seen by their therapists in these locations as part of in vivo exposure. Therapists were also free to exercise some flexibility in settings to meet unusual and temporary needs of a patient. However, this flexibility did not extend to allowing treatment to occur in offbeat places simply because the patient did not feel like coming into the therapist's office.

In contrast to adult patients, adolescents who were highly ambivalent about therapy were accorded more flexibility. Out-of-office sessions in places such as bowling alleys and cars were occasionally helpful in continuing contact through difficult phases. The same end might have been achieved by waiting until the adolescent was ready to come to the therapist's office. However, a research constraint of termination of therapy following four consecutive absences made this degree of flexibility more practical when adolescents were in treatment.

A final but important setting for DBT is the telephone call. Patients are encouraged to call their individual therapists when confronted with difficult stressful situations, both for practice in asking for help effectively and for in vivo practice of coping skills. Thus, multiple calls per month are not uncommon during some stages of treatment.

Patient Characteristics

The borderline patients treated to date with DBT have been diagnosed by both DSM-III-R (American Psychiatric Association 1987) and the Diagnostic Interview for Borderlines (DIB; Gunderson et al. 1981) criteria (the latter was defined by a minimum score of 7) and the requirement of multiple parasuicides with at least one in the 8 weeks prior to treatment. The resulting sample may have demonstrated more severe pathology than patients who just met DSM-III-R criteria alone. However, the treatment as described should apply as well to patients with less severe problems, although there would be a corresponding decrease in the amount of time needed for some of the behavioral targets. The borderline patients treated by Linehan and her associates have included men, but patients in the outcome studies have been exclusively women. Although the treatment as defined theoretically and procedurally may apply equally to men, that application has not been submitted to rigorous testing.

Other exclusionary diagnostic criteria in the research studies, but not in clinical applications, have included those for schizophrenia, bipolar disorder, and organic mental disorders or deficits such as cerebral palsy. The intent in applying these was to maintain homogeneous samples for research purposes. Acute drug or alcohol use that was either the sole precipitating factor for suicidal behavior or severe enough to dominate the patient's life was also grounds for exclusion until appropriate rehabilitation could be completed. More moderate problems that could be addressed within the scope of the treatment were acceptable.

Miscellaneous characteristics that were important in preventing pre-mature terminations from treatment included a local residence, a free choice of DBT treatment over other treatment options, and a willingness to commit to the reduction of suicidal behaviors. Individuals who did not indicate a willingness to take part in the therapy, which has the goal to reduce suicidal behavior, and to commit to a specified time period in therapy (usually 6 to 12 months) were not accepted into therapy. Finally, patients who could not control hostile behavior toward others in a group setting were dropped from group therapy.

Orientation

Treatment is initiated with the negotiation of numerous agreements be-tween patient and therapist. This properly is an orientation phase and must be completed before treatment can begin. This type of explicit negotiation is common in behavior therapy. It has been particularly help-ful when clarification of the ambivalent motivations of one or more of the participants is critical to proceeding, such as in marital therapy (e.g., Jacobson and Margolin 1979). The agreements for the patient include specific agreements about therapy, attendance, suicidal behavior, ther-apy-interfering behavior, skills training, and payment. The basic therapy agreement ordinarily includes details of the time duration, frequency, and conditions under which either the therapist or the patient would unilater-ally terminate it. The most common mode in DBT has been to negotiate for a year at a time, with some specification of what would be required to renew for an additional year. Some patients may insist that they cannot effectively function in a time-limited treatment. The key aspect of the agreement, however, is that treatment is not offered unconditionally. Therapy that proves to be ineffective, for example, will not be continued. Thus, there is a need for periodic reviews and renegotiations.

As part of therapy, the patient must also agree that two of the goals of treatment are the reduction of suicidal behaviors and therapy-interfering behaviors. Patients extremely ambivalent about suicidal behavior may not be able to make its reduction their explicit goal. However, they must at least recognize that its reduction is a goal of treatment and that in order to remain in treatment they will have to change their behavior. Patients must also agree to attend a year of concurrent skills training in order to receive individual therapy.

Besides providing clarity for both patient and therapist about agreements, a primary goal of the orientation is to elicit and strengthen commitment to therapy. A foot-in-the-door technique is used whereby the therapist initially obtains seemingly small commitments, then "ups the ante" slightly by making even more clear the difficulties inherent in therapy, asks again for a commitment, and continues on in this manner.

TREATMENT GOALS

Individual Treatment Goals

As is typical in behavior therapy, DBT goals are described in terms of *behavioral targets*, that is, behaviors that should either be increased or decreased. These targets represent classes of behaviors, such as suicidal behavior, that pertain to a theme or an area of functioning. While each class of behaviors will remain an important focus of treatment over the length of therapy, the specific behaviors within a class will probably change as the most salient problems are resolved and the less important behaviors then rise in priority. For example, within the class of suicidal behavior, high-risk suicidal behaviors (e.g., buying a gun and threatening to use it) and parasuicide, if present, would be the primary behaviors to reduce at the beginning of therapy. Later, after high-risk behaviors and parasuicide had stopped, suicidal urges might be the focus within this behavioral class.

The degree of focus upon a class of behaviors in DBT depends upon the mode of treatment that is employed at any given moment. DBT involves three concurrent modes of treatment for BPD patients: weekly individual sessions, a weekly group specifically for skills training, and telephone contacts primarily with the individual therapist on an as-needed basis.

The six treatment foci in individual therapy are

1. Suicidal behaviors
2. Therapy-interfering behaviors

3. Behaviors that interfere with quality of life
4. Behavioral skills acquisition
5. Posttraumatic stress behaviors
6. Self-respect behaviors

These targets are approached hierarchically and, if a higher-priority be-havior reappears, recursively. It is likely that for patients with significant levels of problem behaviors, early treatment will necessarily focus upon the upper part of the hierarchy. This order makes explicit the DBT contin-gency that parasuicidal behavior must stop and the patient must actively engage in therapy so that she can get on with her life. This is the funda-mental dialectic: that acceptance of current life (rather than rejection by parasuicide and other avoidant behaviors) must precede its change.

Suicidal behaviors.   Because goals in psychotherapy have no meaning for a dead patient, the highest priority in DBT is to address behaviors that are associated with a high risk of suicide. This class of behaviors is *never* ignored, whether or not the therapist believes that suicide is likely. Thus, the therapist must develop the pattern of eliciting this information at the beginning of the session when choices are less constrained. The method of obtaining this information in DBT is by having patients routinely fill out diary cards asking for daily ratings or check-offs about various aspects of suicidal behaviors and mood. In practice, without such cards, therapists soon stop asking about suicidal behavior on a routine basis, especially when frequency of suicidal behaviors decreases.

When opposing such suicidal behaviors in DBT, the therapist must in effect take a stand on the appropriateness of suicide as an option for BPD patients. Given that many borderline patients behave in a manner that pressures the therapist to agree that their lives are not worth living, and also given that at particularly hopeless times a therapist may feel in agree-ment with this pessimistic assessment, the DBT therapist must have a predetermined, nonnegotiable stance against suicide.

Parasuicidal behaviors are also never ignored by the individual DBT therapist. The reasons for this emphasis include the significant association of parasuicide with subsequent suicide, the possibility of accidental death, and the occurrence of cumulative, irreversible physical damage to the patient's body. Furthermore, parasuicidal behaviors are among the most stressful events for a therapist (Hellman et al. 1986; Roswell 1988), and stress reduction lowers the likelihood of therapist burnout and/or rejection of the patient, which clearly is in the best interests of the patient. Therefore, parasuicidal behaviors are neither accepted nor ignored by the individual DBT therapist.

Thus, the first individual session priority following patient parasuicidal behavior is to discuss the behavior and obtain detailed information about both preceding and subsequent events. The aim is to enable the patient to achieve more adaptive problem solutions by applying the problem-solving strategies discussed later and thereby raise the likelihood of three interrelated outcomes. First, the amount of parasuicidal behavior will decrease as the patient replaces parasuicidal behavior with other solutions to the precipitating events. Second, the therapist will communicate that she or he takes the behavior very seriously. Given the invalidating environment frequently associated with borderline patients, this is especially important. Third, a contingency for parasuicidal behavior is established—that is, patients are made aware that they decrease their opportunities to talk about other issues when they engage in parasuicidal behavior (Linehan 1987). Compared with the frequent patient experience in which parasuicide has been largely ignored unless life threatening, this contingency communicates the DBT message that changing these behaviors cannot wait until the patient is less distressed about her circumstances. Instead, the point is made that feeling bad or suicidal is a signal to engage in active coping that has the chance of ultimately improving the patient's life.

Swenson (1989) has said that DBT ignores the intrapsychic events that are seen by many as important in the production of suicidal behaviors in BPD patients. This will always be true regarding metapsychological events whose existence can only be inferred within specific theoretical systems. However, this criticism may also arise through a misunderstanding of the degree of inquiry conducted in DBT. As described under suicidal goals, significant attention is given to all events, intrapsychic or otherwise, that show a relationship to targeted behaviors. The affect and/or impulses associated with these events are also taken very seriously. Indeed, without such attention to the patient's experiences, neither validation of the patient nor a useful behavioral analysis of the determining events can occur. A misunderstanding of the priority scheme for behavioral targets may also equate the intervention selected for control of a problem behavior at a given moment with the therapist's understanding of the original causes of the behavior. For example, trauma associated with sex abuse may be a source of many problematic behaviors, but the choice of a DBT therapist early in treatment may be to ignore the trauma for the moment and teach some short-term distress management techniques. Intrapsychic events can thus be very important, but the emphasis initially may be to reduce suicidal behavior by more direct means.

Therapy-interfering behaviors. The second priority in DBT is to reduce *both* patient and therapist behaviors that interfere with therapy and to increase those behaviors that make therapy more effective and likely to continue. No therapeutic approach is likely to be effective if patient or therapist behaviors attenuate the delivery of the therapy or lead to a premature end. With the chronic nature of borderline patients' problems and the high dropout rate that is traditionally reported, the category of therapy-interfering behaviors is necessarily placed second in priority only to suicidal behaviors.

Patient behaviors that interfere with therapy can be divided into those that directly interfere with receiving the therapy and those that lead to therapist burnout or decrease therapist motivation to work with the patient (Linehan 1992). Those behaviors that directly interfere with therapy include nonattentive, noncollaborative, and noncompliant behaviors. A patient must comply with the proscriptions of therapy for any treatment to work; the amount of patient activity between sessions required by DBT for expanding and practicing coping skills as well as active treatment components such as exposure makes compliance vital for progress. Yet, achieving anything like consistency in following through on these types of assignments is quite difficult for most borderline patients. Noncompliant behaviors such as not completing diary cards properly, not doing or even attempting homework assignments, and breaking agreements with the therapist must be addressed consistently. Shaping, the reinforcement of partial responses, is useful for gradually developing the patient's repertoire of therapy-appropriate behaviors. The dialectic between accepting a current lack of compliance and working to build new responses is important to keep this part of therapy from being a critical failure for the patient and a complete frustration for the therapist. Correspondingly, the patient also needs therapist reinforcement for compliance that did not help the patient.

Patient behaviors that interfere with therapy through an impact on the therapist are seen as part of a dialectical balance of behaviors between therapist and patient. The important point here is that in DBT, safeguarding therapists' personal limits is an important therapeutic strategy. A large part of the DBT success in reducing dropout rate may stem from therapists' being less likely to subtly encourage a patient to drop out of therapy or conclude after an initial period of therapy that a particular patient is "not yet ready," or "inappropriate," for the treatment.

Behaviors that interfere with quality of life. In keeping with the stated objectives of DBT that a patient must work at building a life worth living as well as reduce suicidal behavior, the third goal of individual DBT is the reduction of behaviors (other than suicidal) that seriously interfere with the development of a better life for the patient. The choice of these targets is made, ideally, by the therapist and patient together. However, in instances where a recognition of the problem is itself a significant therapeutic step (e.g., drug or alcohol abuse), the therapist should be careful to target only behaviors that can functionally be related to the patient's quality of life. The supervision group, case presentations, and colleagues are resources that can help a therapist weigh the importance of behaviors in this category.

Behaviors that interfere with the patient's quality of life include substance abuse or addiction, high-risk sexual behavior, severe financial and employment difficulties, and criminal behavior that could expose the patient to significant legal consequences. Other such behaviors are dysfunctional interpersonal behaviors (e.g., selecting or remaining with abusive partners) and failing to take care of health problems. The general guideline for inclusion as a quality-of-life target is that if left unaltered, the behavior in question would either cause the patient's quality of life to deteriorate or be a source of such stress and chaos that the patient would be unable to significantly benefit from gains in other areas.

Behavioral skills. The fourth goal of the individual treatment is to integrate DBT behavioral skills into the patient's daily life and increase the frequency with which they are used. These skills have been selected to address the four areas of borderline problems as specified in DSM-III-R: self-instability (inadequate sense of self, sense of emptiness), behavioral instability (suicidal, impulsive, and self-destructive behaviors), emotional instability (emotional lability and anger problems), and interpersonal instability (chaotic relationships, abandonment fears). The DBT skills are mindfulness, distress tolerance, emotion regulation, interpersonal effectiveness, and self-management skills. Although the DBT group has primary responsibility for teaching these skills, the therapist must be very experienced with their use in order to help the patient substitute them for her maladaptive repertoire.

Mindfulness skills form the core of DBT skills. These skills are divided into what the patient does and how she does it—that is, actions and manner of acting. The mindfulness actions are labeled *observing, describing,* and *participating,* and the manners or ways of doing these are labeled *nonjudgmentalness, one-mindfulness,* and *effectiveness.* However, these simple labels barely hint at the depth and complexity of each action. For example, self-observing entails the ability to observe whatever cognitive, affective, and overt behavioral events are occurring at any specified moment. Observing the environment requires alertness to others and to events outside of one's self, as well as the ability to differentiate events from one's opinions about events. Clearly, this level of awareness is likely to be foreign to patients with frequent impulsive and mood-dependent behaviors. The manner of performing these actions addresses in part the dichotomous, or black-and-white, thinking frequently found in borderline patients. Nonjudgmentalness means not judging and labeling in terms of good and bad. Events and actions can be evaluated in terms of the outcome or effect, but the addition of a judgmental label can be handicapping. Effectiveness concerns what works rather than what might be thought of as the "right" way to do something. Nonjudgmentalness and effectiveness together address the difficulty of the borderline patient in developing her own frame of reference for evaluating both her behavior and that of others. Finally, one-mindfulness pertains to the ability to focus attention, something that most borderline patients appear to have trouble directing.

The other skills—distress tolerance, emotion regulation, and interpersonal effectiveness—are taught in a modular form in the group and blended as needed with self-management skills. The DBT individual therapist must be able to further explain these skills as well as steer patients toward the skill or skills appropriate to a given situation. Therefore, the therapist must know both the techniques and their intended targets.

Distress tolerance skills are taught to help the patient to 1) deal with the slowness with which painful affect can be reduced by treatment, and 2) recognize that it is impossible to eliminate painful experiences from life. Thus, a patient needs the option of enduring a painful time rather than engaging in behaviors that ultimately increase her problems. The distress tolerance skills are broken into six strategies for coping with crises (e.g., distraction and self-soothing) and skills for accepting (not approving of) reality as it is.

Emotion regulation skills are taught to deal with the emotional instability that is typical of patients with the borderline diagnosis. These include strategies for reducing initial vulnerability and techniques for identifying and changing emotions. Both distress tolerance and emotion regulation skills have to be accompanied by much validation of the patient's experience and emotional state. Otherwise, the patient is likely to perceive any hint that she could tolerate or change an emotion as a continuation of her past invalidating environment.

Interpersonal effectiveness skills are taught to help the patient deal with the interpersonal chaos and conflict that are a frequent part of the diagnosis. While borderline individuals often appear to be highly skilled interpersonally, a close assessment of skills and performance across situations will usually reveal that patients have difficulty determining when specific skills are relevant. Inhibited in the use of these skills by inaccurate beliefs about what is possible, these patients have difficulties in managing affect. The interpersonal effectiveness skills target deficits in cognitive and expressive skills as well as in a patient's overt behavioral repertoire. Frequently components from the emotion regulation skills are useful in furthering performance in these three areas. For the therapist, a major mistake to avoid is assuming that the use of a skill under some circumstance indicates that the patient can perform similarly under most relevant circumstances.

In conjunction with the preceding skills, self-management skills are taught as needed. These refer to the skills for learning, maintaining, and generalizing new behaviors as well as the skills for eliminating unwanted behaviors. These skills include setting realistic goals and learning basic behavioral control techniques such as stimulus control. In our experience, borderline patients often have the belief that they should be able to perform new, complex behaviors if they only have enough motivation. They also generally think punishment is the best strategy for changing behavior. Needless to say, DBT therapists need to be much more knowledgeable about behavior change techniques, as they must deal with unrealistic beliefs and teach more useful knowledge before change in behavior can be expected.

Posttraumatic stress behaviors.   Borderline patients very frequently come with a history of childhood abuse, either physical, sexual, or emotional. In a recent sample of patients, the number reporting sexual abuse alone approached 80% (Wagner and Linehan 1989). Two other small studies have cited a similar rate of incest in hospitalized borderline patients (Nelson, unpublished study, cited in Herman and van der Kolk 1987; Stone 1981). Indeed, some authors have suggested that such abuse may play a significant role in the development of BPD either as a posttraumatic stress effect or through a more pervasive effect on the patient and her family environment (Courtois 1988). Because not all patients report childhood events this severe, this can be viewed as the extreme end of the continuum of the invalidating environment hypothesized in Chapter 5. In DBT the therapist does *not* presume that patients who do not recall abuse must have experienced it.

Because of the trauma of dealing with topics related to posttraumatic stress disorder (PTSD) in therapy, its place in the DBT hierarchy of treatment targets follows the reduction of suicidal, therapy-interfering, and serious quality-of-life–interfering behaviors and the development of behavioral skills. Although abuse is not ignored in the early phases of treatment, in DBT the therapist assumes that it cannot be systematically treated directly before the patient is ready. Four goals are highlighted:

1. *Help the patient remember the abuse.* Because many patients remember only fragments of childhood events, it can be a very difficult process to reconstruct the abusive events and associated feelings. At times, even when the abuse is remembered, the individual who never received any validation of the fact of the abuse will have trouble believing her own recollections and, at times, will believe that she has simply made up the

memory. Ferreting out and accepting the probable facts is an important task here.

2. *Help the patient reduce the amount of self-blame, self-invalidation, and stigmatization that stems from the abuse.* The validation strategies are key here in convincing the patient that she caused neither the victimization nor its effect on her.

3. *Interrupt the cycle of denial and intrusion of the abuse that the patient may be experiencing.* The denial phase is similar to the concept of inhibited grieving described in Chapter 5. This has often been the patient's only way of coping with the trauma. It can now be replaced with the DBT behavioral skills in conjunction with longer periods of exposure to the intrusive stimuli to allow the patient to gradually extinguish the intrusive aspects.

4. *Resolve the patient's tendency to view herself and the abuser in black-and-white terms of all bad.* It is often important when the perpetrator was a parent to be able to see some aspects of that person in positive terms, although forgiveness is not a goal with all patients in DBT. Moreover, patients will alternately view themselves as all bad for having been abused. A more dialectical view of the family situation is helpful as an outcome goal.

Self-respect behaviors.   The sixth goal of individual DBT is to focus on patient behaviors that enhance the patient's ability to value, trust, believe, and validate herself. Borderline individuals often have a marked tendency to invalidate their own beliefs, emotions, and actions, looking to others instead for truth and validation. Although they are often able to assert their own values, opinions, and beliefs, they are rarely able to hold onto these beliefs in the face of disagreement from others in their social environment. Their inability to comfortably hold contrary points of view sets up an oscillating cycle between, on the one hand, demanding that others give up their opinions and agree with the patient and, on the other, giving up and giving in to the environment. Ultimately, neither approach works because coercing agreement invalidates the agreement and adopting beliefs that are incompatible with one's own beliefs is experienced as inauthentic.

Thus, a primary goal of DBT is to help the patient learn how to maintain her own opinions, values, emotional reactions, and behavioral decisions in the face of disagreement, disapproval, and invalidation by the environment, including the therapist. Making the transition toward greater self-reliance is a gradual process throughout therapy, but it assumes greater importance in the final stages of treatment. In this stage, the therapist must very consistently reinforce self-validation, self-care, and problem solving independent of the therapist.

Consultation Group Goals

In DBT the consultation group plays a fundamental role. Indeed, DBT is conceptualized as a three-part system including the patient, the therapist, and the consultation group. The consultation group can consist of one other person or many, with the defining characteristic being that all members of the group are attempting to apply DBT, at least to the case at hand. The fundamental dialectic that change is possible only with acceptance is a basic consultation guideline. Thus, a major goal for the supervisor or other members of the consultation group is to balance in time the therapist's emphasis on acceptance versus change.

A second goal is to promote phenomenological empathy in the therapist's understanding of the patient. To this end, the least prejudicial theory consistent with the behavior is advanced. In the many situations where the "true cause" of a behavior cannot be determined, an important part of DBT is to choose the explanation that will raise the likelihood of the therapist liking the patient. For example, patient behaviors that stress the therapist or interfere with therapy are more likely to be explained in DBT as arising from fear and hopelessness rather than excessive aggressive drive, malicious intent, manipulation, or "game playing." Recent data (Shearin 1990; Shearin and Linehan 1991) have validated the importance of this approach with the indication that changes in DBT therapists' liking of patients were inversely related to subsequent suicial behavior.

A final goal of the consultation group is to both validate and problem-solve the therapist's issues and difficulties with the patient. Although the flexible position that DBT takes on personal limits is done both to gain therapeutic efficacy (such as with telephone calls) and to avoid arbitrary positions, DBT has the disadvantage, compared with therapies having clear proscriptions (usually prohibitive), that the therapist's decision making is more difficult. Therapists often have difficulty determining what their personal limits are until these have been exceeded. The consultation group plays an important role here. Given the difficulty of working with borderline patients, the success of DBT may be due, in an important part, to the care and attention that are given to the therapists in these consultation groups.

Empirical Support

There are limited data pertaining to the effect of DBT on the preceding behavioral targets. To date, there have been three studies using random assignment of borderline patients to treatment conditions that have compared the effectiveness of DBT with treatments available in the community. The results of these studies indicate that DBT reduced the parasuicide rate over the course of a 1-year treatment more than did the control treatment condition (Linehan et al. 1991). The DBT patients also had fewer parasuicides that required outpatient medical attention or caused hospitalization for medical treatment. Thus, compared with control treatments, DBT has been shown to be effective for its primary target of suicidal behavior.

The same studies (Linehan et al. 1991) also showed that DBT was more effective than the control treatment in keeping patients in treatment. Whereas the dropout rate for the control treatment condition was comparable to the 50% rate reported in previous studies involving borderline patients (e.g., Waldinger and Gunderson 1984), the DBT dropout rate was under 20%. The DBT patients also had fewer days of psychiatric hospitalization over the year of the treatment. Thus, DBT has also been effective compared with control treatments for its secondary target of therapy-interfering behavior. The remaining categories of targets were not measured in these studies, so the efficacy of DBT for these is currently unknown.

A second study (Linehan et al. 1991) was conducted with patients who were referred to a DBT group therapy program by community psychotherapists. These patients remained in ongoing individual (non-DBT) therapy but supplemented it with the group behavioral skills training component of DBT. These patients did not improve relative to the control group, suggesting that simply adding behavioral skills training to ongoing alternate treatment programs is unlikely to be beneficial.

There are also limited data on the effect of DBT strategies from one process study that followed a small number of DBT patients for part of their first year of treatment (Shearin 1990; Shearin and Linehan 1991). Because these results pertain to the comparative effect of strategies within DBT rather than the overall effect of DBT versus other treatments, they are presented at the end of the following section.

TREATMENT STRATEGIES

Dialectical behavior therapy employs five sets of treatment strategies to achieve the behavioral goals described above:

1. *Dialectical strategies* that permeate and guide all aspects of treatment
2. *Basic strategies* that include validation and problem solving
3. *Stylistic strategies* that define the interpersonal and communication styles that mesh with the treatment
4. *Case management strategies* that guide the therapist in dealing with the patient's social network
5. *Integrated strategies* that proscribe how the therapist responds to the run of problems that arise in the treatment of borderline patients

Dialectical Strategies

The principal dialectic is that change occurs in the context of acceptance of life as it is. The therapist uses this as a guide in two distinct sets of activities (Table 14–1). The first is in the therapeutic relationship to balance the relative emphasis on acceptance versus change strategies and

Table 14–1. Balancing of change and acceptance strategies in dialectical behavior therapy

Emphasis on change	Emphasis on acceptance
Irreverent communication	Reciprocal vulnerability
Consultation	Environmental intervention
Problem solving	Validation
Skill training	
Exposure strategies	
Contingency management	
Cognitive modification	

to move within the current dialectic (e.g., the provision of control versus autonomy) to promote a collaborative relationship. The second is in using dialectical techniques to teach dialectical behavior response patterns to the patient. A key point is that for any position, an opposite or complementary one is also possible. Change can be promoted by pushing acceptance, and acceptance, by pushing change. This may have the therapist joining or moving closer to the patient's position and the patient then paradoxically moving closer to the therapist's starting position. This effect with borderline patients was noted much earlier by Sherman (1961, cited in Seltzer 1986), who commented that "whichever side the therapist aligns himself with, the patient will usually feel impelled to leave" (Seltzer 1986, p. 55). Conversely, a rigid adherence to one position, either in time or opposition to the patient, leads to increased tension and decreased reconciliation and synthesis between therapist and patient.

Several examples may clarify what is embodied in this balancing. In response to a patient's description of how very stressful her low-level jobs were becoming and how impossible it was for her to find other work, the therapist validated her feelings and began a discussion of ways of accepting the current situation. After some minutes of this, the patient switched to a discussion of what obstacles she would face in returning to school and how these could be overcome. In this case, the therapist moved closer to the patient's position that no change was possible in her job status, and the patient then moved to a position of change. It is extremely important that the therapist not do this as a gimmick—that is, emphasize acceptance with the idea that change is the more desirable goal—but rather value acceptance for its own sake. Otherwise, the patient is likely to emerge from the interaction, and rightfully so, with the feeling that she has somehow been manipulated toward the therapist's goal rather than her own, and thus she has been proven wrong once more.

Another example concerns a patient whose repetitive parasuicides had exhausted all her usual treatment resources and who faced an involuntary state hospitalization (not her first) or DBT treatment. During the intake, she was told that she was perfect for the DBT program (i.e., acceptance) and that to be a part of the program she would have to work on changing her parasuicidal behavior (i.e., change). It was explained that she was free to choose the DBT program or not (i.e., autonomy) and that the therapist was also free to choose to work with her or not (i.e., control). It is this explicit interweaving of opposites that is guided by a dialectical stance. Recent data (Shearin 1990; Shearin and Linehan 1991) discussed at the end of the treatment strategies section indicate that it may indeed be this blending of strategies (e.g., emphasizing both control and autonomy) that best reduces suicidal behavior.

In addition to a dialectical stance by the therapist within the therapist-patient relationship, an explicit effort is also made to teach dialectical behavior patterns to the patient. With respect to dialectical thinking, the guiding principle is that the truth of any statement or belief is neither relative nor absolute but rather is constructed or emerges within a specific developmental context. Thus, no statement of truth exists in isolation, and within any statement or belief resides the seeds of its own opposition. In practical application, the DBT therapist typically ignores attempts to prove one viewpoint more "right" or "wrong" than another, instead searching for a way to synthesize or construct a new more general or more useful truth from competing oppositional statements.

The dialectical approach to action and emotional responses is similar and is implemented with two key points in mind. The first key point is that the possibilities for change lie within the contradictions, challenges, and limitations of a particular context rather than outside that context. An example is the conflict between the patient's demand that the therapist save her and the therapist's stance that she or he cannot save the patient. Behaviorally, this is resolved by the therapist's giving the patient the tools to save herself and the patient's acceptance and use of these tools.

The second key point is that extremes and rigid behavior patterns are indications that the dialectic has not been achieved. The use of the behavioral skills illustrates the point. In the response to a stressful event, emotional regulation is balanced with mindfulness—that is, techniques for reducing and altering emotions are combined with observing, describing, and participating in the response. The therapist's role is to constantly guide the patient to include the balancing behaviors (Linehan 1992).

"Entering the paradox" is a strategy for the therapist to highlight the paradoxes inherent in any therapeutic relationship in such a way that the patient is pushed to resolve the dilemma herself.

We have previously reviewed (Linehan 1981; Linehan and Shearin 1988) the literature indicating that suicidal individuals think in terms of absolutes and extremes. This is obviously a failure in dialectical thinking, and when the evidence does not fit the conclusions drawn, it is also a failure in logical thinking. The patient is free to choose her own behavior, but she cannot remain in therapy if she does not improve her behavior. The patient has a right to suicide, but credible threats to act on this right might result in the therapist moving to stop the patient. The patient is taught to achieve greater self-efficacy by learning to better ask for and receive help. The therapist exercises great control to help the patient achieve more autonomy. In highlighting these paradoxical realities, the therapist has frequent opportunities to enter (and reenter) the paradox and thus teach the patient a more dialectical approach. It is with this repeated confrontation and struggle that the patient and the therapist are forced to let go of rigid patterns of thought, emotion, and behavior, and achieve more adaptive and flexible repertories.

The "devil's advocate" technique is a method of addressing dysfunctional beliefs that the patient has expressed or problematic rules that she appears to be following. The therapist presents an extreme version of such a statement or rule that uses the patient's logic and then plays the role of devil's advocate to counter patient attempts to disprove the extreme statement or rule. This must be done with a straight face and a somewhat naive style. An example of such a patient belief might be "I can't say [or do] anything that will offend another person." The therapist proceeds by arguing in favor of the dysfunctional belief, for instance, suggesting that there are people on the freeway who might be offended when the patient will not drive over (or under) the speed limit, so she must drive at higher (or lower) speeds in these circumstances. If the patient agrees, the therapist can then point out that significantly deviating from the speed limit will certainly be offensive to the highway patrol, who will probably ticket her. The therapist then proceeds to work on resolving this problem (how to please everyone), communicating all the while that a resolution is possible.

Basic Strategies

The basic strategies are so called because, in combination with the dialectical strategies, they form the core of the treatment. Four of these sets of strategies—validation, problem solving, skill training, and contingency management—are described below.

Validation. From a DBT perspective, one of the essential problems of borderline patients is their inability to self-validate their own behaviors, emotions, and thoughts. It follows from this premise that a necessary target of any treatment must be to help the patient learn to validate herself. To do this, the therapist must believe in the essential validity of the patient's responses and, together with the patient, search for and highlight the basis of this validity. This search is the basis of the validation strategies in DBT.

Validation of the patient's emotions, thoughts, and behaviors is an active, three-step process. First the therapist must help the patient identify the response patterns of interest. In this step, the therapist's task is to observe carefully, discarding theoretical or attitudinal blinders. Next, the therapist communicates hearing and/or observing accurately the patient's responses (emotions, thoughts, perceptions, or actions). Within the patient-therapist dialogue the task here is to provide feedback to the patient so that she can be sure her emotions, thoughts, or actions have not been distorted by the therapist. Finally, the therapist searches for and highlights for the patient that aspect of the patient's behavior that is a valid response to the events occurring at the time of her behavior. In other words, the therapist suggests that even though information may not be available to understand all the relevant causes, the patient's feelings, thoughts, and behavioral responses make perfect sense in the context of the patient's current experience and life to date.

The validation strategy leads the therapist to search the patient's responses for their inherent validity and appropriateness to the situational context before any consideration of a more functional response is begun. This search is dialectical in that the therapist must find the grain of wisdom and authenticity in the patient's responses that on the whole may have been dysfunctional. Although in DBT the therapist does not assume that borderline patients do not at times distort events, the first line of approach is always to discover that aspect of the event that is not being distorted *and* is producing a response. DBT assumes that distortion of events is often a consequence rather than a cause of emotional dysfunction. In contrast, the usual cognitive therapy approach is to search for and either immediately replace dysfunctional processes (Ellis 1962, 1973) or at least suggest an experimental test of them (Beck et al. 1979). With borderline patients, such a disconfirming approach is also invalidating. Thus, the therapist must function for the patient as the dialectically opposite pole to such invalidation.

Problem solving. Problem solving with borderline patients is a two-step process that is fraught with difficulty. The paradox that acceptance is change is clearly illustrated by borderline patients who find the existence of some problems too painful to acknowledge. The therapist must balance the patient between two extremes in which either the patient sees all problems as her fault and is too ashamed to examine any, or she sees all as the fault of everyone else and as having nothing to do with her. Repeated attempts to deal with both the failures in dialectical thinking that lead to these positions and the accompanying painful emotions may be necessary before the patient can acknowledge the existence of the more painful problems. The validation strategy just described and the irreverent communication strategy described later in this chapter aid this process without reinforcing suicidal behavior.

Problem solving is also difficult because the source of distress that initiated the problematic responses is generally unclear. Thus, the therapist must perform a very detailed inquiry and analysis as described under the suicidal behavior targets in order to identify the cause(s) of any response. Hypotheses of determining variables are advanced, tested, and discarded until the determinants of the patient's behavior are clear. This is repeated as needed until the patient can both articulate and understand the patterns involved.

The second problem-solving step begins with the generation, evaluation, and implementation of alternative solutions that can be made in the future. If the preceding analysis reveals that the patient does not have the necessary skills to cope effectively with the problem, the therapist places more emphasis on skills training. If the patient has the needed skills but is inaccurate in the prediction of response contingencies or is exposed to contingencies that favor dysfunctional over functional behaviors, the therapist uses contingency management. If skills exist but their application is inhibited by emotions or faulty beliefs, exposure or cognitive modification strategies (not described) will be employed. Sometimes case management strategies are needed, and the therapist must function as a consultant to enable the patient to elicit needed help such as hospitalization, medication, or other services from community professionals. Alternatively, environmental intervention by the therapist may be necessary to achieve changes that the patient cannot make. Finally, if other difficulties such as issues in the therapist-patient relationship are the problem source, the therapist employs an appropriate integrated strategy set such as the relationship strategies.

Skills training. Skills training from the viewpoint of the individual therapist means stressing primarily the use of the skills taught in the DBT group. Other basic behavioral skills (e.g., relaxation, stimulus control) described in standard behavior therapy texts (e.g., Goldfried and Davison 1976; Kendall and Hollon 1979) are also candidates if the patient's problems appear to need such skills. However, the individual therapist will usually find that the time constraints of one weekly session prevent the exploration of many additional skills unless a skill trainer is employed. The key activity of the therapist that must be kept in the fore at all times when using this strategy is challenging the avoidant style of the patient. The therapist insists at every opportunity that the patient actively engage in the acquisition and practice of skills needed to cope with her life. Skills training, like problem solving, is squarely at the change pole of the acceptance-change dialectic.

Contingency management. Contingency management requires the therapist to tailor responses to the degree possible to reinforce adaptive, nonsuicidal behaviors while extinguishing maladaptive and harmful behaviors. Because of the life-threatening nature of suicidal behavior, this is necessarily a delicate and somewhat hazardous balance as the therapist attempts to neither excessively reinforce suicidal responses nor ignore them in such a manner that the patient's behavior escalates to a life-threatening level. This approach requires the therapist to take some short-term risks to achieve long-term gains.

A number of guidelines are important in the use of contingency management within DBT. First, natural contingencies are favored over arbitrary ones so that behaviors learned within the therapeutic relationship can be generalized to everyday situations. For example, for the patient who cares about how the therapist feels about her, expressing the emotional impact of the patient's behavior on the therapist (either positive or negative) would be preferred over giving more intellectual feed-

back about the patient's behavior. The therapist's observations and pro-
tections of his or her own personal limits as a therapist are viewed as some
of the most powerful contingencies in working with borderline patients.
Second, reinforcers must be tailored to the patient. What is reinforcing is
evaluated, not assumed. Third, patients must learn to be reinforced by
prevailing reinforcers in the community. The individual who is punished
by praise rather than reinforced will have difficulty in most work and
interpersonal relationships. Fourth, the application of principles of shaping is crucial. A response not in the repertoire cannot be produced by
punishment.

The application of contingency management to suicidal behavior in
DBT is governed by a strict protocol that specifies how to handle both
crisis and noncrisis instances of suicidal threats and overt acts. The dialectical tension arises between the demands of keeping a patient alive and the
demands of teaching the patient those behavioral patterns that will make
staying alive worthwhile. A specific example of contingency management
is the telephone protocol for parasuicidal behavior. Patients are told as
part of orientation that they are expected to call their individual therapist
before they engage in parasuicidal behavior rather than after. Moreover,
they do not have to be suicidal in order to call. The idea here is that
therapists can be more helpful before rather than after attempts to solve
problems via parasuicidal acts. This strategy achieves different effects
depending on the patient's willingness to call the therapist. For those who
find calling the therapist aversive, the strategy offers an opportunity for
learning to replace destructive behavior with asking for help appropriately. Parasuicidal behavior not preceded by attempts to call the therapist
would be viewed as therapy-interfering behavior and thus become a focus
of therapy time. For the patient who finds talking to the therapist comforting, the reinforcing effect of a telephone call increases the likelihood
that behaviors associated with the call will be strengthened. Thus, the
therapist has a choice of reinforcing adaptive behavior or suicidal behavior. A call to the therapist is permitted following 24 hours of nonpara-
suicidal behavior.

Later during treatment, if the patient does call the therapist following
parasuicide, the interaction is limited to the time necessary to determine
the medical risk of the injury. If there is none, the call is ended. If there is
medical risk, the therapist follows standard procedures for responding to

such a crisis. DBT outlines very specific steps for the therapist during and following suicidal behaviors. These can be summarized as follows:

1. Do not reinforce suicidal behavior.
2. Reinforce adaptive nonsuicidal behavior.
3. Evaluate each therapeutic response for its contribution to the risk of suicide versus the risk of the patient not developing a life worth living.

The goal is both to shape the patient toward asking for help while the problems are still manageable and to teach crisis management strategies while the patient is in the crisis state. To this end the therapist must be careful to provide similar time and attention for less crisis-oriented moments as he or she does for peak suicidal periods.

Stylistic Strategies

The *irreverent communication strategy* is a communication style intended to help the patient "jump track" so to speak. Although it is not difficult to recognize, the irreverent communication style has been difficult to describe. The therapist takes a rather irreverent, matter-of-fact attitude toward the patient's dysfunctional behaviors, interacting in a slightly "offbeat" yet very direct style. In these instances, the therapist can be compared to the straight man in the comedy scene. Humor, unorthodox connections, and statement of the facts or of the therapist's opinions in a nonjudgmental, unvarnished way can all contribute to the style. Irreverence is balanced with reciprocal vulnerability.

Reciprocal vulnerability involves the therapist's shifting from a stance of observer to participant in the patient-therapist relationship. Responsiveness to the patient and self-disclosure are the essence of reciprocal vulnerability. The aim, however, is to equalize the distribution of power, at least more than is usual in psychotherapy, and to provide an environment that holds both patient and therapist within the therapeutic enterprise. For example, rather than engage in a power struggle with the patient by continuing a change strategy, the therapist accepts the patient's noncollaborative behavior in a matter-of-fact way that makes his or her own feelings of frustration or impotence part of the agenda to be discussed. For example, the therapist may share with the patient in a nonjudgmental way the effect of the patient's behavior upon the therapist. Another approach in this situation would be for the therapist to share times when he or she has struggled with the same issue, and model ways of coping that the patient may not have considered. A key point in this technique, as in all acceptance strategies, is that the therapist must truly accept the situation. Engaging in this as a change ploy will communicate only that the therapist is still struggling with the patient rather than accepting the moment.

Case Management Strategies

The therapist's contract and agreements, as described in the orientation section, are with the patient, not with other professionals whom the patient may encounter. Health professionals are viewed like any other person in the patient's life. The therapist therefore functions as a consultant for the patient rather than for the patient's network. For problems the patient has with her network, regardless of whether they involve other health professionals, the therapist problem-solves with the patient; the network is then left for the patient to manage. If contacted directly by other professionals, the therapist advises them to follow their normal procedures. Implicit in this approach is belief in the capacities of the patient to learn to interact in a responsible manner as well as validation of the patient's perception that the world is frequently not fair and mental health professionals are often less than perfect. The infrequency of staff splitting both on the DBT treatment team and between the DBT team and other treatment facilities is perhaps a positive outcome of the strategy.

Because DBT has not been used in treating patients younger than 15, the patient's family has also been treated consistently with the consultant strategy. If the therapist thinks communication with the family might be helpful at times, it is advanced, like any other solution to a problem, as something the patient must choose and implement. Family therapy sessions, however, are not inconsistent with DBT and might at times be proscribed. Sessions with family members without the patient present, however, would be inconsistent. The therapist's role is defined as helping the patient understand the reactions of significant others.

The strategy to function as a consultant was chosen with three objectives in mind. A primary consideration was to have a policy that would function as the opposite pole to the borderline patient's preference for avoidance of problem solving. As formulated, the strategy is geared toward consistently requiring active solutions by the patient. This seems essential because therapists cannot solve all environmental problems encountered, either now or in the future, by the patient. A secondary objective is also met by this approach. By remaining in the role of a consultant to the patient, the therapist avoids becoming entangled in the often contradictory positions taken by mental health professionals involved with the patient. Finally, the consultant role promotes respect for the patient and her capabilities that is consistent with the stance of behavior therapy in general.

The consultation strategy has two exceptions. A direct intervention is made when substantial harm may come to the patient from individuals who will not modify their treatment of the patient unless a high-power person intervenes. Situations involving involuntary commitment, public assistance, and insurance claim forms are instances in which this may be necessary. The second exception is the coordination of individual and group therapists. Here, the strategy is modified because patients are discussed when not present. The spirit of the strategy is kept in that therapists do not explicitly intervene with each other on behalf of the patient. Therapists' disagreements over a patient are seen as failures in synthesis and interpersonal process rather than as a characteristic of the patient.

As noted above, we have not used DBT in treating patients younger than 15. For minors, both legal and practical considerations can require that the therapist suspend the role of consultant under certain circumstances when dealing with the patient's family or other individuals with power over the patient. The general guideline that we advocate is the same as just stated: that a direct intervention be made when substantial harm may come to the patient from individuals with control over her who will not modify their treatment of the patient unless a high-power person intervenes. Legal requirements for reporting harm done to the patient generally require that the therapist also contact authorities in all instances of such harm.

Relationship Strategies

The therapist-patient relationship in DBT is best understood as a dialectic. At one pole, the relationship is seen as the means through which the therapist can control and provide therapy. This view is shared with behavior therapy as well as many other therapies (Arnkoff 1983; Beck et al. 1979; Langs 1977, 1982). At the other pole, the relationship is the therapy. Its provision in a specified way provides a foundation from which the patient can autonomously grow and develop to overcome the problems that led her to therapy. This view of the relationship is closest to Rogerian and other humanistic approaches (Rice 1983). Control over behavior and the course of therapy in general is seen as residing primarily with the patient. In contrast, when the relationship is used as the vehicle to bring about therapy, the therapist controls therapy with the consent of the patient. The relationship is then just the means to an end, a way of having sufficient contact and leverage with the patient to cause change and growth.

As with all dialectics in the therapy, the therapist must choose an appropriate balance between these two approaches for each moment. The relationship as therapy facilitates both acceptance of the patient as she is and the patient's autonomy. Therapy through the relationship facilitates therapist control of behavior that the patient cannot control and acquisition of skills, including those necessary for self-reliance, previously unknown or insufficiently generalized. The five groups of relationship strategies specified in DBT can be mapped onto the poles of this dialectic. Relationship validation and relationship problem solving are autonomy/acceptance oriented, whereas relationship enhancement, relationship generalization, and relationship contingency are control/change oriented.

Relationship validation.   Relationship validation focuses upon the process of the therapist's accepting the patient-therapist relationship as it currently exists at each moment. Essentially, it is the process whereby the therapist validates the value and nature of the therapeutic relationship as a real rather than a transferential relationship. As with other acceptance strategies, this cannot be a gimmick or position chosen to achieve change. It is instead an acceptance of the stage of therapeutic progress or lack thereof and of the relationship as it is currently unfolding. At some moments this acceptance may be communicated to the patient, but at all times the strategy is employed, the therapist must explicitly acknowledge it to himself or herself. A high tolerance for criticism and hostile affect, a willingness to tolerate the patient's extreme suffering without immediately trying to get rid of it, and an ability to maintain a nonjudgmental, behavioral approach are extremely important for relationship acceptance. The consultation group is an essential prerequisite to achieving acceptance in the difficult stages of treatment.

Relationship enhancement.   The relationship enhancement strategy involves creating and maintaining a strong therapeutic relationship from the viewpoints of both therapist and patient. At the beginning of treatment, one of the goals is to quickly develop the patient-therapist attachment. Means of achieving and maintaining this include 1) the emphasis upon validation of the patient's affective, cognitive, and behavioral experiences; 2) the clarity of the contract (i.e., ending self-harm and building a life worth living); 3) the focus upon therapy-interfering behavior; 4) outreach and availability through telephone calls; and 5) problem solving of feelings regarding the relationship. Through these, the therapist nurtures the patient's feelings of attachment and trust. The therapist also actively attempts to enhance the patient's beliefs in the therapist's competence and the efficacy of the therapy. Questions about training and expertise are answered, data are given on the treatment's efficacy, and the environment is arranged to communicate credibility. When possible, interventions with a high likelihood of quick effects are used early in the treatment.

Equally important, however, is the therapist's attachment to the patient. If the therapist feels ambivalence or dislike for the patient, this will be communicated through omissions, if not direct actions, and the relationship will suffer. Resolution is facilitated by the focus upon self-harm (which will reduce therapist stress), therapy-interfering behaviors, and feelings about the relationship. Supervision in the consultation group is also vital in helping the therapist see the patient more positively during difficult moments.

Relationship problem solving.   The relationship problem-solving strategy is applicable when the relationship is a source of problems for either member. Patient unhappiness, dissatisfaction, or anger at the therapist and negative feelings of the therapist are treated as signals that the relationship needs problem-solving attention. When addressing the patient's feelings, the therapist must clarify for the patient what she can realistically expect from both the therapist and the treatment, and remain sensitive to moments when the patient appears to be operating on the basis of unreal-istic and probably unverbalized expectations of the therapist. The thera-pist should explore with the patient what aspects of the therapist's own behavior might have contributed to the unrealistic expectations and, when appropriate, validate the patient's legitimate need for more than can perhaps be offered. In a similar fashion, the therapist's unrealistic expec-tations of the patient also need to be clarified, discussed, and changed. Attention to both the patient and the input from the consultation group are important here.

As part of problem solving their own negative feelings, therapists must both be aware of and observe their own limits. The word "observe" is used rather than "set" in DBT to imply a flexible and personal rather than arbitrary, external standard for limits. As discussed above, the bias of DBT is for natural over arbitrary conditions of therapy. In DBT, such natural limits are explained not as if they are good for the patient, but rather as is necessary in the long run for the therapist to continue to perform effective therapy. Therapists' limits, however, are often connected to patient be-havior. For example, limits might expand when the patient is perceived as working hard in therapy or is not excessively demanding. This relation-ship between limits and patient behavior is a legitimate focus of discus-sion and problem solving. Therapist limits are also influenced by many factors other than the specific patient-therapist relationship. Thus, in some respects painful limits may not be amenable to patient influence. The distress and need of the patient in the face of therapist limits are validated and treated as legitimate problems to be solved; the therapist's limits are seen as unfortunate and sometimes at odds with the patient's needs. Therapists must themselves be comfortable with a nonjudgmental approach in order to observe their limits. Once again, the consultation group can facilitate this goal.

Relationship generalization. The relationship generalization strategy guides the therapist as she or he serves as a model to the patient of both how to resolve difficult interpersonal problems and, in general, how to act while in a relationship. Although a therapeutic relationship is not the same as one of the patient's social involvements, there are similarities between therapy and a "real" relationship (Linehan 1988) from which the patient can learn by observation as well as participation. To go beyond the limited effects of modeling, the therapist must search for similarities across relationships that can be addressed during the treatment.

Relationship contingency.   The relationship contingency strategy is one of the most important strategies in the middle phases of therapy but is one of the most difficult strategies to implement effectively. It is implicit in statements to the patient that she must improve to remain in treatment. This strategy involves the use of the contingencies inherent in the patient's attachment to the therapist as the motivation for behavioral changes for which there is little positive or even negative reinforcement in the patient's environment. Behaviors in this category include ending parasuicide, approaching problems rather than avoiding them, and staying out of hospitals. At times, the only contingency available to get control of destructive behaviors is the valence of the therapeutic relationship. In its mildest form, the contingency may only be a communication that the therapist views the behavior as dysfunctional and therefore not altogether desirable. Or, the therapist may simply remind the patient of her agreements in beginning treatment. A bit stronger, and more typical, is the reflection to the patient of the effect of the patient's behavior on the therapist's feelings about working with the patient. For example, the therapist might suggest (if accurate) that when the patient repeatedly refuses to talk in sessions, the therapist feels demoralized, or that when the patient approaches rather than avoids a difficult topic, the therapist feels encouraged or pleased. The strongest contingency, ending therapy, should be a very last resort because a termination of treatment can be used only once.

Three conditions are essential to the successful use of the relationship contingency strategy. Most obviously, there must be a strong patient-therapist relationship. Second, both the therapist and the patient must be clear that the behavioral change is for the greater welfare of the patient and not just for the convenience of the therapist. To achieve this clarity, the therapist may have to appeal to the patient's "wise" sense of what is best for her. Third, the patient must have the capability to make the change. The therapist must know the patient very well because the exact nature of the contingency and other important criteria depend greatly upon the particular patient. With some patients, conditional warmth may be key, but with others, this might be harmful. Finally, therapist skill is

crucial because mistakes in either timing or exact wording can have disastrous effects. We describe the technique here primarily to note its existence and importance within the therapy rather than to provide sufficient
guidelines for its use.

Empirical Support

As noted above, there are also limited data on the effect of DBT strategies
from one process study (Shearin 1991; Shearin and Linehan 1991) that
followed four DBT patients for the first 31 weeks of their initial year of
treatment. In this study, the perceptions that patients and therapists had
of each other were measured weekly and related to subsequent changes in
suicidal behavior and other behavioral targets of the treatment.

Most important from a theoretical viewpoint, dialectics were the most
consistent predictors of changes in suicidal behavior. Suicidal behavior as
measured by suicidal ideation and self-harm urges was lower a week after
patients perceived their therapists to be interacting with them in ways that
combined nurturing behaviors (e.g., teaching, directive support) and the
giving of autonomy. This finding provides some empirical support for the
theoretical emphasis in DBT on balancing change strategies (in this case,
teaching and directive support) with acceptance strategies (e.g., the provision of autonomy).

Relationship effects were also important. The results indicated that
more positive therapist perceptions of the patients were followed by decreased suicidal behavior. Conversely, when patients perceived therapists
to be more critical and less helpful, the patients became more passive in
their approach to problems. These findings are consistent with the DBT
emphasis upon choosing the least pejorative explanations of patient behavior and utilizing the numerous strategies just described to improve the
quality of the therapeutic relationship.

There were also results compatible with previously demonstrated effects of behavioral and social learning treatments. Modeling by the therapist had short-term effects (within the same week) on the behavior of the
patient. When the patients perceived the therapists to be nurturing and
protecting, the therapists also observed patients to be more self-nurturing
and self-protecting. This effect is consistent with the literature on the
efficacy of modeling. The transient nature of it is not surprising so early in

treatment, but it also indicates the need for more attention to generalization strategies.

Given both the small number of subjects and the short period of observation, considerable care must be taken not to overgeneralize these findings. Nonetheless, the consistency of the results with DBT predictions indicates that under specific conditions the components of DBT that were measured appear to work as theoretically postulated. Taken together with the results of the outcome studies described earlier, there is now some empirical evidence that DBT may be helpful to borderline patients and that limited measurements of patient and therapist perceptions are consistent with how the treatment is postulated to operate.

SUMMARY

In the preceding sections we have described the framework, goals, and selected strategies of dialectical behavior therapy, a psychotherapy developed by Linehan and her associates for the treatment of parasuicidal patients with a diagnosis of borderline personality disorder. We have also included a summary of the currently available empirical support for the efficacy of the treatment and its theoretical hypotheses. The implementation of the treatment depends heavily upon a unique theoretical approach involving a dialectical balance between opposites such as acceptance and change. Consistent with behavior therapy in general, the therapy is specified in terms of a hierarchy of behavioral targets that vary in importance depending upon the stage in therapy. However, in DBT the therapist focuses more attention than is common in behavior therapy on the therapeutic relationship itself for strategies to achieve the behavioral targets. We hope that this overview will provide a fresh viewpoint on some possible ways of approaching BPD and parasuicidal behavior in the beginning phases of treatment.

REFERENCES

American Psychiatric Association: Diagnostic and Statistical Manual of Mental Disorders, 3rd Edition, Revised. Washington, DC, American Psychiatric Association, 1987

Arnkoff DB: Common and specific factors in cognitive therapy, in A Guide to Psychotherapy and Patient Relationships. Edited by Lambert MJ. Homewood, IL, Dorsey Professional Books/Dow Jones-Irwin, 1983, pp 85–125

Beck AT, Rush AJ, Shaw BF, et al: Cognitive Therapy of Depression. New York, Guilford, 1979

Courtois CA: Healing the Incest Wound: Adult Survivors in Therapy. New York, WW Norton, 1988

Ellis A: Reason and Emotion in Psychotherapy. New York, Stuart, 1962

Ellis A: Humanistic Psychology: The Rational Emotive Approach. New York, Julian Press, 1973

Goldfried M, Davison G: Clinical Behavior Therapy. New York, Holt, Rinehart & Winston, 1976

Gunderson JG, Kolb JE, Austin V: The diagnostic interview for borderline patients. Am J Psychiatry 138:896–903, 1981

Hellman ID, Morrison TL, Abramowitz SI: The stresses of psychotherapeutic work: a replication and extension. J Clin Psychol 42:197–205, 1986

Herman JL, van der Kolk BA: Traumatic antecedents of borderline personality disorder, in Psychological Trauma. Edited by van der Kolk BA. Washington, DC, American Psychiatric Press, 1987, pp 111–126

Jacobson NS, Margolin G: Marital Therapy: Strategies Based on Social Learning and Behavioral Exchange Principles. New York, Brunner/Mazel, 1979

Kendall PC, Hollon SD (eds): Cognitive-Behavioral Interventions: Theory, Research, and Procedures. New York, Academic, 1979

Langs R: The Therapeutic Interaction: A Synthesis. New York, Jason Aronson, 1977

Langs R: Psychotherapy: A Basic Text. New York, Jason Aronson, 1982

Linehan MM: A social-behavioral analysis of suicide and parasuicide: implications for clinical assessment and treatment, in Depression: Behavioral and Directive Intervention Strategies. Edited by Glazer HG, Clarkin JF. New York, Garland Press, 1981, pp 229–294

Linehan MM: Dialectical behavior therapy for borderline personality disorder: theory and method. Bull Menninger Clin 51:261–276, 1987

Linehan MM: Perspectives on the interpersonal relationship in behavior therapy. Journal of Integrative and Eclectic Psychotherapy 7:278–290, 1988

Linehan MM: Cognitive-Behavioral Treatment for Borderline Personality Disorder: The Dialectics of Effective Treatment. New York, Guilford, 1992

Linehan MM, Shearin EN: Lethal stress: a social-behavioral model of suicidal behavior, in Handbook of Life Stress, Cognition, and Health. Edited by Fisher S, Reason J. Chichester, UK, Wiley, 1988, pp 265–285

Linehan MM, Armstrong HE, Suarez A, et al: Cognitive-behavioral treatment of chronically parasuicidal borderline patients. Arch Gen Psychiatry 48:1060–1064, 1991

Rice LN: The relationship in client-centered therapy, in A Guide to Psychotherapy and Patient Relationships. Edited by Lambert MJ. Homewood, IL, Dorsey Professional Books/Dow Jones-Irwin, 1983, pp 36–60

Roswell VA: Professional liability: Issues for behavior therapists in the 1980s and 1990s. The Behavior Therapist 11:163–171, 1988

Seltzer LF: Paradoxical Strategies in Psychotherapy: A Comprehensive Overview and Guidebook. New York, Wiley, 1986

Shearin EN: Perceptions of borderline personality disorder patients and relationship to treatment progress. Unpublished doctoral dissertation, University of Washington, Seattle, WA, 1990

Shearin EN, Linehan MM: Dialectics and behavior therapy: a meta-paradoxical approach to the treatment of borderline personality disorder, in Therapeutic Paradox. Edited by Ascher LM. New York, Guilford, 1991, pp 255–288

Shearin EN, Linehan, MM: Behavior therapy for parasuicidal borderline women. Paper presented at the of the American Psychiatric Association, New Orleans, LA, May 1991

Sherman MH: Siding with the resistance in paradigmatic psychotherapy. Psychoanalysis and the Psychoanalytic Review 48:43–59, 1961

Stone MH: Borderline syndromes: a consideration of subtypes and an overview, directions for research. Psychiatr Clin North Am 4:3–24, 1981

Swenson C: Kernberg and Linehan: two approaches to the borderline patient. Journal of Personality Disorders 3:26–35, 1989

Wagner A, Linehan MM: Parasuicide: characteristics and relationship to childhood sexual abuse. Poster presented at the annual meeting of the Association for Advancement of Behavior Therapy. Washington, DC, November 1989

Waldinger RJ, Gunderson JG: Completed psychotherapies with borderline patients. Am J Psychother 38:190–202, 1984

CHAPTER 15

Pharmacological Therapies in Borderline Personality Disorder

Paul H. Soloff, M.D.

IN THE PAST DECADE, THE PHARMACOTHERAPY OF BORDER-line personality disorder has moved from being a topic of theoretical controversy to an accepted area for clinical research. The borderline patient is progressively viewed as having *both* biological vulnerabilities (to affective dyscontrol and impulsive behavior) and core characterological pathology. Reliable and valid methods for diagnosing borderline patients have been developed and applied in medication studies using rigorous double-blind, placebo-controlled designs. Pharmacotherapy trials with patients with criteria-defined borderline personality disorder (BPD) now include studies of 1) neuroleptics, both high and low potency; 2) antidepressants, tricyclics and monoamine oxidase (MAO) inhibitors; 3) anticonvulsants; 4) anxiolytics; and 5) lithium carbonate. Case reports extend this literature further with novel approaches to extreme presentations (e.g., opiate antagonists for self-injurious behavior).

This is the "good news." The "bad news" is a growing appreciation of the high prevalence, morbidity, and mortality of BPD and a sense of urgency and frustration around the need to find effective treatments. The prevalence of BPD in the general community has recently been estimated at 1.8% of the population (Swartz et al. 1990). Borderline patients account for a far greater proportion of persons seeking psychiatric attention—up to 11% of outpatients and 23% of inpatients in some psychiatric settings (Widiger and Frances 1989). Half of the borderline patients surveyed in a community sample used outpatient mental health services in the 6 months prior to the survey; 19.5% were hospitalized in the prior year (Swartz et al. 1990). Medical morbidity is substantial. Among a sample of consecutively admitted borderline patients at the University of Pittsburgh, 62.2% gave histories of past suicidal gestures; approximately 50% engaged in self-mutilation. Completed suicide rates for borderline patients average 3% to 9.5% and are equal to rates for affective and schizophrenic disorders (Stone 1989). While the need for effective treatment appears urgent, there is no definitive therapy for the affective dyscontrol or impulsive behavior of the borderline patient.

GOALS OF PHARMACOTHERAPY

Ten years experience has made clear the need to define specific goals for pharmacological interventions in BPD. The clinical problem is to separate biological elements of borderline pathology, which may be responsive to medication, from learned character dynamics. This is difficult in a disorder for which many of the diagnostic criteria are acute symptoms arising from underlying trait vulnerabilities that may be biological in origin (e.g., part of "temperament") or learned (e.g., part of "personality organization"). Which comes first, temperament or personality organization, has been debated fruitlessly for years. The primary goal of pharmacotherapy research in BPD has been to define indications for pharmacological treatment through medication response, independent of the theoretical debate on etiology. A second goal has been to define meaningful subtypes within this heterogeneous disorder through a pharmacological behavioral dissection into medication responsive symptom patterns (Klein 1968).

From the clinician's perspective, the pharmacological approach to the borderline patient is organized around several critical assumptions:

1. The borderline patient has a temperamental (biological) vulnerability to affective dysregulation and to impulsive behaviors.
2. Trait vulnerabilities arise from neurotransmitter pathology, not psychodynamics, and are legitimate targets for pharmacological treatment.
3. Psychodynamics of interpersonal relatedness are not primary targets for pharmacological intervention, although interpersonal behavior may change when symptom severity diminishes. Indeed, some character traits may be revealed as adaptations to chronic affective, anxiety, or cognitive disorders and remit with pharmacological treatment.

In this review we will discuss controlled studies using criteria-defined patient samples. Studies conducted before the advent of formal diagnostic criteria or structured interviews are difficult to reconcile with current diagnostic standards and are subject to considerable misinterpretation. They have been reviewed elsewhere (Cole and Sunderland 1982; Soloff 1981). Open-label reports will be included only when needed to complete the data base or illustrate new directions. Preference is given to the most recent double-blind, placebo-controlled studies in an effort to *update* and not duplicate previous reviews (Soloff 1989).

PHARMACOLOGICAL THERAPIES

Neuroleptics

The usefulness of low-dose neuroleptics in the management of the symptomatic borderline patient has been established by clinical reports and controlled treatment trials (Brinkley et al. 1979; Cowdry and Gardner 1988; Goldberg et al. 1986; Leone 1982; Serban and Siegel 1984; Soloff et al. 1986b). An overview of this literature indicates that there is a broad spectrum of efficacy for neuroleptics in patients with BPD, including therapeutic effects against both affective and cognitive symptoms, perceptual distortions, anger and hostility, phobic anxiety, obsessive-compulsive symptoms, and impulsive behavior. In short, neuroleptics appear to have a beneficial but *nonspecific* mode of action in borderline patients, acting as tranquilizers to blunt symptom severity regardless of symptom content.

The issue of specificity of medication response is critical for any effort at pharmacological dissection into biologically meaningful subtypes and for empirical definition of treatment indications. The early use of neuroleptics in treatment of borderline disorders arose from the hypothesized relationship of schizotypal borderline symptoms (e.g., schizotypal personality disorder [SPD] and BPD) to the schizophrenic spectrum and, theoretically, to dopaminergic neurotransmitter pathology. Recall that one definition of borderline disorder arose as a subschizophrenic diagnosis (e.g., latent, ambulatory, pseudoneurotic schizophrenia). Borderline disorder has been redefined only recently as a subaffective disorder (Stone 1979). Case reports in recent literature define "soft signs" of thought disorder as primary target symptoms for neuroleptic treatment in border-line patients (Brinkley 1980). These target symptoms include schizotypal features such as tangentiality, circumstantiality, off-target and non sequi-tur responses, eccentricities, and magical thinking.

Early comparative studies of low-dose neuroleptics found them to be effective against a broad spectrum of symptoms in BPD, including both cognitive and affective symptom domains, but these studies did not use placebo control groups (Leone 1982; Serban and Siegel 1984). Placebo-controlled studies followed, but these emphasized either the schizotypal or the affective presentation of borderline patients.

Goldberg et al. (1986) studied 50 outpatients with DSM-III (American Psychiatric Association 1980) BPD but required "at least one psychotic symptom" for inclusion in the study. Patients were recruited by advertise-ments outlining criteria from the Schedule for Interviewing Borderlines (SIB) (Baron et al. 1981). The results of this double-blind, placebo-con-trolled trial of thiothixene (mean dose = 8.67 mg) over 12 weeks revealed significant improvement in illusions, ideas of reference, and psychotic-ism, with trend significance in derealization and depersonalization. The more severe the symptom presentation, the better the observed drug response. Despite a bias toward schizotypal pathology, it is noteworthy that obsessive-compulsive and phobic-anxiety symptoms (both as mea-sured by the SCL-90) also improved.

Cowdry and Gardner (1988) studied an affectively biased sample by recruitment of 16 female BPD outpatients, diagnosed by DSM-III and Diagnostic Interview for Borderline Patients (DIB) criteria, who also were required to meet criteria for hysteroid dysphoria and have "extensive his-tories of behavioral dyscontrol." Patients with current diagnoses of major depression were excluded. Although 6 patients (37%) of the sample met criteria for DSM-III SPD, there were no assessment instruments sensitive to cognitive or schizotypal pathology. Cowdry and Gardner reported that only half of the patients (5 of 10) who were given trifluoperazine (average = 7.8 mg/day) completed the 6-week trial, but that those who completed a minimum medication trial of 3 weeks ($n = 7$) showed significant improve-ment in depression, anxiety, and sensitivity to rejection.

Soloff et al. (1986a, 1989), at the University of Pittsburgh, reported the only double-blind, placebo-controlled study of borderline *inpatients*, contrasting a neuroleptic (haloperidol) with an antidepressant (amitriptyline) medication. Their study included 90 consecutively admitted borderline patients who met DIB and DSM-III criteria for BPD and SPD (56.7%), SPD alone (4.4%), or BPD alone (38.9%). These were cooperative but very disturbed inpatients. The medications, which were given for 5 weeks, averaged 4.8 mg/day for haloperidol, with a mean plasma level of 8.66 ± 3.7 ng/ml. Assessment measures were sensitive to a wide spectrum of symptom domains. Significant improvement in global functioning, depression, hostility, schizotypal symptoms, and impulsive behavior was reported for haloperidol compared with placebo. A factor analysis allowed definition of a symptom severity factor independent of symptom content. Haloperidol was significantly superior to both placebo and amitriptyline against symptom severity (Soloff et al. 1986a).

The Pittsburgh group has recently completed a second study comparing haloperidol (up to 4 mg daily) with phenelzine (up to 60 mg daily) in 108 DIB- and DSM-III–defined BPD inpatients (P. H. Soloff, A. George, R. S. Nathan, unpublished manuscript, 1990). In this double-blind, placebo-controlled study, patients participated in an acute treatment trial of 5 weeks duration, followed by a continuation therapy of 16 weeks (for those patients responding to medication). Using identical assessment methods in the same treatment setting, the investigators *failed to replicate* the previously reported efficacy of haloperidol over placebo in the acute treatment across *all* symptom domains. Upon comparison of the two study populations, they found significantly greater acute symptom severity in the haloperidol group, specifically in global impairment, schizotypal symptoms, psychoticism (e.g., perceptual distortions), and impulsive ward behavior, symptoms that statistically predict favorable response to haloperidol (Soloff et al. 1989). The phenelzine group, though less acutely symptomatic, had more severe borderline character pathology (as measured on the DIB) and depressive complaints. Paradoxically, the failure of this 4-year study to replicate the efficacy of haloperidol across all symptom domains in a less severely symptomatic population supports the hypothesis of nonspecificity for neuroleptic action in BPD and the recommendation that neuroleptics be reserved for the more severely symptomatic BPD patient.

Does neuroleptic medication treat the personality disorder itself, that is, the basic vulnerability to affective dyscontrol and impulsive behavior? This question has been raised by Teicher et al. in an ongoing open-label trial of thioridazine in 11 outpatient volunteers with BPD defined by DIB and DSM-III criteria (Teicher et al. 1989). Using a modified version of Gunderson's DIB as a measure of change, the authors noted improvement in the impulse action, affects, and psychosis sections of the DIB following 12 weeks of thioridazine (average dose = 92 mg daily). These symptom domains represent the acute (state) symptoms of BPD but may also reflect chronic (trait) vulnerabilities. Significant improvement was also noted on more traditional change measures—for example, the Brief Psychiatric Rating Scale (BPRS) (Overall and Gorham 1988) and the Hopkins Symptom Checklist–90 (SCL-90) (Derogatis et al. 1973) hostility, paranoid ideation, interpersonal sensitivity and additional depression subscales. The Overt Aggression Symptom Check List, a self-report form devised by the author, showed significant change from baseline to end of trial. Patients completing the study ($n = 6$) did much better than the total sample, with additional improvement in global functioning (GAS, CGI), obsessive-compulsive symptoms (SCL-90), and anxiety (SCL-90). Responding patients are described as "less impulsive, slightly less depressed and less overtly borderline."

There was no change on the interpersonal relations section of the DIB, which measures the chaotic interpersonal style of the borderline patient (i.e., the core of the character pathology). Unfortunately, only 6 of 11 patients completed the neuroleptic trial, severely limiting interpretation of data from this ongoing study.

Predictors of Response

Soloff et al. (1989) performed a factor analysis on all outcome measures (expressed as change scores) in their initial study of haloperidol and amitriptyline in BPD. Three "change factors" were identified, corresponding to symptoms responding as a group to medication: global depression, hostile depression, and schizotypal change factors. Haloperidol was most effective against hostile depression (made up of SCL-90 depression, SCL-90 hostility, SCL-90 general severity index, and the Buss-Durkee Hostility Inventory [BDHI] [Buss and Durkee 1957]). Haloperidol was also superior to amitriptyline on the schizotypal change factor, which was made up of the Schizotypal Symptom Inventory, Perceptual Distortion, and Paranoid Projection subscales of the Inpatient

Multidimensional Psychiatric Scale (IMPS) (Lorr and Klett 1966). Predictors of outcome were derived by regression analysis. Favorable outcomes on hostile depression were predicted by high IMPS scores on paranoid projection, hostile belligerence, suspiciousness, and motor excitement. On the schizotypal change factor, patients with prominent schizotypal symptoms, indirect hostility (BDHI), and multiple subjective complaints (SCL-90, IMPS) had more favorable outcomes on haloperidol. A pattern of intense, unstable relationships (DIB) predicted poor outcomes. These findings for neuroleptics suggest a response against acute symptoms but little effect against chronic character dynamics.

Antidepressants

Depression is ubiquitous in BPD and presents as a reactive mood state, an expression of character, or a comorbid affective disorder. The borderline personality is defined in part by affective instability, depressive "mood crashes," and recurrent suicidal behavior. Biological psychiatrists see in this affective dysregulation a biologically mediated vulnerability to mood disorders (e.g., Akiskal's [1981] subaffective dysthymia or Winokur's [1979] character spectrum depression). Analytic theorists, viewing the personality organization as primary, tend to see the affective displays as reactive epiphenomena to underlying structural pathology (Kernberg 1975). Empirical studies indicate a comorbidity of BPD and Axis I major depression ranging from 14% to 83% depending on method and setting. When methods that account for base rates of depression in control samples are used, the incidence of comorbidity of BPD and major depression in *inpatients* was 45% (Fyer et al. 1988a). In a community sample of over 1,500 persons surveyed with rigorous epidemiological methods, the comorbidity of major depression among BPD patients was 40.7% (Swartz et al. 1990). (Only comorbidity with anxiety disorders was more prevalent, with generalized anxiety disorder found in 56.4% of BPD patients, simple phobia in 41.4%, agoraphobia in 36.9%, social phobia in 34.6%, and panic disorder in 13.1%.)

Does the depressed borderline patient have one disorder or two? Is BPD a depressive disorder or a personality organization uniquely vulnerable to comorbid affective disorders? (See Gold and Silk, Chapter 2.) Can pharmacotherapy studies contribute to the resolution of this debate?

The method of pharmacological behavioral dissection seeks to define meaningful diagnostic subtypes through patients' responses to medication (Klein 1968). However, "dissecting" the affective presentations of borderline patients with antidepressants is a formidable task. *Depression in BPD is not a homogeneous entity,* nor is it easily measured. Soloff et al. (1987b) studied a sample of consecutively admitted borderline inpatients using three diverse constructs for depression and three different assessment methods: a structured interview for Research Diagnostic Criteria (RDC) depressive diagnoses, a self-rated checklist for hysteroid dysphoria, and an observer-rated scale for symptoms of atypical depression. No one method was sufficient to characterize the sample. An RDC depressive diagnosis (major, intermittent, minor, or schizoaffective depression) was found in 64.1%, atypical depression in 41%, and hysteroid dysphoria in 64.1% of the patients studied. Also, 64.1% of patients met criteria for two diagnoses, while 17.9% met criteria for all three depressive disorders.

How valid are diagnoses of depression in BPD? Research diagnoses are typically cross-sectional in nature, based on relatively brief interviews. It is common experience to have the ward staff contradict research diagnoses based on their own longitudinal observation. In fact, Siever et al. (1985) reported the spontaneous resolution of major depression criteria in 17 of 22 (90.9%) patients with personality disorders following 2 weeks of medication-free hospital care.

With this background, the issues of sample definition and research method are critical to interpretation of antidepressant trials in BPD. Placebo-controlled studies (which remain few in number) show some effect, though modest in magnitude, of tricyclics and MAO inhibitors in reducing depression. Soloff et al. (1986b, 1989) studied an inpatient sample of DIB-defined borderline patients administered amitriptyline (average dose = 149 mg/day) compared with groups administered placebo and haloperidol. The authors found significant improvement in self- and observer-rated depression compared with placebo. Scores on the HAM-D-24 decreased 35%, from a mean of 24.8 to 16.1, the latter still in the impaired range for most pharmacotherapy studies of depression. (These effects were not, however, superior to the antidepressant effects of haloperidol.) Soloff et al. (1986b, 1987a) also described a distinct worsening among amitriptyline nonresponders: a behavioral toxicity manifested by increased suicidal threats, paranoid ideation, and demanding and assaultive behavior. Schizotypal symptoms, verbal aggression, and paranoia, common in this inpatient sample, predicted poor outcomes with amitriptyline, whereas indirect hostility, multiple subjective complaints (SCI -90), and histories of manipulative suicide attempts predicted favorable outcomes (Soloff et al. 1989). Depressive measures were not identified as predictors of outcome in this analysis. Indeed, there appears to be a paradoxical *independence* of response to amitriptyline and comorbid diagnosis of major depression in borderline patients. It was therefore not possible to "dissect" out an affective borderline subtype with this medication trial.

Links et al. (1990) has reported on an ongoing placebo-controlled study of desipramine and lithium carbonate in DIB-defined borderline patients in whom affective and impulsive symptoms were prominent target symptoms. Major depression was not an exclusionary criterion. In this crossover study, each medication condition is defined by a 2-week titration period and a 4-week trial. Preliminary data ($n = 17$), including data on both outpatients and inpatients, reveal no significant differences in depression between groups at 3 weeks or 6 weeks into medication trials. A nonsignificant trend favoring lithium over desipramine was noted when comparing their effects on anger and suicidal symptoms. Therapists' ratings of improvement have favored lithium over placebo, most likely in response to decreased irritability, anger, and suicidal symptoms. There was a nonsignificant trend for therapists to favor lithium over desipramine, but not desipramine over placebo. The tricyclic antidepressant had no greater efficacy against depression than did placebo or lithium.

Monoamine oxidase inhibitors. Cowdry and Gardner (1988) reported limited efficacy for the MAO inhibitor tranylcypromine in borderline *outpatients* (defined by DIB criteria) who had hysteroid dysphoria and histories of impulsive behavior. Despite small numbers completing the MAO trial in this double-blind, placebo-controlled crossover study (which used four active medications), some efficacy was reported for tranylcypromine (average dose = 40 mg/day) in reducing depressed mood and related impulsiveness. The presence of major depression was an exclusionary criterion in this functional outpatient sample. Response to tranylcypromine was independent of histories of prior affective illness or family histories of classical affective disorder. The improvement against impulsiveness, though measured only by physician judgment, is noteworthy in light of the failure of other antidepressant medications (e.g., mianserin and nomifensine) to prevent the recurrent impulsive suicidal behaviors of borderline and histrionic patients (Gardner and Cowdry 1986b; Montgomery and Montgomery 1982; Montgomery et al. 1987). Response to tranylcypromine was associated with a history consistent with attention-deficit disorder. Patients with attention-deficit disorder can present with a syndrome similar to BPD. Some suggest that attention-deficit disorder is one of many etiologies for BPD, especially in the rare male borderline patient (Andrulonis et al. 1981). The efficacy of tranylcypromine, a stimulant in such cases, is not surprising.

Phenelzine. Following early reports of efficacy for phenelzine in patients with hysteroid dysphoria and BPD (Liebowitz and Klein 1981; Liebowitz et al. 1984), Soloff et al. (unpublished data) conducted a double-blind, placebo-controlled study of phenelzine and haloperidol among 108 DIB-defined borderline inpatients. As in Soloff et al.'s earlier studies, acute treatment trials were 5 weeks in duration; however, a continuation therapy of 16 weeks was added for medication responders, shifting the emphasis from acute inpatient care to longitudinal outpatient follow-through. Significant changes occurred within each medication group across time in measures of depression, global symptom severity, and schizotypal symptoms. Phenelzine was superior to haloperidol but not superior to placebo on the SCL-90 depression subscale and the Borderline Syndrome Index, a broad measure of borderline pathology. There was no efficacy for phenelzine compared with placebo in reducing atypical depression or scores on the traditional Hamilton Depression Rating Scale or the Beck Depression Inventory. Phenelzine was significantly superior to placebo on the BDHI, a self-report measure of anger and hostility. Thus, subjective depression, "borderline" symptoms, anger, and hostility appear more responsive to phenelzine than do observed symptoms of classical depression, or even atypical depression. Overall, symptom change was modest at best, with residual symptoms the rule.

The study of phenelzine in the treatment of BPD is discouraging in regard to its efficacy against atypical depressive symptoms in the borderline patient. Parsons et al. (1989) recently reported superiority for phenelzine compared with imipramine and placebo in patients with a *primary diagnosis* of atypical depressive disorder (based on Columbia criteria) and a *secondary diagnosis* of BPD. Their study samples consisted of cooperative outpatients, screened for compliance through multiple ambulatory assessments, a sample very different from the inpatient samples in the Pittsburgh studies (P. Soloff, unpublished data). The Columbia sample was homogeneous for atypical depressive disorder, whereas the Pittsburgh borderline samples were heterogeneous in depressive presentation. The differences between the two studies are reflected by the significant *increase* in "mood reactivity" with phenelzine treatment in the Pittsburgh borderline samples, whereas, based on Columbia standards, elevated mood reactivity is generally seen as a pathological symptom. The heterogeneity of depressive presentations in a BPD sample (primary diagnosis) includes many quiet, withdrawn depressed patients whose "reactivity" increases with phenelzine. The applicability of the Columbia findings to general clinical treatment of borderline patients, while promising, requires further study.

Amoxapine.   Jensen and Andersen (1989) used amoxapine, an antidepressant with neuroleptic activity, in an open-label study comparing five inpatients with BPD, as defined by DSM-III and DIB criteria, with five inpatients with SPD and BPD, also as defined by DSM-III and SIB criteria. BPD patients received an average of 200 mg/day of amoxapine, while SPD/BPD patients received 250 mg/day. (Unfortunately, oxazepam was freely used for sedation in both groups.) Treatment averaged 28 days. Depressive symptoms and schizophrenia-like symptoms were assessed weekly with the HDRS, the BPRS, and the Clinical Global Impression Scale (CGI). Patients with SPD plus BPD showed significant improvement in global impression and depressive and schizophrenic-like symptoms, whereas the patients with BPD alone showed *no change*. The efficacy of amoxapine in the SPD/BPD group was attributed to a *neuroleptic effect* on SPD and to the increased severity of symptoms found in the SPD/BPD patients.

Fluoxetine.   The latest and most pharmacologically selective medication under study for treating depression in the BPD patient is fluoxetine, a serotonin reuptake-inhibiting antidepressant. Serotonin has long been postulated to play a role in the etiology of depression. A low level of

5-hydroxyindoleacetic acid (5-HIAA) in the cerebrospinal fluid (CSF) may be a predictor of suicidal behavior, especially violent suicide, and has been correlated with suicidal behavior in patients with affective disorders, schizophrenia, and BPD (Stanley and Mann 1988). In patients with personality disorders (and no affective disorder), low levels of CSF 5-HIAA have also been correlated with syndromes of impulsive aggression and criminal violence (Virkkunen et al. 1989). Borderline patients appear to have diminished central serotonergic activity as demonstrated by low levels of CSF 5-HIAA and blunting of the prolactin response to fenfluramine challenge, a serotonin-mediated response (Brown and Goodwin 1986; Brown et al. 1979, 1982; Coccaro et al. 1989; Gardner et al. 1990). Blunting of the prolactin response to fenfluramine correlates with suicidal behavior in both depressed and borderline patients, but it correlates with impulsive aggression only in borderline patients compared with depressed control subjects (Coccaro et al. 1989). In theory, a drug that enhances central serotonin neurotransmission may demonstrate effects against both depression and impulsive aggression.

Three open-label studies have now reported fluoxetine trials in a total of 35 borderline patients. In a private practice setting, Norden (1989) followed 12 outpatients with BPD based on DSM-III-R (American Psychiatric Association 1987) criteria (and no comorbid major depression) for periods ranging from 5 weeks to 26 weeks on fluoxetine, 5 to 40 mg/day. Although standardized ratings were not used, the author described quantitative improvement (on his own severity scale) in the areas of "rejection sensitivity, anger, depressed mood, mood lability, irritability, anxiety, obsessive-compulsive symptoms and impulsivity, including substance use and over-eating." Improvement for two-thirds of the patients appeared rapidly, in 2 to 5 days—that is, long before the attainment of steady-state plasma levels. Improvement was lost on discontinuation within 4 to 8 days. Seventy-five percent of the patients were assessed as much or very much improved.

Using a systematic research methodology and standardized questionnaires, Cornelius et al. (1990) studied five inpatients meeting DIB and DSM-III criteria for BPD. All patients had failed several trials of other psychotropic agents and were considered "refractory" cases. All were held free of medication for 1 week and met symptom severity criteria for continuation into the medication trial (as defined by a GAS score ≤ 50, and either a HAM-D-24 score ≥ 17 or an IMPS score ≥ 66). As a group, these patients were symptomatically depressed, with a mean HAM-D-24 score of 29.6 and a mean BDI score of 33.8. One patient had a concurrent diagnosis of major depression, and two had dysthymic disorder. Patients received fluoxetine for 8 weeks, starting with 20 mg and increasing to 40 mg in 2 weeks if clinically indicated.

Research ratings obtained weekly revealed significant improvement over time in global symptom severity (GAS, SCL-90), depression (HAM-D-24, BDI, SCL-90 depression), and impulsive ward behavior. Self-reported measures of hostility, paranoid ideation, psychoticism, somatization, and obsessive-compulsive symptoms (as measured by the SCL-90) also showed significant improvement, whereas an observer-based measure of schizotypal symptoms did not. The authors were most impressed by clinical effects on depressive and impulsive symptoms in keeping with the theoretical predictions for this drug.

These observations were extended by Markovitz et al. (1990), who studied 8 outpatients with BPD, 10 outpatients with both BPD and SPD, and 4 outpatients with SPD, all as defined by DSM-III criteria. Major depression was a comorbid diagnosis in 13 of the 22 patients and significant self-mutilation a current clinical problem in 12. Patients had failed multiple other treatment modalities. Patients received fluoxetine, 80 mg/day, for 12 weeks with symptom ratings (by SCL-90-R) taken every 3 weeks. Significant improvement at 12 weeks was noted in all scales of the SCL-90-R (e.g., obsessive-compulsive, interpersonal sensitivity, depression, anxiety, psychoticism, and paranoid ideation), with no differences between the BPD, BPD/SPD, and SPD groups or between patients with ($n = 13$) and without ($n = 9$) major depression. Self-mutilating behavior dramatically decreased, stopping completely in 10 of the 12 patients and decreasing in 2 others. A follow-up evaluation (mean $= 24.7 \pm 15.4$ weeks) showed continued improvement in all patients.

Double-blind, placebo-controlled trials of fluoxetine are needed in depressed and/or impulsive borderline patients to test these uncontrolled findings. Correlation of clinical response to fluoxetine with baseline assessment of central serotonergic function (e.g., CSF 5-HIAA, fenfluramine challenge) will further elucidate the role of serotonin in mediating the affective and impulsive-aggressive behavior of patients with BPD. Caution is warranted until controlled trials are available.

Teicher et al. (1990) have recently reported serious behavioral toxicity with fluoxetine in six cases, manifested by emergence of "intense suicidal preoccupation" in patients otherwise free of *recent* serious suicidal ideation. These patients had very complex histories and multiple diagnoses. The two patients who were diagnosed as having BPD both had major depression, one complicated by temporal lobe epilepsy, the other by episodic alcohol abuse. Both of these patients had prior suicidal symptoms, one with prior attempts, the other with ideation only. Suicidal ideation appeared in the context of a depressive syndrome and progressed markedly during fluoxetine treatment (despite doses of up to 80 mg/day). For the six patients taken as a group, the intense, obsessive suicidal rumination continued an average of 27 days after the drug was discontinued. Progression of depressive illness with resistance to medication is not a new phenomenon, but the intensity of suicidal preoccupation in all six of Teicher's cases suggests a paradoxical drug response. No explanation is evident at present. Fluoxetine also was associated with akathisia in four cases, a possible contributing factor. Nonetheless, patients on fluoxetine for depressive syndromes warrant additional surveillance for the emergence of suicidal ideation.

Minor Tranquilizers

Given the widespread use of minor tranquilizers in psychiatry and their efficacy in stress-related anxiety states, it is remarkable that so few papers describe the use of these medications in treating borderline disorders. The appeal of minor tranquilizers in the borderline patient lies in the rapid and effective relief of anxiety in patients characterized by low frustration tolerance and vulnerability to stress. Faltus (1984) described three male borderline patients defined by DSM-III criteria with marked schizotypal symptoms (including hallucinations in two of the cases) who responded to alprazolam with improvement in the severity of both cognitive and affective features of their disorder. They were less anxious, paranoid, suspicious, angry, and irritable. Also, they were better able to withstand stress without developing further schizotypal symptoms.

Reus and Markrow (1984) reported the first systematic study of alprazolam in 18 hospitalized DIB-defined borderline patients. In a double-blind crossover study, a favorable response occurred in half of the patients treated with alprazolam and was statistically predictable by baseline measures of hostility, suspiciousness (as measured by the BPRS), cognitive and sleep disturbance (as measured by the HDRS), and pathological interpersonal relatedness (as noted on the DIB). A more pessimistic note was sounded by Gardner and Cowdry (1985), who reported a significant increase in behavioral dyscontrol in borderline patients receiving alprazolam compared with control subjects. In a multidrug, placebo-controlled crossover design, 7 of 12 patients (58%) assigned to alprazolam (average = 4.7 mg/day) became overtly suicidal, self-destructive, or assaultive compared with only 1 of 13 patients on placebo (8%). Although serious dyscontrol was a new manifestation of illness for some patients, most had prior lifetime episodes of impulsive behavior and, indeed, were selected for histories of impulsiveness and hysteroid dysphoria. Alprazolam was not associated with overall improvement in global ratings or ratings of mood; however, 2 of 16 patients improved on alprazolam. Several patients demonstrated mood improvement before the episodes of behavioral dyscontrol. Alprazolam appears to have a potentially disinhibiting effect analogous to the disinhibition of aggression reported for other benzodiazepines (e.g., "librium rage").

Case reports by Freinhar and Alvarez (1985–1986) suggest a potential role for clonazepam, a benzodiazepine with anticonvulsant and serotonin-enhancing capacity, as an adjunct to other medications (e.g., thiothixene) in the management of anger, anxiety, and impulsivity in the borderline patient. Daily doses ranged from 4 to 10 mg. The authors suggest that specificity of effect against impulse dyscontrol may be due to the serotonin-enhancing potential of clonazepam.

Wolf et al. (1990) are currently conducting a double-blind, placebo-controlled trial of buspirone in outpatients with BPD based on DSM-III-R criteria. These patients were followed for 8 weeks and treated concurrently with supportive psychotherapy. Buspirone is a unique non-benzodiazepine anxiolytic agent with a high affinity for the serotonin (5-hydroxytryptamine) receptor 5-HT_{1A} and moderate affinity for the brain D_2 dopamine receptor. Eighty-three percent of the subjects found the overall treatment beneficial; 50% felt that the combination of medication and psychotherapy was helpful. Because the analysis of medication effects has not yet been completed, we must withhold judgment on the usefulness of buspirone in treating BPD. Nonetheless, an anxiolytic with no abuse potential (and no street value) warrants further investigation in the borderline patient.

It is the potential for development of pharmacological tolerance and abuse that limits the usefulness of the entire benzodiazepine family in treatment of the borderline patient. Disinhibition of anger and impulsive behavior and exaggeration of depressive mood further increase this risk. Benzodiazepine anxiolytics should be prescribed with great caution in patients with BPD and monitored carefully.

Anticonvulsants

The empirical use of anticonvulsants in borderline patients arises from a neurobehavioral theory of etiology. Are the affective dysregulation, cognitive and perceptual distortions, and behavioral dyscontrol of borderline patients reflections of central nervous system (CNS) pathology? The similarity in presenting symptoms of patients with BPD, of those with complex partial seizures, and those with episodic dyscontrol syndromes suggests the possibility of a common origin for these disorders in subictal limbic discharges, potentially as a predisposing influence toward impulsive behavior and affective or cognitive dyscontrol.

This hypothesis was initially tested through studies comparing the electroencephalograms (EEGs) of patients diagnosed as borderline with those of appropriate control subjects. Cowdry et al. (1985) reported a 46% incidence of abnormal EEG records in clinically defined borderline patients compared with a 10% incidence of abnormality in RDC-defined unipolar depressed control subjects. Snyder and Pitts (1984) found "marginally" or "definitely abnormal" EEGs in 38% of borderline patients compared with 13% in control subjects with dysthymic disorder. However, Andrulonis et al. (1981) failed to find any significant difference in incidence of EEG abnormalities in a borderline group compared with schizophrenic individuals. Cornelius et al. (1986) also failed to show any specificity for EEG abnormalities in borderline inpatients, but the authors did report an occasional individual with grade II or greater dysrhythmia whose case might fit the neurobehavioral hypothesis for BPD.

A second strategy for testing the neurobehavioral hypothesis is through pharmacodynamic challenge studies with agents that arouse the limbic system. Kellner et al. (1987) provoked dysphoric mood states in borderline patients with intravenous procaine, a limbic system–activating agent. They hypothesized that these discharges occur naturally in the borderline patient, resulting in affective dysregulation of neurologic origin. The authors postulated a specific pathophysiology involved in the borderline syndrome that is characterized by a relatively low threshold for arousal in limbic structures such as the amygdala or the hippocampus. It is in pursuit of the neurobehavioral etiology that trials of anticonvulsant agents have been used in patients with BPD.

In a very early clinical report, Davies (1977) described open-label, uncontrolled treatment trials of phenytoin (Dilantin) in 23 clinically defined borderline patients. His diagnostic criteria for borderline disorder included most of the Gunderson-Singer criteria, including affective, schizotypal, and impulsive behavioral features. EEG abnormalities were present in 21 patients, though so subtle as to warrant clinical reading as normal or only mildly abnormal (Cowdry et al. 1985). Patients were placed on phenytoin by clinicians' choice and were different from other borderline patients meeting the same diagnostic criteria, principally in the degree of visual symptoms, dissociative symptoms and, of course, the EEG abnormality. Of the 23 borderline patients placed on phenytoin, 16 "did very well, with good reduction in symptomatology." Davies implied that, in many patients, there was not simply a reduction of symptoms but a change in their interpersonal relatedness.

Gardner and Cowdry (1985) reported a significant clinical superiority for carbamazepine over placebo on the incidence of behavioral dyscontrol in a double-blind, placebo-controlled crossover study of 16 female outpatients meeting DSM-III and DIB criteria for BPD. Patients for this study were outpatients at the National Institute of Mental Health (NIMH) who had "an extensive history of behavioral dyscontrol" and who were free of Axis I schizophrenia, alcoholism, substance abuse, and major depression. Patients received carbamazepine, 200–1,200 mg qd (average = 820 mg) adjusted over a 2-week period to plasma levels of 8–12 g/ml and followed for a total of 6 weeks. Patients were seen weekly and interviewed for evidence of "minor dyscontrol" (defined as angry outbursts or suicidal threats) or "major dyscontrol" (defined as physical violence toward persons or objects, self-damaging acts, suicidal gestures, or suicidal attempts). Of the placebo patients, 64% (7 of 11) were discontinued from the study early because of clinical worsening compared with 7% (1 of 14) of the carbamazepine patients. Of patients completing the paired cross-over trials for both conditions, 91% (10 of 11) had less dyscontrol during the carbamazepine trial as opposed to the placebo trial. Carbamazepine was associated with less severe dyscontrol episodes.

The mechanism of action of carbamazepine in BPD is unclear. Patients in Gardner and Cowdry's (1986b) study were free of EEG abnormality. Procaine challenges on 11 of those patients revealed *no correlation* between the degree of procaine-induced EEG activation and subsequent improvement on carbamazepine (Kellner et al. 1987). Three patients developed melancholic depression as a paradoxical response to carbamazepine therapy. The role of carbamazepine in suppressing mood lability and mania as a thymo   agent may be more directly relevant to its efficacy in BPD than to its anticonvulsant action. (Cowdry's patients did not report subjective mood improvement but were rated by their physicians as significantly improved in mood, an equivocal outcome.) While this issue remains unresolved, carbamazepine represents a useful pharmacological tool against impulsive dyscontrol in BPD.

Lithium Carbonate

Lithium is the neglected stepchild of pharmacotherapy in patients with BPD. A generic salt with serotonergic action, lithium earned some early notoriety as a potentially useful agent against violent aggressive behavior in institutionalized criminal offenders (Sheard 1975; Tupin et al. 1973). In case histories and controlled trials, violent aggressive behavior has decreased with lithium despite diagnostic heterogeneity. The antiaggression efficacy of lithium has been reported for hyperactivity and retardation in children (Campbell et al. 1972; Dostal and Zvolsky 1970); for schizophrenia, abnormal EEG, and sociopathy in adult prisoners (Tupin et al. 1973); for severe personality disorders (Shader et al. 1974); and for episodic violence in adolescent offenders (Sheard 1975). Lithium produces a "reflective delay" between the aggressive impulse and physical action. In normal subjects, lithium increases reaction time. Van der Kolk (1986) suggests that lithium decreases responsivity to environmental stimuli and increases indifference in patients without classical affective indications. It produces an "emotional blunting" that is useful to patients who suffer from intense emotions.

Rifkin et al.'s (1972) early, often-quoted study of lithium carbonate in emotionally unstable character disorder (as defined by DSM-I) showed significant effects against mood lability. Although this disorder is felt by many to be an early label for borderline disorder, the authors maintained that their patients' mood lability was independent of environmental input, which suggests a more formal affective process such as cyclothymia rather than BPD. Nonetheless, mood lability is clearly a target symptom for lithium carbonate and a prevalent presentation in BPD. The major drawback in the use of lithium in treatment of patients with BPD is the narrow margin of safety in dose range and the need for constant monitoring. The risk of lethality with overdose is substantial and must be carefully considered when using this drug in impulsive patients.

The recent literature on lithium in DSM-III borderline patients is limited to case reports and one double-blind, placebo-controlled study comparing lithium to desipramine (Links et al. 1990; see above). In five case reports by LaWall and Wesselius (1982), lithium produced improvement in lability of affect, fluctuation of mood, anger, and suicidality. Links et al. (1990) found a similar trend for lithium in the reduction of irritability, anger, and suicidal symptoms compared with placebo or desipramine. Further study of this useful generic salt is clearly needed.

Novel Directions: Opiate Antagonists

Two related symptom complexes common in BPD have led investigators to the study of the endogenous opioid peptide system: 1) complaints of chronic anhedonia, boredom, and emptiness relieved by substance abuse (or self-injury); and 2) the syndrome of self-injurious behavior associated with topical analgesia, dissociation, and relief of tension. Both syndromes are associated with high levels of plasma opioid peptides in BPD. Two theories have been advanced relating these symptom patterns to endogenous opioid peptides. A "pain hypothesis" suggests that elevated endogenous opiates result in reduced responsiveness to ordinary stimulation (e.g., anhedonia, boredom), requiring extraordinary input via substance abuse (or self-injury) for relief. An "addiction hypothesis" assumes that chronically elevated levels of endogenous opiates are the result of repeated physical injury and produce pleasurable sensations. The patient becomes "addicted" to the endogenous high (Konicki and Schulz 1989). Bonnet and Redford (1982) reported elevated levels of plasma ß-endorphin in five borderline patients with marked boredom, dysphoria, anhedonia, and drug abuse. The authors followed the addiction hypothesis and postulated development of pharmacological tolerance to the endogenous neuropeptide as a biological basis for the patients' anhedonia and drug-seeking behavior. With evidence that dopamine is the tonic inhibitory regulator of pituitary ß-endorphin, these investigators gave L-dopa plus carbidopa (as Sinemet) to increase dopamine levels within the CNS, decreasing the ß-endorphin release and reversing the hypothetical tolerance. The clinical effect was marked reduction in dysphoria, in depressive ideation, in anhedonia, and in drug-seeking behavior.

Coid et al. (1983) found high mean plasma Met-enkephalin concentrations in 10 DSM-III BPD patients who were habitual self-mutilators compared with matched healthy control subjects. Patients had at least three (and up to 100) previous episodes of self-mutilation, and they had at least two episodes characterized by complete absence of pain, derealization or depersonalization, and relief of tension. Five patients who were still symptomatic inpatients had the highest levels of Met-enkephalin, significantly greater than those of five remitting outpatients, indicating that the raised levels of the neuropeptide depended on symptom severity; however, adrenocorticotropin (ACTH), another stress-sensitive peptide, did not differ between groups.

These observations suggest the experimental use of opioid antagonists for self-mutilating patients with BPD, and certainly for the BPD patient abusing narcotics. Naltrexone has been used in self-abusive autistic and retarded children with some success. Sternlicht and Payton (unpublished manuscript, 1989) report a systematic single case study of a 37-year-old patient with DSM-III BPD and a history of polysubstance abuse, multiple impulsive overdoses, chronic depression, and intermittent suicidality. Following a medication-free period in the hospital, the patient received naltrexone, 50 mg, in a double-blind design for 15 days, then crossed to placebo for 4 days, and then crossed again to naltrexone. Improvements that were noted on the SCL-90, the BDI, and the BDHI during naltrexone therapy were lost following the switch to placebo. Measures of borderline psychopathology, hysteroid dysphoria, impulsivity, and impulse control also improved with naltrexone and returned toward pretreatment levels on placebo.

These findings warrant further systematic exploration of the opioid peptide function in BPD and the potential usefulness of opiate antagonists in the treatment of chronic dysphoria, "self-medicating" substance abuse (especially narcotic), and self mutilation in BPD.

CAN WE STUDY, OR TREAT, THE BORDERLINE PATIENT WITH MEDICATION?

Problems that plague research on borderline disorders have a direct relationship to dilemmas faced by the clinician in treating the borderline patient. These problems have been reviewed at length in the literature but bear repeating:

1. The borderline disorder is not a homogeneous entity but is a syndrome, defined by a polythetic criterion menu that allows for multiple and diverse symptom presentations (e.g., the unstable affective borderline, the schizotypal borderline, the impulsive borderline). Medication responses vary greatly with symptom pattern despite the common syndromal diagnosis. Thus, the phrase "pharmacotherapy of borderline disorder" is a misnomer, as we do not treat the disorder itself but only responsive state symptoms and underlying trait vulnerabilities.
2. Comorbidity with Axis I disorders is high. Discrimination of borderline psychopathology from related Axis I affective, anxiety, and cognitive disorder syndromes is often difficult. Comorbidity with affective disorders and substance use disorders is especially significant because the combination is associated with increased rates of suicidal outcomes (Fyer et al. 1988b; Stone 1989). The issue for the clinician is which symptom pattern to treat. *In a hierarchal order, we treat clearly proven, discrete Axis I disorders first.* Having said this, we must also note that pharmacological treatment of comorbid Axis I affective disorders is hindered by the presence of BPD.
3. Many symptoms of patients with BPD are stress related and transient, hence the excellent response to "placebo" in the first 2–3 weeks of controlled medication trials.
4. The compliance of borderline patients with treatment is problematic. Dropout rates in pharmacotherapy studies may be as high as, for

example, 48% in 12 weeks (Goldberg et al. 1986) or 77% in 22 weeks of study (Soloff 1989). These rates are comparable to those in psychotherapy studies in which dropout accounted for 43% over 6 months in Gunderson et al.'s (1989) sample of borderline *in*patients, and 66% over 3 months in Skodol et al.'s (1983) outpatient sample.

5. The literature on treatment of BPD with pharmacotherapy or psychotherapy is heavily biased in favor of cooperative patients. Generalizability of results to the more impaired (i.e., involuntary) population is questionable. This criticism is even more relevant to the large volume of psychoanalytic writings on borderline disorder, derived from the intensive study of relatively few highly cooperative, articulate, and functional patients. How widely applicable are our theories of borderline pathology or treatment when derived from such biased sources?

6. Abuse of medication through noncompliance, excessive dosing, or intentional overdose is a problem in all pharmacotherapies, exaggerated in the borderline case by the opportunity for manipulation of the therapist. Overdose in particular is more feared than observed. The Borderline Disorders Research Clinic at the University of Pittsburgh followed 108 criteria-defined borderline inpatients through double-blind medication trials over a period of 4 years and into open clinical follow-up. Although many patients experienced episodes of dyscontrol (20% readmitted within 8 weeks), there were only *five* overdoses (4.6%), none with significant medical consequences. In 8 years of pharmacological studies involving 225 criteria-defined borderline patients in controlled medication trials in this same clinic, there have been no life-threatening medical consequences of medication abuse or any fatalities. No borderline patient in this clinic has intentionally induced a significant hypertensive crisis while on phenelzine by "overdosing" with cheese or chocolate (a common unspoken fear of therapists.) These data are offered as concrete evidence of the relative safety of pharmacotherapy trials in the borderline patient to offset the resistance of therapists who avoid medication on theoretical grounds (that medication will be used to act out, etc.; see, e.g., Coid et al. 1983). In any setting, medication must be given in the context of a *close doctor-patient relationship*. It is this supportive relationship and the limits surrounding medication prescription and informed consent that inhibit the patient's temptation to abuse medication.

Practical Recommendations

It is apparent from this review that little is firmly established concerning the medication responses of borderline patients. Therefore, our approach to treatment is purely empirical. The following guidelines are based on currently available data:

1. A period of medication-free observation is essential to the accurate diagnosis of the symptomatic borderline patient. When "extreme behaviors" are a risk (e.g., suicidal or assaultive behaviors), this evaluation should be conducted in the hospital. Studies on consecutively admitted borderline patients leave little doubt that many symptoms (including severe depressive states) may resolve in part or completely within 2 to 3 weeks of hospitalization.

2. In any symptom presentation where intensity or severity of symptoms is clinically pressing, independent of content, one may begin with low-dose neuroleptics. When schizotypal symptoms predominate, especially accompanied by anger, assaultiveness, suspicion, or referential thinking, low-dose neuroleptics are the first line of defense. These can be given in an emergency setting with or without full patient cooperation. Response is rapid, within hours to days, and broad in scope.

3. If the predominant symptom pattern is depressive, MAO inhibitors or serotonergic antidepressants are suggested. Patients with atypical depressive presentations (i.e., mood reactivity plus reverse neurovegetative symptoms) should have a trial of MAO inhibitor antidepressants. Anger and hostility may also respond to phenelzine in the affectively impaired patient. Schizotypal features are predictive of poor response to antidepressants and should be "covered" with low-dose neuroleptics where clinically prominent.

4. Impulsive behavior generally does not exist as an isolated symptom in the borderline patient but usually accompanies an acute mood state or transient thought disorder. Carbamazepine and lithium have empirical support as anti-impulse agents and may be useful in combination with other agents when impulsivity fails to remit with primary antidepressant or neuroleptic treatment. Fluoxetine has theoretical promise as an antidepressant with anti-impulse efficacy and warrants empirical consideration.

5. All medication trials in the BPD patient are empirical trials and should be carefully defined for specific desired outcomes and *time limits*. Continuation therapy, especially for neuroleptic medications, must be based on clear empirical evidence of a patient's continuing vulnerability to stress and decompensation. Given the risk of tardive dyskinesia, indefinite maintenance treatment is hard to justify in the borderline patient. The duration of treatment for antidepressant medications should not exceed limits generally applied to more clearly defined affective disorders. In some circumstances (e.g., impulsivity) the question of continuation and maintenance therapy is unresolved, as these medications may address a fundamental biological trait vulnerability. In the absence of any empirical guidelines, clinical judgment should prevail. In general, when the patient is stable in a psychosocial sense, the impulse-controlling agent may be weaned away.

CONCLUSIONS

This review presents the findings of recent systematic studies of criteria-defined borderline patients, a remarkably small foundation on which to base clinical recommendations. Viewed in this light, any conclusions must be considered preliminary.

Nonetheless, several conclusions have become painfully evident:

1. *There is no one treatment of choice for the borderline patient.* The heterogeneity of the borderline syndrome precludes a single pharmacological solution.
2. *Medication effects tend to be modest, with residual symptoms the rule.* Medication effects reduce the intensity of biologically mediated symptom states, leaving a residual core of character pathology.
3. *Medications do not cure character anymore than psychotherapy changes biology.* At the heart of the borderline disorder, we are left with both biological factors (affective dyscontrol, impulse disorder) and a pathological personality organization.
4. *An empirical approach to pharmacotherapy to suppress state symptoms (and trait vulnerability), combined with psychotherapy to address interpersonal dynamics, appears to be the most rational approach to treatment of the borderline patient.*

5. *Treatment expectations should be modest and coupled strongly with social and vocational rehabilitation,* which provides the reality supports and limits so desperately needed in the borderline patient.

Psychotherapy for the borderline patient remains a poorly defined treatment. Despite decades of debate and an extensive clinical literature, there is a paucity of empirical studies of psychotherapy for BPD and no clear proof of general efficacy for one form of treatment over another (e.g., supportive, expressive, behavioral, etc.). At the very least, psychotherapy is "anti-demoralizing" (Donald Klein) and provides our only avenue for reshaping interpersonal dynamics and altering behavior patterns. Effective treatment of the borderline patient is impossible outside of such an interpersonal matrix.

Further research is clearly needed in both pharmacotherapy and psychotherapy of the borderline patient before a more optimistic review can be written.

REFERENCES

Akiskal HS: Subaffective disorders: dysthymic, cyclothymic and bipolar II disorders in the "borderline" realm. Psychiatr Clin North Am 4:25–46, 1981

American Psychiatric Association: Diagnostic and Statistical Manual of Mental Disorders, 3rd Edition. Washington, DC, American Psychiatric Association, 1980

American Psychiatric Association: Diagnostic and Statistical Manual of Mental Disorders, 3rd Edition, Revised. Washington, DC, American Psychiatric Association, 1987

Andrulonis PA, Glueck BC, Stroebel CF, et al: Organic brain dysfunction and the borderline syndrome. Psychiatr Clin North Am 4:47–66, 1981

Baron M, Asnis L, Gruen R: Schedule of interviewing schizotypal personalities: a diagnostic interview for schizotypal features. Psychiatry Res 4:213–228, 1981

Bonnet KA, Redford HR: Levodopa in borderline disorders (letter). Arch Gen Psychiatry 39:862, 1982

Brinkley JR: Haloperidol and other neuroleptics in the treatment of borderline patients, in Haloperidol Update, 1958–1980. Edited by Ayd FJ. Baltimore, MD, Ayd Medical Communications, 1980, pp 117–126

Brinkley JR, Beitman BD, Friedel RO: Low-dose neuroleptic regimens in the treatment of borderline patients. Arch Gen Psychiatry 36:319–326, 1979

Brown GL, Goodwin FK: Cerebrospinal fluid correlates of suicide attempts and aggression. Ann N Y Acad Sci 487:175–188, 1986

Brown GL, Goodwin FK, Ballenger JC, et al: Aggression in humans correlates with cerebrospinal fluid amine metabolites. Psychiatry Res 1:131–139, 1979

Brown GL, Ebert MH, Goyer PF, et al: Aggression, suicide, and serotonin: relationships to CSF amine metabolites. Am J Psychiatry 139:741–746, 1982

Buss AH, Durkee A: An inventory for assessing different kinds of hostility. Journal of Consulting Psychology 21:343–349, 1957

Campbell M, Fish B, Korein J, et al: Lithium and chlorpromazine: a controlled crossover study of hyperactive severely disturbed young children. Journal of Autism and Childhood Schizophrenia 2:234–263, 1972

Coccaro EF, Siever LJ, Klar HM, et al: Serotonergic studies in patients with affective and personality disorders: correlates with suicidal and impulsive aggressive behavior. Arch Gen Psychiatry 46:587–599, 1989

Coid J, Allolio B, Rees LH: Raised plasma metenkephalin in patients who habitually mutilate themselves. Lancet 2:545–595, 1983

Cole JO, Sunderland P III: The drug treatment of borderline patients, in Psychiatry 1982: The American Psychiatric Association Annual Review, Vol 1. Edited by Grinspoon L. Washington, DC, American Psychiatric Press, 1982, pp 456–470

Cornelius JR, Brenner RP, Soloff PH, et al: EEG abnormalities in borderline personality disorder: specific or non-specific. Biol Psychiatry 21:977–980, 1986

Cornelius JR, Soloff PH, Perel JM, et al: Fluoxetine trial in borderline personality disorder. Psychopharmacol Bull 26:151–154, 1990

Cowdry RW, Gardner DL: Pharmacotherapy of borderline personality disorder: alprazolam, carbamazepine, trifluoperazine and tranylcypromine. Arch Gen Psychiatry 45:111–119, 1988

Cowdry RW, Pickar D, Davies R: Symptoms and EEG findings in the borderline syndrome. Int J Psychiatry Med 15:201–211, 1985

Davies R: MBO in borderlines. Grand rounds presentation, Yale University, New Haven Hospital, New Haven, CT, 1977

Derogatis L, Lipman R, Covi L: SCL-90: an outpatient psychiatric rating scale—preliminary report. Psychopharmacol Bull 9:13–17, 1973

Dostal T, Zvolsky P: Anti-aggressive effect of lithium salts in severely mentally retarded adolescents. International Pharmacopsychiatry 5:203–207, 1970

Faltus FJ: The positive effect of alprazolam in the treatment of three patients with borderline personality disorder. Am J Psychiatry 141:802–803, 1984

Freinhar JP, Alvarez WA: Clonazepam: a novel therapeutic adjunct. Intl J Psychiatry Med 15:321–328, 1985–1986

Fyer MR, Frances AJ, Sullivan T, et al: Comorbidity of borderline personality disorder. Arch Gen Psychiatry 45:348–352, 1988a

Fyer MM, Frances AJ, Sullivan T, et al: Suicide attempts in patients with borderline personality disorder. Am J Psychiatry 145:737–739, 1988b

Gardner DL, Cowdry RW: Alprazolam induced dyscontrol in borderline personality disorder. Am J Psychiatry 142:98–100, 1985

Gardner DL, Cowdry RW: Development of melancholia during carbamazepine treatment in borderline personality disorder. J Clin Psychopharmacol 6:236–239, 1986a

Gardner DL, Cowdry RW: Positive effects of carbamazepine on behavioral dyscontrol in borderline personality disorder. Am J Psychiatry 143:519–522, 1986b

Gardner DL, Lucas PB, Cowdry RW: CSF metabolites in borderline personality disorder compared with normal controls. Biol Psychiatry 28:247–254, 1990

Goldberg SC, Schulz SC, Schulz PM, et al: Borderline and schizotypal personality disorders treated with low-dose thiothixene vs placebo. Arch Gen Psychiatry 43:680–686, 1986

Gunderson JG, Frank AF, Ronningstam EF, et al: Early discontinuance of borderline patients from psychotherapy. J Nerv Ment Dis 177:38–42, 1989

Jensen HV, Andersen J: An open, noncomparative study of amoxapine in borderline disorders. Acta Psychiatr Scand 79:89–93, 1989

Kellner CH, Post RM, Putnam F, et al: Intravenous procaine as a probe of limbic system activity in psychiatric patients and normal controls. Biol Psychiatry 22:1107–1126, 1987

Kernberg O: Borderline Conditions and Pathological Narcissism. New York, Jason Aronson, 1975

Klein DF: Psychiatric diagnosis and a typology of clinical drug effects. Psychopharmacology (Berlin) 13:359–386, 1968

Konicki PE, Schulz SC: Rationale for clinical trials of opiate antagonists in treating patients with personality disorders and self-injurious behavior. Psychopharmacol Bull 25:556–563, 1989

LaWall JS, Wesselius CL: The use of lithium carbonate in borderline patients. Journal of Psychiatric Treatment and Evaluation 4:265–267, 1982

Leone NF: Response of borderline patients to loxapine and chlorpromazine. J Clin Psychiatry 43:148–150, 1982

Liebowitz MR, Klein DF: Interrelationship of hysteroid dysphoria and borderline personality dsorder. Psychiatr Clin North Am 4:67–87, 1981

Liebowitz MR, Quitkin FM, Stewart JW, et al: Phenelzine v imipramine in atypical depression: a preliminary report. Arch Gen Psychiatry 41:669–677, 1984

Links PS, Steiner M, Boiago I, et al: Lithium therapy for borderline patients: preliminary findings. Journal of Personality Disorders 4:173–181, 1990

Lorr M, Klett CJ: Inpatient Multidimensional Psychiatric Scale Manual. Palo Alto, CA, Consulting Psychologists Press, 1966

Markovitz PJ, Calabrese JR, Schulz SC, et al: Fluoxetine in borderline and schizotypal personality disorder. Paper presented at the 45th annual meeting of the Society of Biological Psychiatry, New York, May 1990

Montgomery SA, Montgomery D: Pharmacological prevention of suicidal behaviour. J Affective Disord 4:291–298, 1982

Montgomery SA, Roy D, Montgomery DB: The prevention of recurrent suicidal acts. Br J Clin Pharmacol 15:1835–1885, 1987

Norden MJ: Fluoxetine in borderline personality disorder. Prog Neuropsychopharmacol Biol Psychiatry 13:885–893, 1989

Overall JE, Gorham DR: Introduction—the Brief Psychiatric Rating Scale (BPRS): recent developments in ascertainment and scaling. Psychopharmacol Bull 22:97–99, 1988

Parsons B, Quitkin FM, McGrath PJ, et al: Phenelzine, imipramine, and placebo in borderline patients meeting criteria for atypical depression. Psychopharmacol Bull 25:524–534, 1989

Reus MD, Markrow S: Alprazolam in the treatment of borderline personality disorder. Paper presented at the 39th annual meeting of the Society of Biological Psychiatry, Los Angeles, CA, May 1984

Rifkin A, Levitan SJ, Galewski J, et al: Emotionally unstable character disorder: a follow-up study. Biol Psychiatry 4:65–79, 1972

Serban G, Siegel S: Response of borderline and schizotypal patients to small doses of thiothixene and haloperidol. Am J Psychiatry 141:1455–1458, 1984

Shader RI, Jackson AH, Dodes LM: The anti-aggressive effects of lithium in man. Psychopharmacology (Berlin) 40:17–24, 1974

Sheard MH: Lithium in the treatment of aggression. J Nerv Ment Dis 160:108–118, 1975

Siever LJ, Klar H, Coccaro E: Psychobiologic substrates of personality, in Biologic Response Styles: Clinical Implications. Edited by Klar H, Siever LJ. Washington, DC, American Psychiatric Press, 1985, pp 35–66

Skodol AE, Buckley P, Charles E: Is there a characteristic pattern to the treatment history of clinic outpatients with borderline personality? J Nerv Ment Dis 171:405–410, 1983

Snyder S, Pitts WM Jr: Electroencephalography of DSM-III borderline personality disorder. Acta Psychiatr Scand 69:129–134, 1984

Soloff PH: Pharmacotherapy of borderline disorders. Compr Psychiatry 22:535–543, 1981

Soloff PH: Psychopharmacological therapies in borderline personality disorder, in American Psychiatric Press Review of Psychiatry, Vol 8. Edited by Tasman A, Hales RE, Frances AT. Washington, DC, American Psychiatric Press, 1989, pp 65–83

Soloff PH, George A, Nathan RS, et al: Paradoxical effects of amitriptyline in borderline patients. Am J Psychiatry 143:1603–1605, 1986a

Soloff PH, George A, Nathan RS, et al: Progress in pharmacotherapy of borderline disorders: a double-blind study of amitriptyline, haloperidol, and placebo. Arch Gen Psychiatry 43:691–697, 1986b

Soloff PH, George A, Nathan RS, et al: Behavioral dyscontrol in borderline patients treated with amitriptyline. Psychopharmacol Bull 23:177–181, 1987a

Soloff PH, George A, Nathan RS, et al: Characterizing depression in borderline patients. J Clin Psychiatry 48:155–157, 1987b

Soloff PH, George A, Nathan RS, et al: Amitriptyline v haloperidol in borderlines: final outcomes and predictors of response. J Clin Psychopharmacol 9:238–246, 1989

Stanley M, Mann JJ: Biological factors associated with suicide, in American Psychiatric Press Review of Psychiatry, Vol 7. Edited by Frances AJ, Hales RE. Washington, DC, American Psychiatric Press, 1988, pp 334–352

Stone MH: Contemporary shift in the borderline concept from a subschizophrenic disorder to a subaffective disorder. Psychiatr Clin North Am 2:577–594, 1979

Stone MH: The course of borderline personality disorder, in American Psychiatric Press Review of Psychiatry, Vol 8. Edited by Tasman A, Hales RE, Frances AJ. Washington, DC, American Psychiatric Press, 1989. pp 103–122

Swartz M, Blazer D, George L, et al: Estimating the prevalence of borderline personality disorder in the community. Journal of Personality Disorders 4:257–272, 1990

Teicher MH, Glod CA, Aaronson ST, et al: Open assessment of the safety and efficacy of thioridazine in the treatment of patients with borderline personality disorder. Psychopharmacol Bull 25:535–549, 1989

Teicher MH, Glod C, Cole JO: Emergence of intensive suicidal preoccupation during fluoxetine treatment. Am J Psychiatry 147:207–210, 1990

Tupin JP, Smith DB, Clanon TL, et al: The long-term use of lithium in aggressive prisoners. Compr Psychiatry 14:311–317, 1973

van der Kolk BA: Uses of lithium in patients without major affective illness. Hosp Community Psychiatry 37:675, 1986

Virkkunen M, De Jong J, Bartko J, et al: Psychobiological concomitants of history of suicide attempts among violent offenders and impulsive fire setters. Arch Gen Psychiatry 46:604–606, 1989

Widiger TA, Frances AJ: Epidemiology, diagnosis, and comorbidity of borderline personality disorders, in Review of Psychiatry, Vol 8. Edited by Tasman A, Hales RE, Frances AJ. Washington, DC, American Psychiatric Press, 1989, pp 8–24

Winokur G: Unipolar depression: is it divisible into autonomous subtypes? Arch Gen Psychiatry 36:47–52, 1979

Wolf M, Grayden T, Carreon D, et al: Psychotherapy and buspirone in borderline patients. Paper presented at the 143rd annual meeting of the American Psychiatric Association, New York, May 1990

Inpatient Treatment of Borderline Personality Disorder

Daniel Silver, M.D.
Michael Rosenbluth, M.D.

A SUBSTANTIAL NUMBER OF PATIENTS WITH BORDERLINE personality disorder (BPD) will require hospitalization at some time during their outpatient treatment (Gunderson 1984; Skodol et al. 1983; Werble 1970). Yet the management of this phase of treatment, while often crucial, remains quite controversial. Research into the issues of hospitalization of patients with BPD has lagged behind the burgeoning interest in the outpatient treatment of this disorder. This lag reflects the relative lack of formal research into issues of hospitalization in psychiatry and specific difficulties with regard to BPD.

In this chapter we will review some of the basic principles of the hospitalization of BPD patients and discuss the strengths and weaknesses of different treatment approaches.

LONG-TERM VERSUS SHORT-TERM HOSPITALIZATION

One of the controversies involved in the hospitalization of the BPD patient is between those clinicians who favor long-term admissions and those who prefer shorter hospitalizations. One central issue in this controversy is the use or avoidance of regression that frequently occurs with hospitalization and its effect on the subsequent length of stay. This central issue has considerable therapeutic implications whenever the potentially negative effects of hospitalization for these patients are described (Friedman 1969). Related to this issue is the controversy of whether the major goals of inpatient treatment should be stabilization and attachment (Viner 1983) or internalization of new psychic structures (Kernberg 1976). Gordon and Beresin (1983) attempt to summarize the two main approaches as "structural" and "adaptational." The main distinction, perhaps, revolves around the diagnostic and therapeutic implications of the inevitable regression that working with the BPD patient entails.

The literature on hospitalization of BPD patients comes from two traditions, one using a clinically rich descriptive approach and the other drawing on outcome research. In the clinical descriptive approach, the most common strategy has been for interested clinicians to describe their own, often considerable, experience in the hospital treatment of borderline patients. The strength of the clinical approach is the careful observation and documentation of the phenomena that occur and the elaboration of a conceptual framework within which to understand these phenomena. There have been descriptions of transference and countertransference issues (Book et al. 1978; Kernberg 1987), discussion on the role of the hospital as a holding environment (Adler 1977), commentary on the need to set limits effectively (Adler 1973), discussion of outpatient issues as they relate to hospitalization (Bernstein 1980), and a description of the different approaches to the inpatient care of BPD (Brown 1981; Hartocollis 1980; Kernberg 1976; Rinsley 1968; Silver et al. 1983a).

Long-Term Hospitalization

The leading advocate of long-term hospitalization of BPD patients is Otto Kernberg (1976). In his view, hospitalization of the borderline patient fits into a therapeutic approach that is based on a structural conceptualization of borderline psychopathology. He minimizes nonstructural changes in the patient, referring to these changes as merely behavioral. Kernberg views the hospital as a relatively unstructured milieu that presents the patient with a host of possible relationships. In this context, the borderline patient rapidly develops numerous relationships that operate on and reflect his or her primitive object relations. This provides a diagnostic opportunity to view the patient's internal world of object relationships and to gradually change them using analytically informed understanding, confrontation, and clarification. The focus is on the interpretation, in the here and now, of the patient's impact on the social system of the hospital and how it is colored by primitive distortions caused by the patient's past. Thus, the goal of Kernberg's approach is the integration of previously primitive, nonmetabolized object relationships. The diagnosis, interpretation, and resolution of primitive transferences that reflect primitive internalized object relations are seen as resulting in structural intrapsychic change. Because of the centrality of observing and diagnosing these primitive object relationships and transferences, Kernberg takes what may be termed a "pro-regression" position, feeling that a highly regimented hospital routine may block regression and obscure its full observation (Kernberg 1976).

Kernberg has based his view of long-term hospitalization on his clinical experience and on the Psychotherapy Research Project of the Menninger Foundation (Kernberg et al. 1972). The study involved 42 patients in long-term treatment, although it is not clear how many of them met the criteria for BPD. Patients in expressive, insight-oriented psychotherapy were found to do better than those in supportive psychotherapy without hospital treatment. Comparison of long-term and short-term hospitalization was not done. Thus, the subject of this study was the different modes of outpatient psychotherapy, not the effect of hospitalization. Hospitalization is described only as a parameter used in expressive, insight-oriented treatment. Kernberg's (1973) indications for long-term hospitalization are low motivation, severe ego weakness, and poor object relations.

The shortcoming of a clinical approach is that it lacks a standardized vocabulary to describe the issues in the hospitalization of BPD patients. The observational approach all too often focuses on broad issues such as the dynamics, dangers, and length of hospitalization, while the complexities of the variables of hospital treatment and the effect of such treatment on individual patients have been understated. Little consideration has been given to the diagnostic heterogeneity of the disorder or to the considerable modifying factors such as intelligence, social skills, age, ego strength profile, social support systems, and severity of the disorder. Most important, the recommendations of Kernberg have not yet been backed up by research.

Short-Term Hospitalization

The therapeutic implications of regression comprise a crucial problem in treating patients with BPD. Those clinicians favoring longer hospitalization see regression as essential and ultimately positive, whereas those favoring a short hospitalization see regression as counterproductive, non-essential, and perhaps iatrogenic.

Advocates of short-term hospitalization feel that regression to primitive object relationships made manifest and utilized in the transference is undesirable and unworkable. Friedman (1975), developing positions previously taken by Anna Freud and Zetzel, contends that preverbal experience, while of great importance to development, cannot be fully recovered in the transference with successful therapeutic effect. He advocates an approach emphasizing the treatment alliance—not mobilizing negative transference yet clarifying and interpreting it when it develops and using limit setting when necessary. Hospitalization is shorter and focuses on concrete goals rather than on structural change.

Nurnberg and Suh (1980, 1982) also advocate time-limited hospitalization with rapid diagnostic assessment and the establishment of a firm discharge date whereupon transfer or discharge occurs. These authors emphasize the importance of this time-focused approach in combating the borderline patient's ahistoric tendency. Viner (1983) emphasizes the use of brief hospitalization for attachment and not internalization. He focuses on the selfobject function of the hospital and its role in providing a holding environment for the patient. Wishnie (1975) emphasizes the rapid diagnosis of the BPD patient; clear definition of goals, limits, and expectations; and education of staff in terms of consistent responses. Sederer and Thorbeck (1986) have described the dangers of exploratory therapy in a short-term hospitalization.

RESEARCH ON HOSPITALIZATION OF PATIENTS WITH BORDERLINE PERSONALITY DISORDER

The Duration of Hospitalization

Masterson and Costello (1980) described a follow-up study of 31 borderline adolescents. Mean hospitalization duration was 14.5 months. While indicating considerable variation in outcome (from minimal to severe functional impairment), the authors concluded that 58% showed significant improvement at follow-up of approximately 4 years. However, their conclusions are limited by 1) follow-up on only 53% of the original sample; 2) cases treated that were, by the authors' own description, particularly suitable for psychotherapy; and 3) the absence of a control group receiving outpatient treatment and short-term hospitalization. The authors themselves pointed out that their research was designed for hypothesis gathering, and this outcome study is not sufficient to confirm the value of long-term inpatient treatment for BPD. It is interesting to note, particularly in light of Kernberg's indications that more severely disturbed patients are candidates for long-term hospitalization, that Masterson and Costello indicate that it was the healthier borderline patient who benefited from long-term inpatient treatment, not the more severely disturbed borderline patient.

Tucker et al. (1987), in a prospective evaluation of long-term hospital treatment of borderline patients, showed that, after the first postdischarge year, patients hospitalized for more than 1 year were more likely to remain in outpatient therapy and to avoid rehospitalization. However, follow-up after the second postdischarge year showed little difference between those hospitalized for shorter or longer stays.

McGlashan (1986) described the outcome of BPD patients treated with long-term inpatient treatment averaging 2 years in duration. Although not described in detail, the treatment took place in a milieu that was tolerant of regression and that utilized intensive psychotherapy (four times per week). The outcome was assessed as being comparable with that of unipolar affective disorder and significantly better than that of schizophrenia. The author's conclusion regarding long-term inpatient treatment was that its clinical efficacy could not be considered to have been demonstrated by his study because of the absence of clinical trial methodology. However, he felt that further study with controlled clinical trials was indicated. McGlashan (see Chapter 12) found that one of the three most frequent variables predicting poor outcome was longer hospitalization, but this finding may be tautological, in that sicker patients may require longer hospitalization.

Stone (1987) followed up 254 borderline patients treated with intensive hospitalization. Retrospectively, the author felt that only one-third were amenable to expressive psychotherapy. Improvement in the other borderline patients was attributed to supportive therapy, the patients' personality characteristics, good fortune, or a combination of the three. Stone concluded that the efficacy of expressive psychotherapy was difficult to prove. As in McGlashan's study (1986), Stone's work is a study of the natural history of borderline patients treated with intensive hospitalization rather than a clinical trial of the intensive hospitalization of patients with BPD.

These outcome studies raise questions about whether long-term hospitalization should be a primary modality of treatment. They are, however, rather consistent with studies on long-term versus short-term hospitalization in general, which show little effect of length of stay. Global outcome seems to be better correlated with prehospital level of functioning than with length of stay; the amount of aftercare is also a more important determinant of outcome than the length of hospitalization (Cournos 1987).

None of the outcome studies of BPD patients (Fenton and McGlashan 1990; McGlashan 1986; Paris et al. 1987; Plakun et al. 1985; Stone et al. 1987; Werble 1970) really measures the goals of intensive long-term hospitalization. There appears to be a marked dichotomy between what is sought in intensive hospitalization (structural change, internalization of new introjects) and what is measured in follow-up studies (general work and social adaptation, persistence of symptoms, rate of rehospitalization). Silver et al. (1987) have attempted to bridge this dichotomy by noting that even patients who do well on the grosser measures of long-term follow-up appear to have strong remnants of the psychological fragility readily elicited on psychodynamic assessment when followed up years later.

Conclusions

Intensive hospital treatment requires special staffing, skills, interest, and financial support that few facilities have (Klagsbrun et al. 1987; Silver et al. 1987). The absence of firm evidence demonstrating the superiority of longer hospitalization; the heterogeneity of the disorder; its uncertain etiology; and the economic realities of hospital care in the 1990s—all point to short-stay hospitalization as the hospital treatment of choice for borderline patients.

Long-term hospitalization, while useful for learning more about borderline dynamics and teaching psychotherapy (Rosnick 1987; Silver et al. 1983b), should be regarded as heroic treatment best reserved for a very small minority of patients, particularly those who cannot be contained outside of a hospital and for whom no alternative exists. Unfortunately, in practice, longer hospitalizations are more likely to occur when the treatment staff extend the length of stay because of difficulties in discharging an acting-out patient. Thus, the longer stay may be reactive rather than proactive, and active treatment is often sacrificed as staff focuses on discharging the patient.

Because the definitive treatment for BPD patients has not yet been established, it would seem most reasonable clinically to remain eclectic and flexible and to not oversubscribe to the notion of a dichotomy between treatment approaches such as adjustment versus structural change or long-term versus short-term hospital treatment. What is more certain is that the major part of a BPD patient's treatment will occur outside a hospital setting, and hospitalization should be guided by the patient's needs rather than any pronouncements by one therapeutic guru or another.

In summary, for most BPD patients hospitalization should be primarily used for crisis situations. Short-term hospitalization can be most successful when used to help a disorganized BPD patient reintegrate. The particular admixture of vulnerability, irritability, and impulsivity makes the borderline patient prone to need short hospitalizations for crisis intervention during rage attacks, perceived irreparable losses, transient psychotic phenomena resulting from transference issues or other causes, or ruptures in the outpatient treatment for whatever reasons. The inpatient stay, therefore, is planned to help the patient reintegrate and return to the outside therapist as quickly as possible, and patients should continue their regular therapy appointments with their outside therapists either in or out of hospital during their brief hospital stay.

There is a small group of borderline patients, however, who are impaired enough to warrant long-term hospitalization and a major investment of resources. In these cases, there is usually a history of repeated failures of outpatient treatment, the likelihood of continued failures of such treatment, the increasing difficulties in finding suitable therapists to treat them, and serious, increasing risk of self-destructive acting out. The increasingly prohibitive costs of such treatment coupled with the limitations and restrictions of third-party payments make long-term hospital-ization less and less feasible. Nevertheless, as clinicians we must continue to direct our efforts to help provide the kind of care that could ultimately be most beneficial to our patients.

The Role of Hospitalization

In addition to the controversy about length of hospitalization, there is an extensive literature on the role of hospitalization. Important issues include assessing outpatient therapy (Bernstein 1980), stabilizing the patient and the team (Wishnie 1975), choosing a focus (Nurnberg and Suh 1982), combating an ahistoric tendency (Nurnberg and Suh 1980), and using selfobject function for stabilization rather than internalization (Rosenbluth 1987; Viner 1983).

HOSPITALIZATION AND TREATMENT

In the balance of this chapter we will emphasize and elaborate several important aspects of hospital treatment of BPD patients that are not always sufficiently described in the literature. These are the various indications for hospitalization such as suicide risk, diagnostic clarification, and the consultative role of the hospital; family and group modalities of inpatient treatment; particular countertransference issues; and aftercare planning.

Indications for Hospitalizations

Suicide risk. The main indication for hospitalization of any psychiatric patient is suicide risk. However, this is a more complicated issue for BPD patients who may be not only acutely but also chronically suicidal (see Paris, Chapter 17). Acute suicide risk of the borderline patient is probably the most common indication for hospital admission. While in a hospital the usual concerns and difficulties of dealing with suicidality in this patient population continue, but the inhospital context creates new problems.

   The central dilemma is whether the patient is indeed acutely at risk for harming himself or herself, or is seeking caretaking behavior from the therapist (Gunderson 1984). A related concern is whether the suicidal behavior is acute, or whether it is chronic and therefore less likely to be acted upon. In the latter case, protecting the person from self-harm may interfere with the central therapeutic task of the chronically suicidal patient: the transfer of the responsibility for the patient's welfare back to the patient (Gutheil 1982). Failure to do so impedes the therapy and causes treatment to flounder and become preoccupied with suicidal behavior.

In hospital, these issues are colored by what may be termed the "public domain" of hospital care. What was once a dyadic relationship becomes one involving many individuals—the resident, nursing staff, occupational therapists, etc. The consequence is that certain conscious and unconscious determinations enter the decision-making process for the hospitalized BPD patient. Patients expressing suicidal ideation who would be deemed safe to leave the therapist's outpatient office may be placed on constant care or close observation on the ward. Anxiety regarding public scrutiny can interfere with the containing function of the hospital. An overconcern with the sequelae of a patient's self-harming behavior can cause a regression in the therapeutic staff to a controlling, overprotective response or, alternatively, to an abandoning, rejecting response to the patient who may require the setting of limits.

Thus, concerns about how staff will be seen cause primitive fears of exposure and humiliation to increase. This reflects both the consequence of projections from the patient having been inadequately processed and the ambivalent attitude our society has about psychiatric care (e.g., hospital wards are criticized for being too restrictive or too lax). Experiences with previous patients also color staff response. Recent suicides or attempts by other patients, particularly if not sufficiently processed, can increase the countertransference reactivity of treatment staff.

The problem of suicidality frequently becomes more of an issue as discharge nears. The patient who has made considerable progress may suddenly become suicidal. This frequently causes a short hospitalization to become longer, because the team is unable to discharge the patient. Several steps facilitate the staff's response to the suicidal inpatient:

1. It is important for staff to have an understanding of countertransference issues stirred up by the suicidal BPD patient, and a forum to process these feelings in order to distinguish real concerns from patient anxieties projected onto the staff.

2. A screening process is essential so that more severe BPD patients who might undergo malignant regressions are identified and receive a more structured approach in order to avoid regression to unworkable levels.

3. Contracting (Bloom and Rosenbluth 1989) can be useful to spell out consequences of self-harm behaviors. Transfers to another institution can occur if the patient's self-harm behavior does not stop. Often, a clear statement about the possibility of transfer acts as an effective limit, resulting in a decrease in the patient's self-harm behavior (Friedman 1969).

4. In order to diminish the suicidal potential of BPD patients, it is crucial to identify the main issues of the discharge phase such as separating from hospital (i.e., leaving behind significant figures) and reentry into the outside world (i.e., building and repairing relationships). Separation and reentry challenge the equilibrium achieved by patients in the hospital, once again threatening them with painful feelings, and may lead to an increase in suicidal ideation (Silver et al. 1987). A mutually agreed-upon initial discharge date is set, with staff realizing that it may not be met. This first discharge date is set so that the anticipated regression and acting out can be worked through, particularly the attendant separation and abandonment feelings and some of the anticipatory anxiety about reentry. Anticipating this occurrence diminishes the staff's disappointment and permits them to help the patient with the feelings evoked rather than to confirm the patient's fears of abandonment and rejection. A second firm discharge date frequently goes more smoothly.

5. A very important aspect of discharge planning is to facilitate the transition of continuity of therapeutic care. In those units where the inpatient staff take total charge of treatment during the patient's stay, resumption of therapy with the outpatient treaters should begin either in hospital or outside prior to the discharge date to help deal with both the anxieties of separation and any feelings of abandonment. Aftercare planning must also be concerned with addressing social and vocational issues and the patient's chronic sense of inner alienation from the community that he or she must reenter.

Diagnostic clarification. Usually reassessing diagnostic classification occurs during a hospitalization necessitated by suicidality or other crises such as transient psychosis or severe self-destructive acting-out behavior. There are two main diagnostic functions that a hospital can fulfill. One is clarifying Axis I and Axis II diagnostic issues. The other is to assess and determine the patient's suitability and/or capacity for various modalities of treatment such as individual psychotherapy, family therapy, group therapy, or pharmacotherapy, or any combination of these.

Frequently, borderline patients' Axis I diagnoses are overlooked in the chaos of the clinical situation and/or when there is an inclination to be preoccupied with the Axis II diagnosis. While the patient is in the hospital, it is important to identify the presence of a coexisting Axis I disorder such as major affective disorder, an anxiety disorder such as panic disorder, or a substance abuse disorder. Treatment of previously unidentified Axis I disorders can have important impact on a patient's overall course.

Another diagnostic role of hospitalization is the identification of a previously unidentified Axis II disorder. This is the converse of the previous situation. That is, because of the centrality of the Axis I pathology (e.g., severe affective disorder and/or an inclination to be preoccupied with biological disorders), an Axis II disorder is overlooked. In this instance, the hospital milieu acts as a culture bringing out previously overlooked signals of BPD such as splitting, projection, or the regression to which the BPD patient is subject. The presence of BPD comorbidity is important to ascertain and has implications for the course of hospital treatment and the aftercare provided for the patient.

Finally, once hospitalized, the patient may require examination of the psychodynamic profile to determine whether or not psychotherapy is a feasible undertaking and, if so, in what form. Not all borderline patients can benefit from an intensive psychotherapeutic approach (Waldinger and Gunderson 1984). A determination of whether the patient is suitable for psychotherapy should be influenced by developmental variables such as whether the patient has had a positive relationship in the past or present; whether he or she demonstrates some capacity to empathize with the experiences of important others; whether he or she has a history of being able to be soothed by something or someone; and how close the patient is able to get to others before withdrawing—if there is a relationship thermostat that is set on "too distant" (Silver et al. 1988). The severity of early deprivation and/or serious abuse is another very important factor in determining the kind of therapy that is likely suitable for a given patient. More generally, hospitalization can also help by educating patients in the work of psychotherapy, increasing their awareness that much of their behaviors and feelings are determined by processes that are not always available to them at a conscious level, and that words rather than action can be used to convey feelings.

The consultative role.   Patients with BPD are frequently prone to regression in therapy, resulting in increasingly primitive acting out and suicide attempts. A large number of admissions to a hospital can follow the development of various severe strains on the outpatient therapeutic relationship. For example, Maltsberger and Buie (1974) have described the "transference onslaught" upon the therapist and have detailed the countertransference reactions to suicidal patients. They stress the temptation to abandon the patient as a defense against countertransference hate. This can easily lead to a suicidal crisis admission. At this point, hospitalization provides among other things a consultative opportunity as well as a therapeutic holiday for the patient and the therapist. Most often, within the safety and structure of the hospital and availability of interested and supportive colleagues for discussion and consultation, outpatient therapy can resume in a rejuvenated way. Occasionally, however, a mutual consensus can arise among hospital staff, patient, and therapist, who may decide that termination of therapy with the current therapist is in the best interests of the therapeutic process. In such cases, the hospital can be very useful in helping plan alternative outpatient follow-up care.

A great deal of tact, respect, and sensitivity must be exercised at all times between the staff and the referring therapist. The staff must be careful not to judge the competence of the outside therapist by accepting at face value the patient's initial devaluation of the psychotherapeutic process prior to hospitalization. Often, not always, this may be his or her way of defending against an abandonment depression by quickly idealizing the potential relationships with various hospital staff members. The patient's early compliance is often misinterpreted as an indication of mismanagement by the outside therapist that precipitated the hospitalization. Thus, it is frequently in collusion with the patient's denial that the staff sometimes prematurely blame the patient's difficulties on the outside therapist's incompetence, a family's overintrusiveness, or the unfortunate rupture of an important relationship.

Jacobs et al. (1982), in discussing the role of hospital consultation, note special rare situations that are usually not described in the literature—for example, the impaired therapist, a therapist who may be experiencing his or her own acute crisis, or the therapist whose work is either not up to standard or too inexperienced or unprepared to deal with some of the more difficult BPD patients. In such cases, discreet and sensitive meetings and discussions by the most senior psychiatrist on the team can effect a reasonable resolution to the problem in question or can be used to arrange for smooth transfer of patient care to another therapist when necessary.

Countertransference Issues

A crucial aspect of the hospital care of the BPD patient is the full and effective use of the countertransference processes that are elicited. Considerable attention has been given to what can be learned about the inner world of the BPD patient by examining and understanding the feelings induced in the therapist and inpatient treatment team (Adler 1977; Book et al. 1978; Kernberg 1976). The main theme of this literature has been the effects of splitting on the patient-team interaction, with the emphasis on integrating the split and avoiding the acting out of the patient's inner world by the team.

There are other uses of countertransference that have been insufficiently emphasized. In addition to understanding the patient's inner world, the response of treatment staff to the patient can be used to clarify outpatient countertransference problems and the family's interaction with the patient. Friedman (1975) has discussed the signal function of countertransference in the dyadic outpatient setting. This concept can be elaborated to yield a new conceptualization and use of countertransference for the inpatient setting.

Attention to the feelings induced in the treatment team may reveal important information about general system features such as the team's history, needs, and capacity. This signal function may also be important in increasing the team's understanding of the patient's diagnosis and management. The first step in using the countertransference is to learn how it reflects the individual patient's dynamics. The second step is to ascertain what reflection of general system factors is occurring.

A consideration of the system aspects of the inpatient setting permits an elaboration of the traditional views of countertransference. While the content of the feelings engendered in the team may be used to increase the understanding of the patient's dynamics, the rapidity and intensity of the countertransference response may raise more general questions about the patient-ward interaction and the patient.

Mental health professionals who have a broad concept of counter-transference can more thoroughly utilize the feelings engendered in them when working with troubled and difficult patients. This awareness permits better patient care with a difficult patient population by facilitating a more thorough involvement with each patient. In addition, over time, it permits the team as a whole to continue to work with difficult patient populations, such as those with BPD, in an ongoing, creative manner. Failure to develop a means for the full identification and utilization of countertransference leads to increased staff turnover, burnout, and a less effective therapeutic involvement with each patient.

The countertransference response may reflect unresolved issues in the team's history of working with a certain kind of patient. The response not only may be indicative of one patient's dynamics but may also be a signal that there are unresolved feelings within the team from previous patients that are being transferred to the current patient. These responses could elicit particular feelings or might disclose more general attitudes about working with certain kinds of patients such as the patient with BPD.

The countertransference response may disclose important aspects of the team's capacity to be therapeutic as well as reflect the dynamics of the individual patient. The treatment staff, both individually and collectively, need to feel that their therapeutic contributions are acknowledged, respected, and valued. The relationship between the team, team leader, and the institution may serve to fulfill or heighten this need. The response to an individual patient may reflect and/or be prejudiced by the team's global response to the particular inpatient population at the time. The countertransference noted may partially demonstrate that there are simply too many difficult patients with which the team must work in a therapeutic manner.

Not only may the presence of an intense or unexpected countertransference response reflect the individual dynamics of the patient, but it also may be a signal that there is a malignant regression occurring. Balint

(1968) has described this situation as occurring when the patient seeks gratification, not understanding, and when the neediness, rather than the psyche, of the patient grows. The patient's object hunger is increased rather than satisfied.

Dealing with such a situation depends on the team's treatment philosophy and may call for rapid patient and team stabilization so that this regression can be appropriately managed and not be allowed to remain malignant. The response to this signal countertransference is an examination of how the patient and the team are interacting. Insufficient structure for the patient may promote regression that is beyond a workable level. Increased attention must be given to the therapeutic alliance rather than to the transference. Responses include addressing clinical administration issues, such as passes and privileges, as well as defining the goals and expectations of the patient more clearly (Gutheil 1982).

Family Involvement

The family of the BPD patient often needs to be stabilized. Demoralized and drained by the efforts of dealing with what they see as a tyrannical individual, members of the family may require treatment or at least some guidelines for relating to the patient. It is beneficial to help the family develop ways of providing the external control the patient requires, rather than provoking and perpetuating negative behaviors.

The literature suggests that there are two major family patterns in BPD. There are 1) families that exclude the borderline patient and 2) families that are enmeshed and overinvolved (Gunderson and Englund 1981). Patterns similar to those relating to the therapist's countertransference may be noted in the family's involvement with patients. The axis of involvement may revolve around either masochistic submission to or inappropriate distancing and abandonment of the patient. In either case, attention to the connection of the patient to the family and the role of the family in the aftercare of the patient can contribute to aftercare stabilization. This involves clarification of the interactive dynamics of the patient and family. It may also include helping the family achieve an appropriate degree of involvement.

In an excellent review of the role of family therapy in the treatment of BPD patients, Aronson (1989) asserts that the psychopathology usually

subscribed to the patients in the literature is "inconsistent, probably because most are uncontrolled, unsystematic, anecdotal reports that rarely
specify the study setting, the methods of data collection or the number of
cases seen" (p. 523). Even more striking is the absence of borderline cases
in the family therapy literature.

Desperate and confused parents, spouses, or other relations would
benefit from a psychoeducational approach. All too often, hospital staff in
particular are too ready to side with the BPD patient as the victim and to
see all others as the victimizers. This, of course, reflects countertransference effects whereby the staff are filled with the projections of the BPD
patient and resort to the same splitting mechanisms as the patient. Relatives are entitled to know more about the current state of our knowledge
of borderline patients, and aftercare requires their cooperation

Group Therapy

The group therapy process serves many funtions on an inpatient unit,
whether it is a long-term or short-term treatment facility. Hospitalized
BPD patients are usually in group therapy for much shorter periods of
time than they would be as outpatients. The aims of the group therapy
process for BPD inpatients are therefore quite different. Rarely is there
enough time to establish a solid therapeutic alliance, and the opportunities for working through are very limited (Leszcz 1992).

Nevertheless, there are some realistic goals that may be achieved. For
example, the group can provide support and identification, link behavior
to affect, support the notion that talking and engaging can be rewarding
and safe, and clarify interpersonal distortions as they occur on the ward or
in other modalities of treatment (i.e., individual, case work, occupational
therapy, pharmacotherapy) (Leszcz et al. 1985). As the group process
continues, even on a short-term basis, the patient is aware that this form
of treatment is integrally linked to the total inpatient experience and does
not occur in isolation. This helps to support reality testing and define
boundary limits, and can decrease the patient's feelings of estrangement
and isolation (Kibel 1978, 1981).

A major thrust of inpatient group therapy with borderline patients is
employing here-and-now strategies that are structured to be supportive.
This can be useful in deintensifying affect, particularly in the more prim-

itive borderline patient, so as to increase receptivity to other modalities of treatment. In inpatient group therapy, group members continue to interact with one another on the ward, and therefore it is important to limit destructive interactions within the group. It is also emphasized (Kibel 1978, 1981) that it is vital to protect patients from the disorganization that would occur if confronted too forcefully with their rage in group therapy.

The staff person conducting the group therapy should be an integral part of, and involved in, team meetings in which patient care is discussed or milieu processes examined. It is important that the group staff person not be one of the administrative heads of the unit if self-congratulatory experiences are to be avoided. By regular attendance and meetings, the head of group therapy not only can provide important input regarding patient care but can be extremely helpful in observing and commenting on staff dynamics.

Aftercare Planning

Aftercare planning is a central feature of hospitalization. Reentry into and reconnecting with outside social, work, and therapeutic relationships must be a major concern of good aftercare planning. As has already been noted, treatment with the outside therapist should always resume prior to discharge.

A realistic sense of BPD course, one in which readmissions are accepted and not viewed as signs of failure, permits the patient to reach out appropriately for help when difficulties are encountered in the postdischarge phase. Hospital units that have formal mechanisms such as holding beds for brief readmissions, or informal mechanisms such as the patient returning to the ward for brief visits, facilitate the discharge process.

The borderline patient, who has been described as ahistoric, has difficulty looking beyond the present (Hartocollis 1978; Miller 1964). The same problem exists in the literature on hospital care of patients with BPD. Rather than taking a longitudinal view of the borderline course, one can be preoccupied with the index admission and pay insufficient attention to issues that arise from numerous rehospitalizations that affect the patient, the family, and the hospital staff (Rosenbluth 1987).

The development of the outcome research on BPD (McGlashan 1986; Paris et al. 1987; Plakun et al. 1985; Stone et al. 1987) offers an opportunity to remedy this situation by stressing the need for a longitudinal approach and by underlining how frequent hospitalization can be in the course of the BPD. Not only must hospitalization concern itself with the stabilization of the borderline patient, but it must also address the problems of the system into which the patient returns. Thus, a longitudinal rather than cross-sectional orientation underlines issues of aftercare. These issues include stabilization of the patient but may also require help for the referring therapist, stabilization of the family, and augmentation of the supporting social, vocational, and/or therapeutic structure.

Hospitalization provides an opportunity for outpatient therapy to be reviewed. Outpatient therapy of the borderline patient is often a difficult and demanding enterprise for the patient and the therapist. A longitudinally informed view of the inpatient treatment of the borderline patient implies examination and stabilization of outpatient therapy and helps stabilize the therapist's relationship with the patient so that treatment is not disrupted. Occasionally, the task is to aid in achieving termination when the therapy cannot proceed.

The inpatient team can check for signs of strain and countertransference problems in the outpatient therapist. Signs of therapist strain include change in the frequency of the sessions, missed or changed therapy hours, the therapist's sudden vacation with little notice, or an alteration in the manner in which the therapist speaks to and about the patient (Bernstein 1980). The critical countertransference constellations include the polarities of masochistic submission to the patient's aggression, alternating with an inappropriate and excessive distancing from the patient (Kernberg 1975).

In assessing the state of the therapeutic relationship, a tendency to devalue the outpatient therapist or to accept the ongoing therapy uncritically and uncreatively must be avoided (Adler 1977). The time the patient is in the hospital may help the outpatient therapist to take stock and clarify any countertransference. On other occasions, the patient and/or therapist may refuse to continue with treatment, resulting in termination and a transfer. Ongoing outpatient therapy may benefit from clarification of Axis I diagnosis and/or the addition of auxiliary therapeutic structures such as day hospital, drug clinics, or drop-in centers.

Therapist burnout can be diminished if the therapist is in contact with other mental health workers involved in the care of the patient. This could involve ongoing postdischarge contact by the referring therapist with the inpatient psychiatrist aimed at minimizing transference/countertransference whirls that result in rehospitalization. This in turn can reinforce the therapist's involvement and capacity to contain the patient and to ensure that the patient's disappointment and reactive rage are kept in workable proportions. Winnicott (1965) has described mothers who have the capacity to provide good-enough care and who can be enabled to do better by being cared for themselves in a way that acknowledges the essential nature of their task. Outpatient therapists of BPD patients are similar in this regard, and ongoing postdischarge checking by the inpatient psychiatrist of the therapeutic situation protects the therapy.

An aftercare contract can be an aid in stabilizing the postdischarge course, particularly for the patient with a past history of several admissions. This involves a review of previous interim functioning and treatment planning to determine the nature of the problems. Past failures of treatment are reviewed and analyzed, and a future-oriented plan is emphasized. Those patients who have had several admissions in the last few years prior to the index admission are invited to plan, with the staff's aid, an improvement in this pattern based on an understanding of what contributed to previous readmissions. An attempt is made to help the patient form realistic goals and objectives for the next few years. The possibility of readmissions during that period is recognized. Assurance is given that such backup and support can be counted on.

In addition to defining goals, the expectations of the patient are also defined as much as possible. Particularly, readmission criteria are explicitly discussed. These may include spelling out the patient's responsibility for taking medication, attending various programs, being involved in family meetings, and/or decreasing certain self-destructive behaviors. The target behaviors chosen as readmission criteria depend on a realistic reading of what can be expected of the patient at that point in treatment. Also, the patient and the aftercare system are aided in differentiating between the true need for readmission and the patient's regressive wish to escape the pressures of daily life.

Careful limit setting that takes into consideration the patient's capacities and deficits stabilizes the aftercare and mobilizes the patient. Planning over time tends to help patients to develop a future orientation and a broader sense of their responsibility in treatment.

Community reentry issues. While the patient is in the hospital, attention must be paid to the social, vocational, and therapeutic networks of the patient outside the hospital. From the beginning of the hospitalization, these networks are assessed so that contacts are maintained during the hospitalization and not jeopardized as the patient recedes into the cocoon of the hospital. The patient is encouraged to maintain external structures, such as returning to school or to a job as soon as possible and continuing with outpatient therapy. This helps stem excessive inpatient regression. Attempts are made, while the patient is in the hospital, to coordinate the different agencies that are involved in maintaining aftercare stabilization by making some of the agencies aware of the presence of others or by discontinuing redundant efforts. The role of the day hospital as an alternative to future hospitalization and as a mainstay of the aftercare program can be considerable (Pildis et al. 1978). Stable vocational, educational, and therapeutic structures are seen as important components of a holding environment.

SUMMARY

The hospital care of the patient with BPD can be an opportunity to protect the patient from his or her self-destructive impulses. It can be a time when the entire therapeutic enterprise is reappraised, with attention given to outpatient treatment, social and vocational supports, intervention with the family, and clarification of diagnostic, psychodynamic, and psychopharmacological issues. Or it can mark the end of a therapeutic enterprise characterized by acting out, transference/countertransference whirls, malignant regression and/or premature discharge, and dropping out of treatment. Rather than a beginning, hospitalization may then be just another failed opportunity in the patient's search for peace, stability, and constancy in his or her life.

In this chapter we have described critical issues in hospital care—issues that may determine which path is taken. Concerning the controversy on short- versus long-term hospitalization, consideration of the clinical and research experience suggests that in the majority of cases short-stay treatment is the preferred modality of hospital care of patients with BPD. Long-term treatment, while useful for learning more about borderline dynamics and teaching psychotherapy, should be regarded as a treatment best reserved for a very small minority of patients, particularly those who cannot be contained outside of the hospital and for whom no alternative exists.

The indications for and the role of hospitalization have been reviewed and guidelines for the stabilization of the patient suggested. Countertransference issues are important in inpatient treatment. Considerable attention must be paid to the aftercare system to which the patient is discharged.

The hospital treatment of the borderline patient is never easy. A consideration of the premises and core issues of hospitalizations may facilitate the patient's more successful engagement in treatment in the hospital and after discharge.

REFERENCES

Adler G: Hospital treatment of borderline patients. Am J Psychiatry 130:32–36, 1973

Adler G: Hospital management of borderline patients and its relation to psychotherapy, in Borderline Personality Disorders: The Concept, the Syndrome, the Patient. Edited by Hartocollis P. New York, International Universities Press, 1977, pp 307–323

Aronson TA: A critical review of psychotherapeutic treatments of the borderline personality: historical trends and future directions. J Nerv Ment Dis 177:511–528, 1989

Balint M: The Basic Fault: Therapeutic Aspects of Regression. London, Tavistock, 1968

Bernstein SB: Psychotherapy consultation in an inpatient setting. Hosp Community Psychiatry 31:829–834 1980

Bloom H, Rosenbluth M: The use of contracts in the inpatient treatment of the borderline personality disorder. Psychiatr Q 60:317–327, 1989

Book HE, Sadavoy J, Silver D: Staff countertransference to borderline patients on an inpatient unit. Am J Psychother 32:521–532, 1978

Brown LJ: A short-term hospital program preparing borderline and schizophrenic patients for intensive psychotherapy. Psychiatry 44:327–336, 1981

Cournos F: Hospitalization outcome studies: implications for the treatment of the very ill patient. Psychiatr Clin North Am 10:165–176, 1987

Fenton WS, McGlashan TH: Long-term residential care: treatment of choice for refractory character disorder? Psychiatric Annals 20:44–49, 1990

Friedman HJ: Some problems of inpatient management with borderline patients. Am J Psychiatry 126:299–304, 1969

Friedman HJ: Psychotherapy of borderline patients: the influence of theory on technique. Am J Psychiatry 132:1048–1052, 1975

Gordon C, Beresin E: Conflicting treatment models for the inpatient management of borderline patients. Am J Psychiatry 140:979–983, 1983

Gunderson J: Borderline Personality Disorder. Washington, DC, American Psychiatric Press, 1984

Gunderson J, Englund DW: Characterizing the families of borderlines: a review of the literature. Psychiatr Clin North Am 4:159–168, 1981

Gutheil TG: On the therapy in clinical administration, Part I: introduction and history; administration and its relation to psychotherapy. Psychiatr Q 54:3–25, 1982

Hartocollis P: Time and affects in borderline disorders. Int J Psychoanal 59:157–163, 1978

Hartocollis P: Long-term hospital treatment for adult patients with borderline and narcissistic disorders. Bull Menninger Clin 44:212–226, 1980

Jacobs DH, Rogoff J, Donnelly K, et al: The neglected alliance: the inpatient unit as a consultant to referring therapists. Hosp Community Psychiatry 33:377–381, 1982

Kernberg OF: Discussion of Hospital treatment of borderline patients (by Adler G). Am J Psychiatry 130:35–36, 1973

Kernberg OF: Borderline Conditions and Pathological Narcissism. New York, Jason Aronson, 1975

Kernberg OF: Object-Relations Theory and Clinical Psychoanalysis. New York, Jason Aronson, 1976

Kernberg OF: Projective identification, countertransference, and hospital treatment. Psychiatr Clin North Am 10:257–272, 1987

Kernberg OF, Burstein E, Coyne L: Final report of the Menninger Foundation's Psychotherapy Research Project: psychotherapy and psychoanalysis. Bull Menninger Clin 34:263–268, 1972

Kibel HD: The rationale for the use of group psychotherapy for borderline patients on a short-term unit. Int J Group Psychother 28:339–358, 1978

Kibel HD: A conceptual model for short-term inpatient group psychotherapy. Am J Psychiatry 138:74–80, 1981

Klagsbrun SC, Reibel JS, Piercey MC: Cost-effective tertiary care. Psychiatr Clin North Am 10:207–218, 1987

Leszcz M: Group psychotherapy of the borderline patient, in The Handbook of Borderline Disorders. Edited by Silver D, Rosenbluth M. New York, International Universities Press, 1992, pp 435–470

Leszcz M, Yalom ID, Norden M: The value of inpatient group psychotherapy: patients' perceptions. Int J Group Psychother 35:411–433, 1985

Maltsberger JT, Buie DH: Countertransference hate in the treatment of suicidal patients. Arch Gen Psychiatry 30:625–633, 1974

Masterson JF, Costello JL: From Borderline Adolescent to Functioning Adult: The Test of Time. New York, Brunner/Mazel, 1980

McGlashan T: The Chestnut Lodge follow-up study, III: long-term outcome of borderline personalities. Arch Gen Psychiatry 43:20–30, 1986

Miller MH: Time and the character disorder. J Nerv Ment Dis 138:534–540, 1964

Nurnberg HG, Suh R: Limits: short-term treatment of hospitalized borderline patients. Compr Psychiatry 21:70–80, 1980

Nurnberg HG, Suh R: Time-limited psychotherapy of the hospitalized borderline patient. Am J Psychother 36:82–90, 1982

Paris J, Brown R, Nowlis D: Long-term follow-up of borderline patients in a general hospital. Compr Psychiatry 28:530–535, 1987

Pildis MJ, Soverow GJ, Salzman C, et al: Day hospital treatment of borderline patients: a clinical perspective. Am J Psychiatry 135:594–596, 1978

Plakun EM, Burkhardt PE, Muller JP: Fourteen-year follow-up of borderline and schizotypal personality disorders. Compr Psychiatry 26:448–455, 1985

Rinsley DB: Theory and practice of intensive residential treatment of adolescents. Psychiatr Q 42:611–638, 1968

Rosenbluth M: The inpatient treatment of the borderline personality disorder: a critical review and discussion of aftercare implications. Can J Psychiatry 32:228–237, 1987

Rosnick L: Use of a long-term inpatient unit as a site for learning psychotherapy. Psychiatr Clin North Am 10:309–323, 1987

Sederer LI, Thorbeck J: First do not harm: short-term inpatient psychotherapy of the borderline patient. Hosp Community Psychiatry 37:692–697, 1986

Silver D, Book HE, Hamilton JE, et al: The characterologically difficult patient: a hospital treatment model. Can J Psychiatry 28:91–96, 1983a

Silver D, Book HE, Hamilton JE, et al: Psychotherapy and the inpatient unit: a unique learning experience. Am J Psychother 37:121–128, 1983b

Silver D, Cardish RJ, Glassman EJ: Intensive treatment of characterologically difficult patients: a general hospital perspective. Psychiatr Clin North Am 10:219–245, 1987

Silver D, Cardish RJ, Glassman EJ: The assessment of the capacity to be soothed: clinical and methodological issues, in The Solace Paradigm: An Eclectic Search for Psychological Immunity. Edited by Horton PC, Gewirtz H, Kreutter KJ. Madison, CT, International Universities Press, 1988, pp 91–119

Skodol AE, Buckley P, Charles E: Is there a characteristic pattern to the treatment history of clinic outpatients with borderline personality? J Nerv Ment Dis 171:405–410, 1983

Stone MH: Psychotherapy of borderline patients in light of long-term follow up. Bull Menninger Clin 51:231–247, 1987

Stone MH, Hurt SW, Stone DK: The PI 500: long-term follow-up of borderline inpatients meeting DSM-III criteria, I: global outcome. Journal of Personality Disorders 1:291–298, 1987

Tucker L, Bauer SF, Wagner S, et al: Long-term hospital treatment of borderline patients: a descriptive outcome study. Am J Psychiatry 144:1443–1448, 1987

Viner J: An understanding and approach to regression in the borderline patient. Compr Psychiatry 24:49–56, 1983

Waldinger RJ, Gunderson JG: Completed psychotherapies with borderline patients. Am J Psychother 38:190–202, 1984

Werble B: Second follow-up study of borderline patients. Arch Gen Psychiatry 23:3–7, 1970

Winnicott DW: On security, in The Family and Individual Development. London, Tavistock, 1965, pp 30–33

Wishnie HA: Inpatient therapy with borderline patients, in Borderline States in Psychiatry. Edited by Mack JE. New York, Grune & Stratton, 1975, pp 41–62

Management of Acute and Chronic Suicidality in Patients With Borderline Personality Disorder

Joel Paris, M.D.

S UICIDALITY IS A CHARACTERISTIC FEATURE OF THE BORDER-line syndrome. In fact, the clinical challenge of managing chronic suicidality could be one of the main reasons why clinicians and researchers have written so much about BPD. But suicidal patients are stressful for clinicians, and chronically suicidal patients even more so. Some of us handle that stress by writing about and investigating borderline personality. However, there are other possible reactions. Therapists may avoid treating patients with BPD because they do not want to have this sort of worry and responsibility. There are also clinicians who are attracted to suicidal patients, possibly because of the chance of actually saving lives. Unfortunately, being involved in rescue operations can lead to early burnout.

As pointed out by Fine and Sansone (1990), there are really two kinds of suicidality in BPD. *Acute suicidality*, as in other psychiatric disorders, is managed with protection through hospitalization. *Chronic suicidality* is a problem relatively unique to the borderline syndrome and seems to require a very different management. The problem for the clinician is in deciding whether a suicidal threat represents an acute risk or is part of a chronic risk. As clinicians well know, borderline patients are sensitive to

I would like to acknowledge Dr. John Gunderson, who read an earlier version of this chapter and made important suggestions for revision.

rejection and may act out when they perceive an empathic failure. It is not uncommon for patients to blame their therapist for a suicide attempt, further raising the pressure on beleaguered clinicians attempting to make a rational decision. As pointed out by Maltsberger and Buie (1974) in a classic paper, the countertransference engendered by these situations can be sufficient to make the therapist begin to wish that the patient would in fact commit suicide.

The decision as to whether to hospitalize a borderline patient carries risks either way. On the one hand, the patient may feel engulfed or controlled by the therapist; on the other hand, he or she may feel neglected or abandoned. To compound the problem, there have been a number of reports that borderline patients can get worse in the hospital (Dawson 1988). This dilemma corresponds dynamically with what borderline patients tell us about their parents: that they are both overprotective and neglectful (see Paris and Zweig-Frank, Chapter 7).

IMPLICATIONS OF OUTCOME RESEARCH

Can the empirical literature on BPD provide insight into these thorny management issues? There are a number of important questions that are open to investigation. First of all, how often do borderline patients actually complete suicide? Second, are there any predictors of which patients are most at risk? Finally, is there any evidence that intervention prevents suicide in these patients?

We now have a reasonable idea of the long-term risk for suicide in BPD (Paris 1988). These data come from long-term outcome studies (McGlashan 1986; Paris et al. 1987; Stone 1990) in which borderline patients were followed for 15 years. McGlashan's (1986) reported suicide rate of 3% is probably atypically low. The patients in his study were admitted to a residential facility for long-term treatment after failing to respond to management in general hospitals; therefore the most suicidal patients could have been screened out in the referral process. In two other studies, by Stone (1990) and Paris et al. (1987), the rate of completed suicide over the long term for BPD was closer to 9%. In Stone's follow-up of a large number of borderline individuals admitted to a long-term psychotherapy unit at Psychiatric Institute in New York, the reported rate of suicide completion (9%) is supported by the high rate of location (93%) of the cohort. Paris et al. (1987, 1988, 1989) examined a cohort of patients from a general hospital, which increases the generalizability of the findings because all social classes were represented in the sample. The suicide rate among locatable subjects was 8.5%, and since the publication of these data, further suicides among the surviving patients have increased the rate to 9.5%. In another study still in progress, Silver and Cardish (1991) also found a 10% suicide rate among 70 borderline patients followed for a mean of 10 years after residential treatment. It therefore seems reasonable to conclude that in most clinical settings, about 1 out of 10 borderline patients can be expected to eventually complete suicide.

This is certainly a high rate, approaching those described for schizophrenia (Wilkinson 1982) and affective disorder (Guze and Robins 1970). Can we identify which subgroups of borderline patients have a particularly high suicide risk? In Stone's (1990) study, comorbidity of substance use was significantly associated with a risk of completion. Although these findings were not confirmed by Paris et al., Stone had a higher location rate for his sample, and substance abusers are more likely to have been lost to follow-up. Furthermore, the association makes clinical sense, because we know that there is a strong relationship between substance abuse and youth suicide (Rich et al. 1988).

Paris et al. used the items of Gunderson's Diagnostic Interview for Borderlines (DID) (Gunderson et al. 1981) to distinguish suicides from survivors, but only previous attempts were significantly related to eventual completion. Therefore, previous attempts, even if "manipulative," have to be taken seriously in terms of long-term risk, a finding replicated by Kullgren (1988). Because the sample in Paris et al.'s study varied in socioeconomic background, it was possible to show that suicide completion was more common with higher education. This finding, although not replicated by Kjelsberg et al. (1991), parallels those of Drake and Gates (1984) in schizophrenia, where increased education and higher expectations in life were risk factors for suicide in patients with a disabling mental disorder. In parallel with this finding, Paris et al. (1988) also showed that the borderline individuals who committed suicide had scored lower on an index of developmental problems during childhood than had those who survived, again demonstrating the effect of crushed expectations.

Although there are a number of statistically significant findings on prediction of suicide in BPD, it is not clear if we have a clinically useful profile. In general, the outcome of BPD is not readily predictable (Paris 1988). However, 75% of borderline patients who survive recover after 15 years (Paris et al. 1987). Completed suicide in BPD peaks around the age of 30 and seems to be rare thereafter (Paris et al. 1987; Stone 1990). Frances (1985) and Gunderson (1984) have argued that it is worth keeping patients alive through prevention of suicide until the disorder burns itself out. This view assumes that we can in fact prevent suicide in patients with BPD and that our interventions really do keep these patients alive.

Is there any empirical evidence that treatment prevents suicide in patients with BPD? Only a randomized clinical trial with a 15-year follow-up could hope to answer this question. Although there are prospective studies of long-term BPD outcome under way (Links et al. 1988; Perry 1985), they have not been designed to study treatment. One comparison of interest is that the suicide rates in the Stone (1990) and Silver and Cardish (1991) studies, in which patients received long-term psychotherapy and residential care, were the same as in the Paris et al. study, in which the patients received intermittent crisis intervention. Although differences between the samples make any conclusions doubtful, we can say that the effectiveness of treatment to prevent suicide in the long term remains undemonstrated.

It is even possible that the suicide rate for BPD is increasing. This was the finding of a Swedish study by Kullgren et al. (1986), who reviewed psychiatric suicides over the period 1961 to 1980. This period is the same as the one that saw the tripling of youth suicide in North America (Sudak et al. 1984). There has been much speculation about the meaning of this dramatic epidemiological shift, ranging from the size of the cohort (Easterlin 1980) to the effects of rapid social change (see Millon, Chapter 10). It is worth noting that in the San Diego suicide study (Rich et al. 1988), completion was strongly associated with substance abuse among the young, suggesting a potentially borderline picture. In three recent studies (Lesage et al. 1992; Rich et al. 1990; Runeson and Beskow 1991), blind diagnostic ratings of information drawn from psychological autopsies on a sample of male youth suicides showed that 30% of such cases could be identified as having had BPD. The question of whether the youth suicide epidemic reflects an epidemic of BPD (Paris 1991) or an increase in the lethality of BPD requires further investigation.

MANAGEMENT IMPLICATIONS

The concerned clinician treating a borderline patient will find little comfort in this review of empirical data on suicide. Borderline patients do suicide, with some frequency, and not very predictably, and it is unclear whether intervention makes a difference. Nevertheless, our very uncertainty about our ability to prevent suicide provides a way out of the impasse.

As reviewed by Fine and Sansone (1990), a number of clinicians who are experienced with BPD have suggested communicating to borderline patients that because their potential suicide cannot be prevented, treatment should proceed without making suicide the primary concern. Schwartz et al. (1974) have described the phenomenon of the suicidal character. Chronic suicidality may be necessary to some borderline patients. To be suicidal is a coping strategy that gives one some control over one's world. Borderline patients who feel powerless and victimized in their lives require one where they feel empowered. Until they feel empowered in other, more constructive ways, they need to retain suicide as an option.

Clinical Example

A woman working in the mental health field was in psychotherapy between the ages of 22 and 26. For the first 3 years she was continuously suicidal. The possibility was discussed in almost every session, and the therapist never felt sure he would see the patient the following week. Although hospitalization was discussed, she always rejected the idea, ostensibly because of scandal in the professional community. There were nonetheless several overdoses in the course of treatment, at which time the patient would call the therapist, induce vomiting, then come to his office and discuss what happened in an emergency session.

The patient had a very traumatic childhood in which she was abandoned by both her parents and was raised in a severe and unempathic foster home. She vowed never to trust anyone and concentrated on developing her career and helping others. In her early 20s, after several disappointments in intimate relations, she decided that if she was not feeling better by the age of 25, she could always commit suicide. This idea, which was retained for most of the course of therapy, was empowering and comforting for her. She was always enraged when the therapist suggested he would try and stop her if he could. Toward the end of treatment, when her interpersonal relationships became more satisfying, she simply stopped talking about suicide. On 10-year follow-up she is functioning well and has not been suicidal since termination.

Hospitalization of borderline patients for suicidal threats can have a number of negative effects (Dawson 1988). Terms such as "malignant regression" have been used to describe them. What happens is that hospitalization actually worsens the suicidality. Clinicians will not be unfamiliar with the patient who responds to admission with an escalating series of acting-out behaviors, such as self-mutilation. Why this happens is a matter of conjecture, but one possible explanation is that borderline individuals feel at once object hunger and engulfment, much as they do in object relationships outside the hospital (Melges and Swartz 1989). A number of side effects may ensue, ranging from extended admissions to precipitate and angry discharge. Silver and Rosenbluth, in Chapter 16, offer strategies to limit regression in hospitalized borderline individuals, but the problems are not always avoidable.

Clinical Example

A 25-year-old woman working in a home for the mentally handicapped was a frequent visitor to the emergency room. She would usually come in agitated, threatening suicide, and would become quickly aggressive, hitting or throwing things at the examining doctor. As a result, she would frequently be held overnight for observation. Each time this was done, the nursing staff would be faced with an escalating series of actions, particularly wrist slashing. When sent to the psychiatric ward, she was often physically frightening to the staff and would be put into seclusion or restraints. Eventually she would be discharged, after which she would not attend follow-up but would turn up in the emergency room a month later. This cycle repeated itself several times before the chief of emergency psychiatry sent around a memo asking that she be seen only briefly and not held over. Although never engaged in outpatient therapy, her behavior extinguished over time. On 10-year follow-up, she was unemployed and living a marginal life but was not suicidal.

The controversy over long-term versus short-term hospitalization is reviewed by Silver and Rosenbluth in Chapter 16. There is little evidence at present to support the value of long-term admission for borderline individuals, although McGlashan (1986) suggests that it deserves a clinical trial. Given the cost of residential care, such a trial is unlikely to be carried out, and it would seem reasonable to place the burden of proof on those advocating more labor-intensive methods of treatment.

Most clinicians would support the recommendations of Silver and Rosenbluth for short-term hospitalization of acutely suicidal borderline individuals. There is, however, more controversy about the use of the hospital for chronic suicidality. It is not clear that hospitalization is effective for managing repeated suicidal threats. It has also been suggested that admissions can be used to establish a therapeutic alliance (Kernberg 1975). However, in a follow-up of hospitalized borderline patients by Gunderson et al. (1989), 60% of the discharged patients had dropped out of psychotherapy within 6 months.

Although Dawson (1988) has suggested avoiding hospitalization entirely, the intermediate position of Fine and Sansone (1990) probably represents the consensus among clinicians experienced with BPD. These authors advocate "traditional management" in acute situations but non-hospitalization for chronic risk. Brief hospitalization, if used conservatively, retains a role in the armamentarium of the therapist treating BPD patients (see Chapter 16).

Clinical Example

A 17-year-old high school student became suicidal on the anniversary of the suicide of her best friend. The friend, who was also diagnosed borderline, had jumped off a bridge after the patient refused to join her in a suicide pact. The patient felt intensely guilty and thought of leaping off the same bridge so that she could rejoin her lost friend. At the same time she had intense fantasies that her life was unreal and that she existed in another reality she could only enter when she was dead. She was hospitalized for 3 weeks. The hospital provided a holding environment that carried her over the dangerous anniversary. In addition, she benefited from a low-dose phenothiazine and from work with her family. She then resumed outpatient psychotherapy. Although there were other suicidal crises, she was not readmitted and eventually recovered. On 15-year follow-up, she is married, has two children, and runs a small business.

Although hospitalization is useful for acute risk, there is no clear boundary between acute, subacute, and chronic suicide risk. This is what makes the decision not to hospitalize and accept the risk so difficult. Gunderson (1984) suggests that patients should be told that the therapist has a limited ability to prevent suicide and that work on the underlying difficulties will continue. Kroll (1988) takes a similar view, advocating exploration of the reasons for suicidality and acknowledging that the patient retains suicide as an option.

If held firmly and consistently, this approach to management of the chronically suicidal borderline has the potential to make therapy manageable. In general, a direct attempt to stop suicidal threats and gestures is not practicable. Asking borderline patients to contract not to overdose or self-mutilate amounts to asking them to give up their symptoms before the therapy starts to work. Although Shearin and Linehan (see Chapter 14) suggest specific methods to bring suicidal behavior under control, suicidality still has to be tolerated until the treatment alliance starts to work. When borderline patients get better, suicidality disappears. Until then, suicidal threats and ideation can be treated as indications of distress that require exploration of underlying issues and conflicts.

Obviously, normal therapeutic work cannot be carried out in an atmosphere of overconcern or panic. In order to work successfully with suicidal borderline patients, the therapist has in most circumstances to simply accept the chronic risk and proceed with the treatment. To be derailed by chronic suicidality is to lose sight of the real work of psychotherapy. Paradoxically, only by tolerating its chronicity can borderline suicidality be successfully treated.

Suicide during therapy is always a possibility, but, by and large, patients engaged in a working alliance will postpone completion, usually presenting gestures and threats in the context of a stormy transference. The presence of a working alliance in which both patient and therapist explore issues is the most secure preventative of suicidal acting out, no matter how disturbing suicidal ideation may be. Suicide attempts reflect a break in that alliance or may demonstrate that it was more tenuous than previously realized (Adler 1979).

It could be argued that the above position carries medicolegal risks. Obviously, no one can feel entirely safe from litigation by suicidal patients or their families. However, it makes no sense not to treat such patients or to treat them inadequately out of fear. There are a number of common-sense precautions that can be taken, from careful documentation to discussing the risk openly with family members. Given the consensus of many experts on BPD that chronic risk should not be managed by repeated hospitalization, and given reasonable overall management, the position of a therapist who loses a borderline patient to suicide is unhappy but legally defensible.

There is a bright side to the treatment of the suicidal borderline patient. If therapy is successful, the personal rewards for the clinician are great. Unlike other cases where one is left in doubt about the efficacy of treatment, the recovered borderline patient who no longer considers suicide as an option provides a dramatic and convincing result. This recovery will not happen in every case, but when it does, the therapist feels amply recompensed for having struggled for years with a patient whose very life hung in the balance.

REFERENCES

Adler G: The myth of the alliance with borderline patients. Am J Psychiatry 136:642–645, 1979

Dawson DF: Treatment of the borderline patient, relationship management. Can J Psychiatry 33:370–374, 1988

Drake RE, Gates C, Cotton PG, et al: Suicide among schizophrenics: who is at risk? J Nerv Ment Dis 172:613–617, 1984

Easterlin RA: Birth and Fortune: The Impact of Numbers on Personal Welfare. New York, Basic Books, 1980

Fine MA, Sansone RA: Dilemmas in the management of suicidal behavior in individuals with borderline personality disorder. Am J Psychother 44:160–171, 1990

Frances A: Discussion. Symposium on Long-Term Outcome of Borderline Personality Disorder, at the 138th annual meeting of the American Psychiatric Association, New York, May 1985

Gunderson JG: Borderline Personality Disorder. Washington, DC, American Psychiatric Press, 1984

Gunderson JG, Kolb JE, Austin V: The diagnostic interview for borderline patients. Am J Psychiatry 138:896–903, 1981

Gunderson JG, Frank AF, Ronningstam EF, et al: Early discontinuance of borderline patients from psychotherapy. J Nerv Ment Dis 177:38–42, 1989

Guze SB, Robins E: Suicide and primary affective disorders. Br J Psychiatry 117:437–438, 1970

Kernberg OF: Borderline Conditions and Pathological Narcissism. New York, Jason Aronson, 1975

Kjelsberg E, Eikeseth PH, Dahl AA: Suicide in borderline patients—predictive factors. Acta Psychiatr Scand 84:283–287, 1991

Kroll J: The Challenge of the Borderline Patient. New York, WW Norton, 1988

Kullgren G: Factors associated with completed suicide in borderline personality disorder. J Nerv Ment Dis 176:40–44, 1988

Kullgren G, Renberg E, Jacobsson L: An empirical study of borderline personality disorder and psychiatric suicides. J Nerv Ment Dis 174:328–331, 1986

Lesage AD, Vanier C, Morisette R, et al: Diagnosis and use of services in suicide victims. Paper presented at the 145th annual meeting of the American Psychiatric Association, Washington, DC, May 1992

Links PS, Steiner M, Offord DR, et al: Characteristics of borderline personality disorder: a Canadian study. Can J Psychiatry 33:336–340, 1988

Maltsberger JT, Buie DH: Countertransference hate in the treatment of suicidal patients. Arch Gen Psychiatry 30:625–633, 1974

McGlashan TH: The Chestnut Lodge follow-up study, III: long-term outcome of borderline personalities. Arch Gen Psychiatry 43:20–30, 1986

Melges FT, Swartz MS: Oscillations of attachment in borderline personality disorder. Am J Psychiatry 146:1115–1120, 1989

Paris J: Follow-up studies of borderline personality disorder: a critical review. Journal of Personality Disorders 2:189–197, 1988

Paris J: Parasuicide, personality disorders, and culture. Transcultural Psychiatric Research Review 28:25–39, 1991

Paris J, Brown R, Nowlis D: Long-term follow-up of borderline patients in a general hospital. Compr Psychiatry 28:530–535, 1987

Paris J, Nowlis D, Brown R: Developmental factors in the outcome of borderline personality disorder. Compr Psychiatry 29:147–150, 1988

Paris J, Nowlis D, Brown R: Predictors of suicide in borderline personality disorder. Can J Psychiatry 34:8–9, 1989

Perry JC: Depression in borderline personality disorder: lifetime prevalence at interview and longitudinal course of symptoms. Am J Psychiatry 142:15–21, 1985

Rich CL, Fowler RC, Fogarty LA, et al: The San Diego Suicide Study, III: relationships between diagnoses and stressors. Arch Gen Psychiatry 45:589–594, 1988

Rich CL, Runeson BS, Fowler RC: Axis I and II comorbidity among young suicides in Sweden and U.S. Paper presented at the Third European Symposium on Suicidal Behavior and Risk Factors, Bologna, October 1990

Runeson B, Beskow J: Borderline personality disorder in young Swedish suicides. J Nerv Ment Dis 179:153–156, 1991

Schwartz DA, Flinn DE, Slawson PF: Treatment of the suicidal character. Am J Psychother 28:194–207, 1974

Silver D, Cardish RJ: BPD outcome studies: psychotherapy implications. Paper presented at the 144th annual meeting of the American Psychiatric Association, New Orleans, May 1991

Stone MH: The Fate of Borderline Patients: Successful Outcome and Psychiatric Practice. New York, Guilford, 1990

Sudak HS, Ford AB, Rushforth NB (eds): Suicide in the Young. Boston, MA, John Wright, 1984

Wilkinson DG: The suicide rate in schizophrenia. Br J Psychiatry 140:138–141, 1982

Treatment of Borderline Personality Disorder: A Critical Review

John Gunderson, M.D.
Alex N. Sabo, M.D.

P SYCHOANALYTICALLY INFORMED EXPLORATION OF DYADIC relationships over the past 60 years has offered clinically useful ways of conceptualizing the psychopathology and treatment of patients with borderline personality disorder (BPD). Over the past two decades, the added advantages of scientific method and empirical research have been brought to bear on this task. In fact, empirical research published over the past 5 years has brought us to a watershed overlooking the psychoanalytic and empirical sources for our understanding of patients with BPD. The multiple follow-up studies tracing the clinical course of hundreds of borderline patients over a 2- to 32-year follow-up period have given us significant data about the life course of borderline patients and what sorts of outcome are possible given various forms of treatment, or even no treatment at all (see McGlashan, Chapter 12). These follow-up studies are complemented by a new series of studies documenting the important role of physical and sexual abuse in the development of the disorder in many patients (see Perry and Herman, Chapter 6). It is now possible to see BPD as a final common pathway emerging from different sources (see Paris and Zweig-Frank, Chapter 7). Beyond this, there have been intensive, focused research efforts into psychopharmacological (see Soloff, Chapter 15) and cognitive-behavioral treatment strategies (see Shearin and Linehan, Chapter 14).

The lifetime risk of suicide in BPD has been reported to be between 3% and 10% (McGlashan 1986; Paris 1990; Stone 1990), and the majority of those suicides occurred early in the course of the disorder. The outcome for patients able to survive those first 5 years is highly variable, but many of these patients attain a better level of adaptation and experience improvement in their suffering during subsequent years of development.

The growing awareness of the sequelae of physical and sexual abuse in borderline patients has had implications for the conceptualization of treatment (Braun 1984; Herman 1981, 1986; Kluft 1985; Moses 1978; Stone 1990; van der Kolk 1987). Many borderline patients are being conceptualized as having dissociative disorders, and their treatments are focusing largely on this symptom as the sequela of traumatic experiences of childhood.

There is a clearly emerging need to integrate useful earlier concepts of BPD with the more recent data and formulations. In this chapter we will review these developments and indicate how empirical data and clinical experience support some forms of treatment over others.

PSYCHOTHERAPIES

Individual Psychotherapy

In practice, individual psychotherapy remains the cornerstone of most treatments for patients with BPD. In the vast literature on vis-á-vis psychotherapies with borderline patients there are a number of controversies, but also areas of agreement. From this literature the following areas of agreement regarding essential components of treatment can be identified (Waldinger and Gunderson 1987):

1. Providing a stable treatment framework
2. Having highly active/involving therapists
3. Establishing a connection between the patient's actions and feelings
4. Identifying adverse effects of self-destructive behaviors
5. Paying careful attention to countertransference feelings

In addition to these areas of consensus, there is also very strong evidence indicating that, regardless of the therapeutic approach or the therapists's level of experience, most individual psychotherapies end with the borderline patient's dropping out (Gunderson et al. 1989; Skodol et al.

1983; Waldinger and Gunderson 1987). This is usually due to the patient's sense of being misunderstood or mistreated but is also often due to antagonism toward therapy on the part of the borderline patient's significant others.

Most borderline patients behave in self-destructive ways, and psychotherapists need to develop a means for differentiating nonlethally motivated self-harm from true suicidal intentions. Paris (see Chapter 17) has argued convincingly that the lifetime risk of suicide in borderline patients is quite high (i.e., 10%). Stone (1990, p. 45) has identified a small subsample of BPD patients with major affective disorder and alcoholism and estimates the 5-year survival for this subgroup at only 58%—even after 1 to 2 years of inpatient psychoanalytically oriented treatment!

Based on the literature and our clinical experience, a number of simple principles are useful. First, therapists should identify, confront, and treat a comorbid substance abuse disorder or clear-cut major depression. Second, while establishing from the outset that safety is an important issue, the therapist should stress that psychotherapy is a collaborative enterprise. It must be made clear to the patient that the therapist is neither omnipotent nor omniscient. Third, therapists can safeguard against suicidality by paying careful attention to the hatred that can be evoked by the patient (Maltsberger and Buie 1974; Winnicott 1947/1975). Fourth, and implied by all of the above, therapists should set a low threshold for seeking consultation.

Psychoanalytic Psychotherapy

Since Knight's (1953) early descriptions, it has generally been accepted that formal psychoanalysis is a form of psychotherapy that is contraindicated for most borderline patients. Some case reports of psychoanalysis have been published (Abend et al. 1983; Volkan 1987), but the patients in these samples would not be considered borderline by current criteria. The reason for this relative contraindication is the proclivity for psychotic transferences and uncontrolled acting out in an unstructured treatment like psychoanalysis. For the occasional exception to this rule, careful consideration and expert consultation should be prerequisite.

Within the domain of psychodynamic psychotherapy, controversy exists about the role of early interpretation and the management of negative transference. Kernberg (1968, 1976) was most articulate in identifying the need for early confrontation and interpretations of primitive transferences in here-and-now situations. Kernberg (Kernberg 1968; Kernberg et al. 1989), Masterson (1976), and Gunderson (1984) all emphasize the need to identify the aggressive motives that exist in the here and now so as to make their inappropriateness visible and dystonic. At times, this involves drawing patients' attention to the sadistic and controlling motives behind their manipulative behaviors. Because interpretations are often transformed or experienced as attacks, linking statements that anticipate such reactions are often needed.

The approach just outlined emerges from a two-person psychology in which one person is assumed healthy and neutral and the other sick and expected to form a transference neurosis. The new trauma data now impel a revision in this approach. First, the aggression of the borderline patient may be understood in terms of an immature self, rightly full of rage at the parent or parent-substitutes who have failed to respectfully provide for its survival and developmental needs and who indeed have even used its body as an object for venting their own rage and for gratifying their own sexual desires. The therapist using this framework is more likely to make a statement that will validate the patient's experience. The patient feels held rather than attacked. The aggressive, manipulative behaviors of these patients still occur, but they are understood in the light of adaptations made in response to past trauma. The therapist still has the task of confronting these behaviors and making them ego-dystonic in order to promote the safety of the patient and to explain the disruptive effects of these behaviors on other aspects of the patient's life such as work and personal relationships. Yet, the paradigm derived from trauma data calls for therapists not to ascribe sadism or manipulativeness to the borderline patient but rather to ascribe such behaviors to the unfortunate survival techniques that resulted from mistreatment.

Kohut (1971), Guntrip (1975), and, later, Buie and Adler (1982–1983) anticipated in many ways the paradigm shift suggested by the trauma data. Guntrip wrote that "psychoanalytic psychotherapy . . . is . . . the provision of a reliable and understanding human relationship of a kind that makes contact with the deeply repressed traumatized child in a way that enables one to become steadily more able to live, in the security of a new real relationship" (p. 155). This statement reflects a broader shift in the conceptualization of psychoanalytic action that suggests a more interactive model, emphasizing the creation of a relationship over interpretive technique (cf. Langs 1976; McLaughlin 1981; Sandler 1976). More specifically for borderline patients, Buie and Adler (1982–1983) and Chessick (1982) argued that interpretations of aggressive themes are at best ineffectual and at worst harmfully disruptive in the early phase of treatment. Consistent with the self-psychology school of Kohut (1971), Buie and Adler emphasized the need to validate the real role of bad parenting in the patient's past as a motivating force for the patient's aggression. These authors advocate reserving transference interpretation to the development of intolerance-of-aloneness themes.

Those who have written about psychoanalytic psychotherapy with borderline patients agree that basic personality change is a legitimate goal. They also agree that such changes require three or more therapy sessions a week conducted by people with psychoanalytic training or supervision to help manage the inevitable countertransference issues. Successful therapies can be expected to last a minimum of 4 years, and usually considerably longer. Though the results of such treatment are not well documented, a detailed exposition of five successfully completed therapies has validated the potential for basic changes (Waldinger and Gunderson 1987): diminution of impulsive behaviors, an improved stability in relationships, and greater affective range and expressiveness were observed. Such basic shifts in their personality enabled the borderline patients to assume independent functioning without ongoing therapies even though in some instances problems in identity formation and self-esteem persisted.

Supportive Psychotherapy

Despite the enormous literature about psychoanalytic psychotherapy with borderline patients, this kind of therapy constitutes a small fraction of the treatment actually given to borderline patients. Most borderline patients are seen in *supportive psychotherapy* (Rockland 1989), usually a once-weekly individual psychotherapy in which the primary focus is on the reality problems of daily life, and there is relatively little opportunity to examine and work through primitive transferences. Nevertheless, within this less intensive and more supportive form of psychotherapy, the same demands for saving interventions and the same accusations of cruel with-holding are predictable strains on the therapists. Again, psychotherapy is expected to last for a long time, generally tapering off into an as-needed schedule after 3 to 5 years. The goals of this psychotherapy are not explic-itly directed at changing personality but at improving the patients' adap-tation to their life circumstances and diminishing the likelihood of self-destructive responses to expectable interpersonal frustrations.

A recent report from the Menninger Outcome Study has cast the role of supportive psychotherapy in a new light for borderline patients (Wallerstein 1986). This work shows that even when analysts start with intensive interpretive strategies, they shift toward a more supportive strat-egy and that, despite this shift, supportive treatments are able to bring about basic changes in personality—changes of the types that have gener-ally been expected to result only from more intensive, exploratory, trans-ference-based treatment. Such observations are in line with the current redefinition of psychoanalytic psychotherapy described earlier, a redefini-tion that recognizes the essential role of supportive strategies and nonspe-cific actions. Such observations cast doubts on accounts of psychoanalytic psychotherapy that propose that change relies on insight without recog-nizing the corrective role of such nonspecific "supportive" interventions (Kolb and Gunderson 1990).

Short-Term or Time-Limited Psychotherapy

Early advocates for the use of short-term psychotherapy specifically ex-cluded borderline patients as suitable for such treatment (Mann 1973; Sifneos 1972). The intense and chaotic personality issues of such patients would not be expected to change over the course of the 10 to 20 sessions usually offered in short-term therapy. Despite the prevailing consensus, however, clinics with training functions are often forced to adopt time-limited (6 to 12 months) strategies for borderline patients to conform with rotation of trainees. These time-limited psychotherapies are focused on specific situational or interactional problems, and the likelihood that a regressive transference will develop is diminished. Because of the time-limited focus and the consequent lack of transference-gratifications in-herent in such treatment, many borderline patients drop out. Those who remain can profit, however, and may subsequently return for further "doses" of similarly circumscribed treatment. This sort of strategy (i.e., with specific time limits and focused subjects) may be particularly well suited for borderline patients who have a history of dropping out of more ambitious treatments and for those who present with concerns about being engulfed, being overwhelmed, or becoming too dependent. Some patients move from short-term treatment into a long-term therapy for which they were initially unmotivated. Silver (1983, 1985) has written of short-term, intermittent therapy offered on a long-term basis.

As such clinical experiences have accumulated, the initial pessimism about the role for short-term psychotherapy with borderline patients has given way, and the approach is gaining advocates (Krupnick and Horowitz 1985; Leibovich 1981, 1983).

Family Therapy

Although borderline psychopathology can arise from many different types of family background, there are two patterns of family involvement that can help clinicians plan family interventions (Gunderson et al. 1980).

One pattern is characterized by *overinvolvement*. Borderline offspring of such families are often actively struggling with dependency issues by denial or by anger at their parents. Whether denied or reviled, these needs for dependency are often being actively gratified by the family (Shapiro et al. 1975). Such a family requires active, ongoing family participation in treatment. To exclude the family from involvement in the index borderline person's treatment leads the parents to withhold support and, moreover, causes the patient to feel as if participation in therapy is disloyal to the parents and will lead to abandonment.

Borderline patients also come from families characterized by *abuse* (violent or incestuous) or *neglect* (Gunderson 1990). In this pattern, the parents are likely to be angry at their offspring for having either sought or been sent for treatment. These parents will be overly resentful of treatment efforts that require their involvement in an examination of the family interactions. Meetings with the parents alone may be required in order to solicit their support for the borderline person's treatment. In such meetings, it is useful to be formally educative about the nature of the offspring's illness and to attempt to reassure the parents that the treatment is directed toward helping the patient develop more independence and, specifically, that it is not directed at blaming them.

Sometimes zealous treaters take the stance that hate should be directed against the person of the abuser. While it is important that the patient's anger and hate be recognized and the reasons validated, with borderline patients, unlike patients with posttraumatic stress disorder, the hated abusers are often ambivalently regarded, and hate directed at them may lead to self-directed hate and self-destructive actions.

These guidelines for using either the family therapy approach per se or a more supportive, educational approach directed toward the parents separately apply to both inpatients and outpatients. Regardless of the family pattern, family interventions may be necessary to maintain an outpatient psychotherapy as long as the borderline patient remains emotionally or financially dependent on his or her parents. At present, there is no reason to believe that family treatment by itself can be sufficient.

Conjoint family therapy is usually conducted in 90-minute sessions once weekly but may be more frequent. The educative, supportive interventions for parents alone usually involve sessions lasting an hour or less. Sessions may be conducted either by the patient's therapist or by someone who works collaboratively with but independently of the therapist. Such meetings are likely to take place on an as-needed basis for an indefinite period until the patient has achieved sufficient autonomy from the parents for the other parts of the patient's treatment plan to be safely stable.

Conjoint sessions in which both a family therapist and the individual therapist meet with patient and family can decrease the amount of distortion and reduce the tendency for parents to develop paranoid attitudes toward their family member's individual treatment. Protestations by patients that they do not want such a treatment is in the service of their not recognizing their own ambivalence. Despite the protests, these patients are often enmeshed with their parents, and the patients' and parents' ability to see themselves safely working together more often stabilizes rather than hinders treatment.

Group Therapy

It is widely accepted that group therapy is useful for borderline patients. Yet, most clinicians find that it is difficult for borderline patients to enter and remain in such treatment. The chances of entering and remaining in group therapy are enhanced if participation is made a contingency from the beginning of an individual therapy.

The presence of peers in a group therapy has a number of benefits not available in individual therapy. Peers are more able than a therapist to confront maladaptive and impulsive patterns without being written off as trying to control the patient. Groups are also very effective in identifying dependent or manipulative gratifications and making them more dystonic. At the same time, the group provides a set of peers with whom communication of feelings and personal problems can be experienced without harmful repercussions. Groups provide a field to study others' methods of coping, and borderline patients often find that it is easier to identify a maladaptive pattern of coping in another person rather than in oneself. Groups also provide a very supportive function that may extend to the development of new and better relationships outside of, as well as within, the therapy.

A controversy exists about the relative advantages of having multiple borderline patients within the same group (Wong 1980). The issue is debated because such patients place major strains on a group's functioning, and the strain can dissolve a group or intimidate other members. Most people agree that concurrent individual therapy is required. These patients are immature and, much like preschool children, have not yet developed the capacity to obtain nurturance and satisfaction from solely triadic relationships.

Clinical experience has shown that many borderline patients have been helped by 12-step self-help groups such as Alcoholics Anonymous (AA), Narcotics Anonymous (NA), and Overeaters Anonymous. Stone's data (1990) indicate a low 5-year survival rate when a patient has BPD, a major affective disorder, and a severe substance abuse disorder. AA and NA not only offer a treatment sometimes capable of interrupting a lethal substance abuse disorder but also provide 24-hour-a-day telephone support, daily group meetings, and a simple, coherent philosophy well-suited to the recovering substance abuser and to patients with BPD. In fact, in Stone's sample (1990), those BPD patients with alcoholism who had achieved sobriety through AA and who continued to participate in the AA program achieved Global Assessment Scores (GAS) 10 points higher at follow-up than the mean scores at follow-up for BPD patients as a whole.

BEHAVIOR THERAPY

Borderline patients present with behavior that constitutes serious management problems that would seem likely targets for systematic positive and negative reinforcement. And yet the explicit use of behavioral techniques with such patients has not been widely advocated. The behavioral literature does focus on problems common to borderline patients such as impulsivity, self-destructiveness, and expression of aggression, and it does offer promising techniques for addressing these problems (Liberman et al. 1981; also see Shearin and Linehan, Chapter 14). As will be described later, the failure of inpatient settings to appreciate what constitutes positive and negative reinforcements for borderline patients and to implement these can aggravate the destructive acts they wish to extinguish. Linehan (1987a, 1987b) has developed a manual-guided behavioral strategy for the treatment of self-destructiveness in a largely borderline cohort of parasuicidal women. She has developed a number of behavioral and cognitive strategies specifically adapted to the problems of borderline patients (Linehan 1989). Patients participate in both individual and group therapy. Linehan's method involves a collaborative effort with the patient and emphasizes the importance of breaking targeted goals into component tasks. The presence of clear time-limited techniques to accomplish these tasks in BPD patients is revolutionary.

Linehan (1989) reports that of 11 patients who began a 1-year dialectical behavioral treatment, none dropped out of therapy, compared with 50% who dropped out of a treatment as usual in a community control group. In addition, the behaviorally treated patients showed reduced medical severity and a lower frequency of parasuicide when compared with the control group. The full report on this promising study is eagerly awaited, but the preliminary data set clear standards against which other treatment approaches can be measured.

BIOLOGICAL THERAPIES

Pharmacotherapy is a commonly employed form of treatment for BPD. Neurochemical models of behavior and empirical pharmacotherapy trials have brought into focus trait vulnerabilities such as loss of control in four

areas: cognition, affect, impulse, and anxiety. These various trait vulnerabilities may involve different neurotransmitters, and the traits may be
amenable to treatment with different pharmacological agents (Soloff
1990, also see Chapter 13). We agree with Soloff that such an approach
may make the overall personality disorder more amenable to change
through psychotherapy.

The trait vulnerabilities and pharmacological approaches to their
treatment are as follows:

1. Cognitive control problems such as depersonalization, derealization,
   illusions, ideas of reference, and brief paranoid states are common in
   borderline patients. These symptoms are best treated with low-dose
   neuroleptic medication. This claim is substantiated by a large body of
   research data (Goldberg et al. 1986; Leone 1982; Serban and Siegel 1984;
   Soloff et al. 1986b).

2. The affective control problems of borderline patients include depression
   and dysregulation of mood and anger. When a borderline patient clearly
   suffers from endogenous depression that is persistent and that does not
   respond to psychosocial interventions such as hospitalization or relief
   of stressors in the environment, a tricyclic antidepressant may be useful.
   Yet, the majority of depressions in borderline patients are of a different
   nature. Liebowitz and Klein (1981) have suggested that such core borderline features as chronic emptiness, boredom, discomfort in being
   alone, and impulsivity might be responsive to monoamine oxidase
   (MAO) inhibitors. Somewhat discouraging has been the report that
   responses to tricyclic antidepressants do not appear to be particularly
   closely linked to initial levels of depressive disturbance, and that these
   drugs may increase behavioral dyscontrol for some patients (Links et al.
   1990; Soloff et al. 1986a). Soloff (1990) has even suggested that "major
   depression in the context of severe personality disorder may represent
   a different syndrome than major depression alone" (p. 235). Soloff cites
   Siever et al. (1985), who reported the "spontaneous" resolution of major
   depression in 90% of a sample of hospitalized patients with personality
   disorders following 2 weeks of drug-free care. Soloff (1986b) also cites
   his own study of amitriptyline and Cowdry and Gardner's (1988) study
   of tranylcypromine to conclude that severity of depression does not
   predict response to these drugs in borderline patients.

Soloff joins Liebowitz and Klein in advocating the use of an MAO inhibitor rather than a tricyclic to treat the depressive symptoms in most borderline patients. Clinically, many borderline patients require both an MAO inhibitor and a low-dose neuroleptic, and this suggests that at least two neurotransmitter systems are involved. Soloff (1990) suggests that when both psychotic-like symptoms and depressive symptoms are present in a borderline patient that the clinician address the psychotic-like symptoms with a low-dose neuroleptic prior to treating the depressive symptoms. This advice derives from his own data that has shown a worsening of referential thinking and increased suicidal and assaultive behavior in borderline patients treated with amitriptyline (Soloff et al. 1986a).

The complicated question of whether BPD represents an early form of a bipolar disorder is beyond the scope of this brief review, but a few comments are in order. Soloff et al. (1987) reported 41% comorbidity of bipolar type II disorder or atypical depression in a sample of borderline patients. Links et al. (1990) reported no significant treatment response for depressive symptoms in borderline patients treated with lithium versus placebo and desipramine versus placebo. Stone (1990) retrospectively studied 205 borderline patients for 25 years, and 17 of those patients (8%) went on to develop bipolar illness. Stone states that particularly in cases with a family history of bipolar disorder, BPD may be a phenotypic expression of bipolar disorder risk. Many borderline patients report symptoms of major depression and brief, hypomanic episodes often lasting only a few hours. Some psychopharmacologists are diagnosing rapid-cycling bipolar disorder in borderline patients. Systematic studies are needed to differentiate these disorders and to provide guidelines for treatment.

Intense anger and disabling hostility are symptoms of disordered affective control and are targets for pharmacological treatment. Low-dose neuroleptics have been most effective (Soloff et al. 1989). Schatzberg and Cole (1981) suggested benzodiazepines for these symptoms in borderline patients, and occasionally benzodiazepines do work (Cowdry and Gardner 1988). Yet, the clinician is cautioned that benzodiazepines, particularly the short-acting ones, may actually disinhibit a large number of borderline patients, causing more severe hostility, self-destructiveness, and assaultiveness. Gardner and Cowdry (1985) report such an untoward outcome among 8 of 15 borderline patients in a crossover study of alprazolam.

3. Impulsivity expressed in actions such as recklessness, binging, promiscuity, and impulsive suicide attempts is a significant problem in patients with BPD that sometimes is amenable to pharmacological treatment. A growing literature demonstrates the relationship between low cerebrospinal fluid (CSF) 5-hydroxyindoleacetic acid (5-HIAA) and a history of suicide attempts and aggression (Åsberg et al. 1976; Brown et al. 1982). Coccaro et al. (1989) reported diminished central serotonin responsiveness in borderline patients to fenfluramine challenge, suggesting that increasing serotonin neurotransmission might decrease impulsive suicide attempts and aggression.

Controlled trials studying aggression and suicidality in borderline patients treated with serotonergic reuptake inhibitors (i.e., fluoxetine, fluvoxamine, zimelidine) need to be carried out. There have been at least four favorable open trials with fluoxetine (Coccaro et al., in press; Cornelius et al. 1990; Markovitz et al. 1990; Norden 1989). On the other hand, some patients may paradoxically respond to fluoxetine treatment with an increase in suicidality (Teicher et al. 1990) and/or self-mutilation. Moreover, clinicians must balance the conceptual appeal of such agents against the already existing empirical documentation of a useful role for neuroleptics in reducing the impulsive, self-destructive behavior of borderline patients, both in the short term (Soloff et al. 1989) and over the long term (Montgomery and Montgomery 1982). Neuroleptics are most helpful with the most severely symptomatic patients (see Soloff, Chapter 15). The long-term risks of tardive dyskinesia must also be considered in these decisions.

Angry affect and hair-trigger impulsive action may also respond to a trial of lithium carbonate or carbamazepine. Rifkin et al. (1972) demonstrated the benefit of lithium carbonate in treating emotionally unstable character disorders, and Turpin et al. (1973) demonstrated the efficacy of lithium in treating aggression in patients with personality disorders. The enthusiasm encouraged by these reports should be tempered by the recent, and only, controlled trial of lithium with borderline patients. Links et al. (1990) found only slight evidence for benefits of lithium beyond those of placebo. Another lead, carbamazepine, also has shown promise of helping borderline patients control discharge of angry impulses (Cowdry and Gardner 1988; Gardner and Cowdry 1986).

4. Severe anxiety is a major problem for many borderline patients. Soloff (1990) describes two types of anxiety: somatic and psychic. *Somatic anxiety* is experienced in the body and is associated with impulsivity and a stimulus-seeking pattern of behavior. It is most frequently associated with antisocial behavior and a histrionic cognitive style. This type of anxiety is best treated with a MAO inhibitor or by catecholaminergic drugs. *Psychic anxiety* is associated with patients who have a low tolerance to stimulation and a high anticipation of harm. These patients use obsessional cognitive styles, and this type of anxiety is best treated with a benzodiazepine. These concepts are mentioned to alert the clinician to developing paradigms for subtyping anxiety.

In summary, the clinician should be able to identify the four trait vulnerabilities and know something of the data base that has established a pharmacological approach to each of them. We encourage pharmacotherapists to engage their borderline patient as an ally who will study along with the pharmacotherapist his or her responses to the various pharmacological agents that might be helpful. This approach has the advantage of a) making somewhat modest claims on what may be accomplished through the pharmacotherapy, b) encouraging the patient to step back and identify his or her own behavior and symptom pattern, and c) encouraging the patient to develop a collaborative rather than an adversarial relationship with the pharmacotherapist.

RESIDENTIAL THERAPIES

Role, Indications, Types

Patients with BPD constitute between 8% and 25% of inpatient admissions—easily the most common form of personality disorder found in psychiatric hospitals.

The overall role of the hospital in the treatment of borderline patients usually involves management of regressions or crises (see Silver and Rosenbluth, Chapter 16) and seldom involves long-term inpatient care—as long as the patient has an ongoing outpatient psychotherapy. For a patient not in psychotherapy, one of the major functions of the hospital is to complete an evaluation and to initiate and consolidate some form of outpatient therapy program. For a patient hospitalized in the context of an already ongoing psychotherapy, the hospital serves to diminish transference distortions, to intervene in response to self-destructive or antisocial acting out, or to allow needed diagnostic, pharmacotherapeutic, or family consultations to occur (Sederer 1986). Misuse of admission includes therapists who use it to cover a reluctance to confront or interpret the manipulative purposes behind suicidal gestures or threats and a reluctance to address the secondary gain issues related to being hospitalized. Stone (1990, p. 55) and McGlashan (see Chapter 12) have advocated a low threshold to hospitalize suicidal borderline patients. While hospitalization is sometimes necessary, we advocate a careful assessment of the clinical situation and weighing the risks and benefits of hospitalization with the patient. Paris (see Chapter 17) has approached this complex problem in a manner consistent with our views.

Even though utilization of a hospital may not be necessary for all borderline patients, access to a hospital and the readiness to employ this approach are essential before undertaking outpatient treatment. The mere presence of a hospital helps diminish the countertransference feelings of helplessness or anger.

The decision about length of treatment depends less on the severity of psychopathology than on the degree to which a given borderline patient has ongoing social structures and supports. Hence, the most common reason to depart from the usual reliance on short-term hospitalization is the presence of unpredictable or abusive social contexts, such as a household that patently stimulates an adolescent's destructive actions toward self or others. There are other rationales for long-term treatment, but they rest largely on the patient's having an established track record of nonresponse to less ambitious and restrictive treatment strategies, including short-term hospitalizations. Whereas until recently some institutions offered the option of long-term hospitalization, this option is now extremely rare. This is due in part to the impact of limited willingness by third-party payers. This is also due in part to the serious questions about the value of this option. Whatever the causes, there is clearly a need for longer-term residential supports for many borderline patients. In view of the general scheme of such options, we advocate (and have created) a less costly stepdown set of services between hospitalization and outpatient care.

Day/night treatment.   Day/night treatment often provides stabilizing and life-sustaining functions for borderline patients with less intensive staffing than hospitalization and the option of using either the day or the night component separately or together. The potential for regression is also greatly reduced. Day treatment programs offer therapeutic supports and structures along with the opportunity for corrective relationships with staff and peers. Good day treatment programs offer active vocational rehabilitation programs that are of value to the many borderline patients with histories of academic or vocational failures.

Halfway houses.   Often, borderline patients who are in outpatient psychotherapy can be managed better in a halfway house than in a hospital. Halfway houses offer distance from toxic family or other social situations. They also offer social relationships with peers without the potential for regressive functioning that is common in inpatient settings.

General Principles of Residential Therapies

Hospitalization contains the danger of nontherapeutic regressions. Common expressions of regressive behavior are angry, negativistic behaviors vis-á-vis the controls imposed by the hospital, and the development of a childlike or even psychotic demand for dependent gratification. There are three common causes for these regressions: 1) the failure to sustain a focus on the situation that precipitated the admission; 2) the failure to address the extratherapeutic context from which the patient seeks asylum; and 3) the unwitting reinforcement of dysfunction rather than function.

Regressive behaviors require early and consistent imposition of limits. Limits do not necessarily mean restrictions, which often signify being "held." Rather, limiting access to a facility or staff in response to behaviors judged to be controllable but destructive is usually more effective. Limits are used to enforce the expectation that patients will collaborate to the best of their abilities, which means they must accept the realistic limitations of the staff's availability.

Staff conflicts ("splits") often complicate the hospital experience for borderline patients. There is general agreement about the content of these conflicts, namely, the contrast between viewing borderline patients as helpless waifs in need of nurturance or as angry manipulators in need of limits. Those whose views of borderline psychopathology emphasize the latter characteristics (i.e., their aggressiveness) see the borderline patient's projections as a cause for disagreements (i.e., they "split" the staff). More important, in our view, is the degree to which staff with more nurturing countertransference reactions are bound to disagree with staff having more angry countertransferences. Here, the staff members are "split" by what they themselves bring to bear on the borderline patient.

Several characteristics are required in any effective hospital, day treatment, or halfway house. One is that these milieu programs rely heavily on structure. Borderline patients need a full schedule of activities that organize their time and place, that is, where they are to be and what they are to do. A second characteristic is that they set a tone of high behavioral expectation. Patients are expected to act as collaborators in their own treatment, and failure to do so can be used as a reason for "therapeutic discharge." That is, patients who insistently regress within the hospital are informed of the program's failure to be helpful and are discharged on this account, with the stipulation that they can return when they feel motivated to work toward common goals with the treatment staff. A third characteristic of milieu programs is that they routinely identify maladaptive interpersonal patterns and provide new strategies for managing the frustrations inherent in interpersonal involvement. A fourth characteristic of communities that are therapeutic for borderline patients is that they focus on adaptation to life in the community. Groups focusing on family problems, abuse experiences, vocation, or transitions that start within inpatient units can diminish regressions, structure patient time, and also serve the valuable function of confronting maladaptive interpersonal behaviors to make them more dystonic. As in our McLean program specializing in treatment for borderline patients, it is very desirable to sustain such groups through gradually reduced levels of care and into the outpatient setting.

Summary

The literature indicates that, regardless of modality, treatment of borderline patients is difficult, severe countertransference problems are common, and the results are uneven. Individual psychotherapy remains the backbone of most treatment strategies for borderline patients. The potential use of behavioral and psychopharmacological modalities is being evaluated and offers hope for more diverse and effective treatment in the future. The role of family and group therapies can be critical but is quite variable. Likewise, the need for hospitalization is variable, but hospitalization is always a resource that should be made available in the overall treatment program. Residential and halfway house treatments are often useful. Drawing upon the past half-century of dynamic work with borderline patients, informed clinicians are bringing to bear the empirical data of the past two decades. The overriding effect of the new data (see McGlashan, Chapter 12) is to suggest a more sober appraisal of what is possible in the treatment of borderline patients, a respect for the healing effects of time, and the importance of initially engaging these difficult patients into their treatments.

REFERENCES

Abend SM, Porder MS, Willick MS: Borderline Patients: Psychoanalytic Perspectives. New York, International Universities Press, 1983

Åsberg M, Träskman L, Thorén P: 5-HIAA in the cerebrospinal fluid: a biochemical suicide predictor? Arch Gen Psychiatry 33:1193–1197, 1976

Braun BG: Towards a theory of multiple personality and other dissociative phenomena. Psychiatr Clin North Am 7:171–193, 1984

Brown GL, Ebert MH, Goyer PF, et al: Aggression, suicide, and serotonin: relationships to CSF amine metabolites. Am J Psychiatry 139:741–746, 1982

Buie DH, Adler G: The definitive treatment of the borderline personality. International Journal of Psychoanalytic Psychotherapy 9:51–87, 1982–1983

Chessick RD: Intensive psychotherapy of a borderline patient. Arch Gen Psychiatry 39:413–419, 1982

Coccaro EF, Siever LJ, Klar HM, et al: Serotonergic studies in patients with affective and personality disorders: correlates with suicidal and impulsive aggressive behavior. Arch Gen Psychiatry 46:587–599, 1989

Coccaro EF, Astill JL, Herbert J, et al: Fluoxetine treatment of impulsive aggression in DSM-III-R personality disorder patients. J Clin Psychopharmacol (in press)

Cornelius JR, Soloff PH, Perel JM, et al: Fluoxetine trial in borderline personality disorder. Psychopharmacol Bull 26:151–154, 1990

Cowdry R, Gardner D. Pharmacotherapy of borderline personality disorder: alprazolam, carbamazepine, trifluoperazine and tranylcypromine. Arch Gen Psychiatry 45:111–119, 1988

Gardner DL, Cowdry RW: Alprazolam induced dyscontrol in borderline personality disorder. Am J Psychiatry 142:98–100, 1985

Gardner DL, Cowdry RW: Positive effects of carbamazepine on behavioral dyscontrol in borderline personality disorder. Am J Psychiatry 143:519–522, 1986

Goldberg SC, Schulz SC, Schulz PM, et al: Borderline and schizotypal personality disorders treated with low-dose thiothixene vs placebo. Arch Gen Psychiatry 43:680–686, 1986

Gunderson JG: Borderline Personality Disorder. Washington, DC, American Psychiatric Press, 1984

Gunderson JG: New prospectives on becoming borderline, in Family Environment and Borderline Personality Disorder. Edited by Links PS. Washington, DC, American Psychiatric Press, 1990, pp 151–159

Gunderson JG, Kerr J, Englund DW: The families of borderlines: a comparative study. Arch Gen Psychiatry 37:27–33, 1980

Gunderson JG, Frank AF, Ronningstam EF, et al: Early discontinuance of borderline patients from psychotherapy. J Nerv Ment Dis 177:38–42, 1989

Guntrip H: My experience of analysis with Fairbairn and Winnicott. International Review of Psycho-analysis 2:145–156, 1975

Herman JL: Father-Daughter Incest. Cambridge, MA, Harvard University Press, 1981

Herman JL: Histories of violence in an outpatient population: an exploratory study. Am J Orthopsychiatry 56:137–141, 1986

Kernberg OF: The treatment of patients with borderline personality organization. Int J Psychoanal 49:600–619, 1968

Kernberg OF: Borderline Conditions and Pathological Narcissism. New York, Jason Aronson, 1976

Kernberg OF, Selzer MA, Koenigsberg HW, et al: Psychodynamic Psychotherapy of Borderline Patients. New York, Basic Books, 1989

Kluft RP: Childhood Antecedents of Multiple Personality. Washington, DC, American Psychiatric Press, 1985

Knight R: Borderline states. Bull Menninger Clin 17:1–12, 1953

Kolb JE, Gunderson JG: Psychodynamic psychotherapy of borderline patients. International Review of Psycho-Analysis 17:515–516, 1990

Kohut H: The Analysis of the Self. New York, International Universities Press, 1971

Krupnick JL, Horowitz MJ: Brief psychotherapy with vulnerable patients: an outcome assessment. Psychiatry 48:223–233, 1985

Langs R: The Bipersonal Field. New York, Jason Aronson, 1976

Leibovich M: Short-term psychotherapy for the borderline personality disorder. Psychother Psychosom 35:257–264, 1981

Leibovich M: Why short-term psychotherapy for borderlines? Psychother Psychosom 39:1–9, 1983

Leone NF: Response of borderline patients to loxapine and chlorpromazine. J Clin Psychiatry 43:148–150, 1982

Liberman RP, Eckman T: Behavior therapy vs insight-oriented therapy for repeated suicide attempters. Arch Gen Psychiatry 38:1126–1130, 1981

Liebowitz MR, Klein DF: Interrelationship of hysteroid dysphoria and borderline personality disorder. Psychiatr Clin North Am 4:67–87, 1981

Linehan MM: Dialectical behavior therapy: a cognitive behavioral approach to parasuicide. Journal of Personality Disorders 1:328–333, 1987a

Linehan MM: Dialectical behavior therapy in groups: treating borderline personality disorders and suicidal behavior, in Women's Therapy Groups: Paradigms of Feminist Treatment. Edited by Brody CM. New York, Springer, 1987b, pp 145–162

Linehan MM: Cognitive and behavior therapy for borderline personality disorder, in American Psychiatric Press Review of Psychiatry, Vol 8. Edited by Tasman A, Hales RE, Frances AJ. Washington, DC, American Psychiatric Press, 1989, pp 84–102

Links PS, Steiner M, Boiago I, et al: Lithium therapy for borderline patients: preliminary findings. Journal of Personality Disorders 4:173–181, 1990

Maltsberger JT, Buie DH: Countertranference hate in the treatment of suicidal patients. Arch Gen Psychiatry 30:625–633, 1974

Mann J: Time-Limited Psychotherapy. Cambridge, MA, Harvard University Press, 1973

Markovitz PJ, Calabrese JR, Schulz SC, et al: Fluoxetine in borderline and schizotypal personality disorder. Paper presented at the 45th annual meeting of the Society of Biological Psychiatry, New York, May 1990

Masterson J: Psychotherapy of the Borderline Adult. New York, Brunner/Mazel, 1976

McGlashan T: The Chestnut Lodge follow-up study, III: long-term outcome of borderline personalities. Arch Gen Psychiatry 43:20–30, 1986

McLaughlin JT: Transference, psychic reality, and countertransference. Psychoanal Q 50:639–664, 1981

Montgomery SA, Montgomery D: Pharmacological prevention of suicidal behaviour. J Affective Disord 4:291–298, 1982

Moses R: Adult psychic trauma: the question of early predisposition and some detailed mechanisms. Int J Psychoanal 59:353–363, 1978

Norden MJ: Fluoxetine in borderline personality disorder. Prog Neuropsycho-pharmacol Biol Psychiatry 13:885–893, 1989

Paris J: Completed suicide in borderline personality disorder. Psychiatric Annals 20:19–21, 1990

Rifkin A, Quitkin F, Carillo C, et al: Lithium carbonate in emotionally unstable character disorder. Arch Gen Psychiatry 27:519–523, 1972

Rockland LH: Supportive Therapy: A Psychodynamic Approach. New York, Basic Books, 1989

Sandler A: Countertransference and role-responsiveness. International Review of Psycho-analysis 3:43–48, 1976

Schatzberg AF, Cole JO: Benzodiazepines in the treatment of depressive, borderline personality and schizophrenic disorders. Br J Clin Pharmacol 11:175–225, 1981

Sederer LL: Inpatient Psychiatry: Diagnosis and Treatment. Baltimore, MD, Williams & Wilkins, 1986

Serban G, Siegel S: Response of borderline and schizotypal patients to small doses of thiothixene and haloperidol. Am J Psychiatry 141:1455–1458, 1984

Shapiro ER, Zinner J, Shapiro R, et al: The influence of family experience on borderline personality development. International Review of Psycho-analysis 2:399–411, 1975

Siever LJ, Klar H, Coccaro E: Psychologic substrates of personality, in Biologic Response Styles: Clinical Implications. Edited by Klar H, Siever LJ. Washington, DC, American Psychiatric Press, 1985, pp 35–66

Sifneos PE: Short-term Psychotherapy and Emotional Crisis. Cambridge, MA, Harvard University Press, 1972

Silver D: Psychotherapy of the characterologically difficult patient. Can J Psychiatry 28:513–521, 1983

Silver D: Psychodynamics and psychotherapeutic management of the self-destructive character-disordered patient. Psychiatr Clin North Am 8:357–375, 1985

Skodol AE, Buckley P, Charles E: Is there a characteristic pattern to the treatment history of clinical outpatients with borderline personality? J Nerv Ment Dis 171:405–410, 1983

Soloff PH: What's new in personality disorders? An update on pharmacologic treatment. Journal of Personality Disorders 4:233–243, 1990

Soloff PH, George A, Nathan RS, et al: Paradoxical effects of amitriptyline on borderline patients. Am J Psychiatry 143:1603–1605, 1986a

Soloff PH, George A, Nathan RS, et al: Progress in pharmacotherapy of borderline disorders: a double-blind study of amitriptyline, haloperidol, and placebo. Arch Gen Psychiatry 43:691–697, 1986b

Soloff PH, George A, Nathan S, et al: Characterizing depression in borderline patients. J Clin Psychiatry 48:155–157, 1987

Soloff PH, George A, Northam RL, et al: Amitriptyline versus haloperidol in borderlines: final outcomes and predictors of response. J Clin Psychopharmacol 9:238–246, 1989

Stone MH: The Fate of Borderline Patients: Successful Outcome and Psychiatric Practice. New York, Guilford, 1990

Teicher MH, Glod C, Cole JO: Emergence of intense suicidal preoccupation during fluoxetine treatment. Am J Psychiatry 147:207–210, 1990

Turpin JP, Smith DB, Clanon TL, et al: The long-term use of lithium in aggressive prisoners. Compr Psychiatry 14:311–317, 1973

van der Kolk BA: Psychological Trauma. Washington, DC, American Psychiatric Press, 1987

Volkan V: Six Steps in the Treatment of Borderline Personality Organization. New York, Jason Aronson, 1987

Waldinger R, Gunderson J: Effective Psychotherapy With Borderline Patients. New York, Macmillan, 1987

Wallerstein R: Forty-two Lives in Treatment: A Study of Psychoanalysis and Psychotherapy. New York, Guilford, 1986

Winnicott DW: Hate in the contertransference (1947), in Collected Papers. New York, Basic Books, 1975, pp 194–203

Wong N: Combined group and individual treatment of borderline and narcissistic patients: heterogeneous versus homogeneous groups. Int J Group Psychother 30:389–404, 1980

Index

Note: Page numbers in **boldface** type refer to figures and tables.